the essential guide to

Women's Herbal Medicine

Cyndi Gilbert, ND
with contributions from Fraser Smith, ND

Robert
ROSE

For complete cataloguing information, see page 371.

Disclaimer

This book is a general guide only and should never be a substitute for the skill, knowledge and experience of a qualified medical professional dealing with the facts, circumstances and symptoms of a particular case.

The medical and health information presented in this book is based on the research, training and professional experience of the author, and is true and complete to the best of her knowledge. However, this book is intended only as an informative guide for those wishing to know more about herbal medicine; it is not intended to replace or countermand the advice given by the reader's personal physician. Because each person and situation is unique, the author and the publisher urge the reader to check with a qualified health-care professional before using any herbal medicines. The author and the publisher are not responsible for any adverse effects or consequences resulting from the use of the information in this book. It is the responsibility of the reader to consult a physician or other qualified health-care professional regarding his or her personal care.

This book contains references to products that may not be available everywhere. The intent of the information provided is to be helpful; however, there is no guarantee of results associated with the information provided. Use of brand names is for educational purposes only and does not imply endorsement.

The names of the patients discussed in the case studies have been changed to protect their privacy.

Caution

Before using any of the herbal medicines described in this book, consult with your health-care professional about a safe dosage. Herbal medicines, like pharmaceutical medicines, should not be self-administered.

Design and production: Daniella Zanchetta/PageWave Graphics Inc.
Editor: Bob Hilderley, Senior Editor, Health
Copy editor: Sue Sumeraj
Proofreader and indexer: Gillian Watts
Cover image: Herbal tea with clover flowers © istockphoto.com/OlgaMiltsova
Back cover images: Ginkgo leaves © istockphoto.com/AlpamayoPhoto and Dried calendula flowers © istockphoto.com/Elenathewise

The publisher gratefully acknowledges the financial support of our publishing program by the Government of Canada through the Canada Book Fund.

Published by Robert Rose Inc.
120 Eglinton Avenue East, Suite 800, Toronto, Ontario, Canada M4P 1E2
Tel: (416) 322-6552 Fax: (416) 322-6936
www.robertrose.ca

\ted and bound in Canada

4 5 6 7 8 9 MI 23 22 21 20 19 18 17 16 15

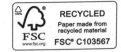

"The plants have long been our teachers and healers. The Cherokee and Creek understood this long ago. It was said among them that the plants took pity on the suffering of their offspring, the human beings, and that each plant offered up a remedy to heal one of the diseases of humankind."

— Stephen Harrod Buhner

Contents

Preface

The botanical and medical information presented in this book combines the best herbal wisdom from several medical traditions with the most recent evidence-based scientific research. The medical traditions include traditional Chinese medicine, Ayurvedic medicine and indigenous North American medicine, as well as "Western" disciplines such as homeopathy, eclecticism, flower essence therapy and naturopathic medicine. The scientific research focuses on contemporary studies in phytochemistry and pharmacognosy, big words for a growing field of complementary botanical and pharmaceutical exploration.

This information is drawn from a variety of highly credible sources: double-blind, placebo-controlled trials reported in respected botanical and medical journals; phytotherapy research, physiomedicalism and eclectic school textbooks; materia medica from homeopathic, traditional Chinese medicine and Ayurvedic traditions; and the work of naturopathic physicians Francis Brinker, Bill Mitchell, Jillian Stansbury, Tori Hudson, John Sherman and, especially, my instructors in the science and art of botanical medicine at the Canadian College of Naturopathic Medicine, Paul R. Saunders and Anthony Godfrey, as well as my colleague Fraser Smith at the National University of Health Sciences.

There is no shortage of good botanical medicine resources. On the contrary, there are several substantial, authoritative reference books, notably *Herbal Medicines* from Pharmaceutical Press in the United Kingdom; *Principles and Practices of Phytotherapy* by Kerry Bone and Simon Mills; *Herbal Drugs and Phytopharmaceuticals*, adapted from the German Commission E monographs; *The ABC Clinical Guide to Herbs* from the American Botanical Council; David Hoffman's *Medical Herbalism*; *55 Most Common Medicinal Herbs* by Heather Boon and Michael Smith; and the standard *PDR for Herbal Medicines*. Despite their authority and reliability, these are professional reference books designed for the laboratory, clinic or classroom. *The Essential Guide to Women's Herbal Medicine*, on the other hand, is designed to make challenging information easy to access, and to encourage the reader to explore the long history, effectiveness and safety of herbal remedies.

A Holistic Approach

I take a holistic approach to treating women with herbal medicines and teaching young naturopathic doctors to continue this practice. When I was a child playing in my yard and garden, our house backed onto a hydro easement with long grass and more diversity of plant life and weeds than the majority of the well-manicured yards of the neighboring suburban landscape. I have wonderful memories of the smell of the cedar hedge that formed a natural fence around the yard, and of the pops of color from dandelions and red clover in the grass. As a young adult, I rekindled my relationship with medicinal plants through food and foraging. I threw myself wholeheartedly into the study of plant identification, wildcrafting and herbal medicine-making. Living and working with medicinal herbs and traditional herbalists taught me about plant energetics, intelligence, communication and connection. I began to understand the relationships between plants and people in a whole new way. I found myself flooded with the awe and wonder of my childhood herbal experiences. Most importantly, I started talking to, and listening to, plants once again.

As my connection to plants flourished, I learned the language of plant chemistry and phytopharmacological actions. I enrolled in a naturopathic college to study the science of herbal medicine and the impact of herbs on human physiology. Synthesizing traditional knowledge and scientific research, I have gained a more complete, nuanced picture of herbal medicine through clinical trials and phytotherapeutic studies. As a result, my approach to medicinal herbs is holistic — ancient, practical, wise, earth-centered, plant-loving, evidence-based, spiritual, complementary and research-oriented.

Women's Health Conditions

The history of herbal remedies is rich in women's lore. In most foraging societies, women were largely responsible for wildcrafting: collecting and preparing plants as both food and medicine. Details on the culinary and medicinal power of these herbs were, and continue to be, passed down from generation to generation, from woman to woman. Your mother or grandmother may have suggested a specific herb for a specific condition, such as an herb to avoid pain and discomfort during menstruation or an herb to help promote a healthy pregnancy. Considerable work has been done in this field, with Susun Weed and Rosemary Gladstar leading the way with their women's herbal books, while Dr. Tori Hudson has studied women's medical lore with scientific rigor.

However, most of the information on herbal treatment for women's health conditions has been reduced to questions of gynecological and reproductive health. While no two women are the same, women do experience certain health conditions more frequently than men. For example, women are at greater risk for depression and autoimmune conditions. Because women's health is about more than just hormones and uteruses (and some women have neither female hormones nor uteruses, just as some people with uteruses do not identify as female), this book includes conditions that are common in women but not directly related to gynecological health, such as heart disease, diabetes and arthritis. I have attempted to use gender-neutral language where possible to reflect the broad range of people who may find this book useful, including cis-women, trans women and trans men.

It's important to emphasize that every woman is different, and everyone experiences and defines health and disease from their own context and perspective. What is a concern for one person may not be for another. Personal ideas about health may sometimes even appear to be at odds with medical definitions of health and disease. Where discrepancies arise, talk to your health-care provider to learn what course of action may be best for you.

How to Use This Book

After a brief introduction to the history and science of herbal medicine, *The Essential Guide to Women's Herbal Medicine* profiles thirty-five common conditions, from acne and anemia to urinary tract infections and vaginitis, and discusses herbs that have proven to be safe and effective for treating those conditions. Information about the signs, symptoms and prevalence of each condition is provided, along with lists of associated conditions, common herbal combinations and conventional medical treatments. Clinical case histories, intriguing folklore tidbits and easy herbal recipes are interspersed throughout.

Part 3 profiles sixty-six herbal medicines, from ashwagandha and barberry to witch hazel and yarrow. Each profile describes the herb's most common medicinal uses today, as well as its historical and energetic uses, then reviews the research evidence and current safety information available on the herb, as related to the health conditions discussed in the book. The chemistry of the plant is often explained, to provide further insight into how botanical medicine works.

Throughout the book, you'll find information on traditional Chinese, Ayurvedic and Native American medicine practices, homeopathic symptom pictures, flower essence characteristics and Doctrine of Signatures qualities. No other book on botanical medicine offers this reach into different but equally successful approaches to herbal medicine.

The Essential Guide to Women's Herbal Medicine is intended as a guide that will enable readers to have a more informed discussion with a regulated health practitioner about how best to use herbs medicinally to benefit their health. Before appropriate herbs or other treatments are determined, a successful treatment plan takes into account an individual's health history, family history, medications, allergies and goals. Caution is strongly advised about using herbal medicines to self-treat without input from a licensed health-care professional.

Acknowledgments

To the plants, who have been my best teachers, and to my family, friends and colleagues, who have supported me in countless ways in the pursuit of what I love: working with, talking about and teaching herbal medicine.

I'd also like to thank my students at the Canadian College of Naturopathic Medicine, who cheered me on and provided some early research support to get the ball rolling on making this book a reality.

Quick Guide to Herbal Treatments for Women's Health Conditions

Health Condition	Page	First-Line Herb	Therapeutic Action	Other Herbal Treatments
Acne	43	Tea tree oil	Antimicrobial	Barberry Calendula Green tea
Anemia	47	Nettle	Nutritive	Dandelion Dang gui
Anxiety	51	Lavender	Nervine	Chamomile Kava Lemon balm Passionflower
Arthritis (osteoarthritis)	58	Cayenne pepper	Circulatory stimulant, counterirritant	Boswellia Devil's claw Nettle
Arthritis (rheumatoid)	63	Evening primrose	Anti-inflammatory	Ginger Turmeric Willow
Breast cancer	68	Soy	Phytoestrogenic	Ashwagandha Barberry Ginger Green tea Red clover Turmeric
Cervical dysplasia	74	Green tea	Antioxidant	Echinacea Licorice
Depression	77	St. John's wort	Antidepressant, nervine	Rhodiola Lavender Saffron
Diabetes mellitus	82	Cinnamon	Hypoglycemic, carminative	Barberry Fenugreek Gymnema Milk thistle
Endometriosis	87	Turmeric	Antioxidant, anti-inflammatory	Green tea Yarrow
Fibrocystic breast changes	91	Chaste tree	Hormonal regulator	Evening primrose

Health Condition	Page	First-Line Herb	Therapeutic Action	Other Herbal Treatments
Fibroids	94	Castor oil	Anti-inflammatory	Black cohosh Cinnamon Yarrow
Genital warts	100	Green tea	Antioxidant	Echinacea Lemon balm St. John's wort
Herpes	103	Lemon balm	Antiviral	Echinacea Propolis St. John's wort
High blood pressure and heart disease	107	Garlic	Hypotensive	Dandelion leaf Green tea Hawthorn Motherwort Yarrow
Hypothyroidism	115	Ashwagandha	Adaptogen	Seaweed
Infertility	118	Raspberry	Uterine tonic	Berberine Black cohosh
Menopause	122	Black cohosh	Hormonal regulator	Dang gui Red clover Sage St. John's wort Soy Valerian
Menstrual Irregularities				
Amenorrhea and oligomenorrhea	130	Dang gui	Hormonal regulator	Black cohosh Chaste tree Licorice and peony Red clover Yarrow
Dysmenorrhea	135	Ginger	Anti-inflammatory, antinauseant	Cramp bark Fennel Valerian Wild yam
Menorrhagia	139	Yarrow	Astringent	Chaste tree Cinnamon Dang gui Geranium Shepherd's purse
Osteoporosis	144	Soy	Phytoestrogenic	Black cohosh Milk thistle Red clover

Health Condition	Page	First-Line Herb	Therapeutic Action	Other Herbal Treatments
Polycystic ovarian syndrome (PCOS)	148	Cinnamon	Hypoglycemic	Berberine Chaste tree Green tea Licorice Spearmint
Pregnancy and Breastfeeding				
Constipation	154	Dandelion	Laxative	
Heartburn	156	Slippery elm	Demulcent	Licorice
Hemorrhoids	158	Horse chestnut	Astringent	Ginkgo Witch hazel Yarrow
Low milk supply	162	Fenugreek	Galactagogue	Chaste tree Fennel Milk thistle and blessed thistle Nettle Shatavari
Morning sickness	166	Ginger	Antinauseant	Peppermint
Varicose veins	169	Horse chestnut	Astringent	Calendula Ginkgo Witch hazel
Weaning	172	Sage	Astringent	Peppermint
Premenstrual syndrome	174	Evening primrose	Anti-inflammatory	Chaste tree Dandelion Ginkgo St. John's wort
Sexual dysfunction	180	Ginseng	Adaptogen	Dang gui Evening primrose Ginkgo Shatavari Tribulus
Stress	186	Rhodiola	Adaptogen	Ashwagandha Eleuthero Schisandra
Urinary tract infections	191	Cranberry	Urinary antiseptic	Corn silk Dandelion Goldenseal Nettle Uva ursi
Vaginitis	197	Garlic	Antimicrobial	Goldenseal Tea tree oil

Quick Guide to Women's Medicinal Herbs

Common Name	Page	Botanical Name	Women's Health Conditions
Ashwagandha	203	*Withania somnifera*	Breast cancer Hypothyroidism Stress
Barberry	206	*Berberis vulgaris*	Acne Breast cancer Diabetes mellitus
Berberine	209	n/a	Diabetes mellitus Infertility Polycystic ovarian syndrome (PCOS)
Black cohosh	212	*Actaea racemosa*	Amenorrhea/ oligomenorrhea Fibroids Infertility Menopause Osteoporosis
Blessed thistle	216	*Cnicus benedictus*	Low milk supply
Boswellia	218	*Boswellia serrata*	Osteoarthritis
Calendula	220	*Calendula officinalis*	Acne Varicose veins
Castor oil	222	*Ricinus communis*	Fibroids
Cayenne pepper	224	*Capsicum frutescens*	Osteoarthritis
Chamomile	226	*Matricaria recutita*	Anxiety
Chaste tree	228	*Vitex agnus-castus*	Amenorrhea/ oligomenorrhea Fibrocystic breast changes Low milk supply Menorrhagia Polycystic ovarian syndrome (PCOS) Premenstrual syndrome

Common Name	Page	Botanical Name	Women's Health Conditions
Cinnamon	232	*Cinnamomum verum* (true or Ceylon cinnamon) *Cinnamomum cassia* (cassia cinnamon)	Diabetes mellitus Fibroids Menorrhagia Polycystic ovarian syndrome (PCOS)
Corn silk	235	*Zea mays*	Urinary tract infections
Cramp bark	236	*Viburnum opulus*	Dysmenorrhea
Cranberry	238	*Vaccinium macrocarpon*	Urinary tract infections
Dandelion (leaf and/ or root)	240	*Taraxacum officinale*	Anemia Constipation High blood pressure and heart disease Premenstrual syndrome Urinary tract infections
Dang gui (dong quai)	243	*Angelica sinensis*	Amenorrhea/ oligomenorrhea Anemia Menopause Menorrhagia Sexual dysfunction
Devil's claw	246	*Harpagophytum procumbens*	Osteoarthritis
Echinacea	248	*Echinacea pallida* (pale purple coneflower) *Echinacea purpurea* (purple coneflower) *Echinacea angustifolia* (narrow-leaved coneflower)	Cervical dysplasia Genital warts Herpes
Eleuthero	251	*Eleutherococcus senticosus*	Stress
Evening primrose	253	*Oenothera biennis*	Fibrocystic breast changes Premenstrual syndrome Rheumatoid arthritis Sexual dysfunction
Fennel	256	*Foeniculum vulgare*	Dysmenorrhea Low milk supply
Fenugreek	258	*Trigonella foenum-graecum*	Diabetes mellitus Low milk supply

Common Name	Page	Botanical Name	Women's Health Conditions
Garlic	260	*Allium sativum*	High blood pressure and heart disease Vaginitis
Geranium	263	*Geranium maculatum*	Menorrhagia
Ginger	265	*Zingiber officinale*	Breast cancer Dysmenorrhea Morning sickness Rheumatoid arthritis
Ginkgo (maidenhair tree)	269	*Ginkgo biloba*	Hemorrhoids Premenstrual syndrome Sexual dysfunction Varicose veins
Ginseng	272	*Panax ginseng*	Sexual dysfunction
Goldenseal	274	*Hydrastis canadensis*	Urinary tract infections Vaginitis
Green tea	276	*Camellia sinensis*	Acne Breast cancer Cervical dysplasia Endometriosis Genital warts High blood pressure and heart disease Polycystic ovarian syndrome (PCOS)
Gymnema	282	*Gymnema sylvestre*	Diabetes mellitus
Hawthorn	284	*Crataegus laevigata* (English hawthorn) *Crataegus monogyna* (common hawthorn)	High blood pressure and heart disease
Horse chestnut	286	*Aesculus hippocastanum*	Hemorrhoids Varicose veins
Kava	288	*Piper methysticum*	Anxiety
Lavender	291	*Lavandula angustifolia*	Anxiety Depression
Lemon balm	293	*Melissa officinalis*	Anxiety Genital warts Herpes

Common Name	Page	Botanical Name	Women's Health Conditions
Licorice	295	*Glycyrrhiza glabra* (licorice) *Glycyrrhiza uralensis* (Chinese licorice)	Amenorrhea/ oligomenorrhea Cervical dysplasia Heartburn
Milk thistle	299	*Silybum marianum*	Diabetes mellitus Low milk supply Osteoporosis
Motherwort	301	*Leonurus cardiaca*	High blood pressure and heart disease
Nettle	303	*Urtica dioica*	Anemia Low milk supply Osteoarthritis Urinary tract infections
Passionflower	306	*Passiflora incarnata*	Anxiety
Peony	308	*Paeonia lactiflora*	Amenorrhea/ oligomenorrhea
Peppermint	310	*Mentha x piperita*	Morning sickness Weaning
Propolis	313	n/a	Herpes
Raspberry	315	*Rubus idaeus*	Infertility
Red clover	317	*Trifolium pratense*	Amenorrhea/ oligomenorrhea Breast cancer Menopause Osteoporosis
Rhodiola	321	*Rhodiola rosea*	Depression Stress
Saffron	323	*Crocus sativus*	Depression
Sage	325	*Salvia officinalis*	Menopause Weaning
St. John's wort	327	*Hypericum perforatum*	Depression Genital warts Herpes Menopause Premenstrual syndrome
Schisandra	330	*Schisandra chinensis*	Stress

Common Name	Page	Botanical Name	Women's Health Conditions
Seaweed	332	*Fucus vesiculosus* (bladderwrack) *Sargassum* spp.	Hypothyroidism
Shatavari	334	*Asparagus racemosus*	Low milk supply Sexual dysfunction
Shepherd's purse	336	*Capsella bursa-pastoris*	Menorrhagia
Slippery elm	337	*Ulmus fulva*	Heartburn
Soy	339	*Glycine max*	Breast cancer Menopause Osteoporosis
Spearmint	342	*Mentha spicata*	Polycystic ovarian syndrome (PCOS)
Tea tree oil	344	*Melaleuca alternifolia*	Acne Vaginitis
Tribulus	346	*Tribulus terrestris*	Sexual dysfunction
Turmeric	348	*Curcuma longa*	Breast cancer Endometriosis Rheumatoid arthritis
Uva ursi (bearberry)	350	*Arctostaphylos uva-ursi*	Urinary tract infections
Valerian	352	*Valeriana officinalis*	Dysmenorrhea Menopause
Wild yam	354	*Dioscorea villosa* (wild yam) *Dioscorea opposita* (Chinese yam)	Dysmenorrhea
Willow	356	*Salix alba* (white willow) *Salix nigra* (black willow)	Rheumatoid arthritis
Witch hazel	358	*Hamamelis virginiana*	Hemorrhoids Varicose veins
Yarrow	360	*Achillea millefolium* (yarrow) *Achillea biebersteinii* Afan. (yellow marabou)	Amenorrhea/ oligomenorrhea Endometriosis Fibroids Hemorrhoids High blood pressure and heart disease Menorrhagia

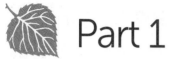 Part 1

Introduction to Herbal Medicine

Herbalism Through the Centuries

The use of plants as medicine is as old as the history of medicine, perhaps human civilization itself. Found at the center of many ancient-world and modern-day medical systems, botanical medicine is interwoven with everyday life in many cultures. There is considerable evidence of disparate cultures, without any communication between them, employing herbs in exactly the same manner and for the same purpose.

Prehistoric Times

The earliest known record depicting the use of plants as medicine comes from cave paintings in Lascaux, France, which date from 13,000 to 25,000 BCE. Botanical knowledge acquired in early tribal communities was protected by and passed down through shamans, medicine men and women, and various kinds of healers unfortunately referred to as witch doctors, primarily orally but later in medical texts, or materia medica. Over the years, ancient peoples developed extensive herbal medicines based on the local flora.

Eastern Traditions

Some of the earliest known written descriptions of medical treatment with herbs are found in Chinese, Mesopotamian and Egyptian texts. Chinese emperor Shen Nong's *Pen Ts'ao Ching*, recorded in 2800 BCE, lists 365 herbs, including *Ephedra sinica*, still in use today. Sumerian cuneiform tablets dating to 2600 BCE specify the use of cypress, cedar, myrrh, licorice and opium poppy. The Edwin Smith Papyrus from Egypt, dated to 1700 BCE but thought to originate from a manuscript written by Imhotep in 3000 BCE, includes treatment protocols using willow and sycamore leaves.

While Ayurvedic medicine is believed to trace its origins to the Vedas, in particular the *Atharvaveda*, around 3000 BCE, Vedic lore had been passed on orally for thousands of years.

Vitalism and Energetics

Vitalistic approaches, such as traditional Chinese medicine (TCM) and Ayurvedic medicine, match patterns of disharmony in the patient with specific energetic qualities of plants. For example, the TCM understanding of a botanical includes its taste (bitter, salty, sweet, sour, astringent, bland, spicy), temperature (cold, cool, neutral, warm, hot), organ/meridian affinities (lung, liver or kidney, for example) and action (cools fire, drains dampness and moves qi, for example). Similarly, Ayurvedic medicine describes herbs in terms of their taste, temperature, *guna* (one of three fundamental qualities: *sattva*/purity, *rajas*/change or *tamas*/inertia), *vipaka* (post-digestive effect), *prabhava* (special properties, including auric action, astral effects, magnetic effects and radiation) and action on doshas (for example, pacifies *pitta*, balances *tridosha* or increases *kapha*).

The first printed medical treatise is believed to be the *Sushruta Samhita*, written in the sixth century BCE, which contained an herbal pharmacopoeia listing over 700 medicinal plants.

Western Traditions

In ancient Greece, the first complete botanical text was likely the *Historia Plantarum*, written by Theophrastus (a successor of Aristotle in the fourth century BCE), which attempted to classify plants taxonomically. *De Materia Medica*, produced in 65 CE by Dioscorides, a surgeon in the Roman army, became one of the best-known and most authoritative works, referenced to this day and widely used up until the Renaissance. In 77 CE, Pliny the Elder published *Naturalis Historia*, an encyclopedia dealing with herbs and other aspects of nature, including information on the Doctrine of Signatures (see box, page 20).

The most influential works for the next 1,500 years were written by two authors, Galen (131–200 CE) and Ibn Sina (980–1037 CE), or Avicenna, as he was known outside the Arab world. Galen, a physician to the gladiators and later to a succession of Roman emperors, evaluated plants in terms of their effects on the four Hippocratic humors (blood, bile, phlegm and choler) and their energetics (hot/cold, dry/moist), creating near-mathematical classifications of herbs. His schematic approach, as well as his preference for complex preparations over simple infusions of two or three herbs, marked the beginning of the distinction between the professional physician and the folk healer, where the latter was considered inferior and unskilled.

Did You Know?

Peter Rabbit

Herbal knowledge has been preserved in the names of plants and passed down in stories, mythology and literature. For example, in *The Tale of Peter Rabbit*, Beatrix Potter reminded readers of an important use for chamomile. After Peter eats too many radishes and runs for his life from Mr. McGregor, his mother sends him to bed with chamomile tea, an herbal remedy that eases digestive upset and gently calms the nerves.

Did You Know?

Hildegard von Bingen

During the Middle Ages in Europe, monks and monasteries preserved medical knowledge, translating and copying earlier herbal texts. Hildegard von Bingen, a German Benedictine nun famous for her visions and musical compositions, also wrote two medicinal texts, one specifically on the medicinal use of plants, animals and precious stones. She expanded upon Galen's theories, superimposing four elements (fire, air, earth and water) on Galen's four humors.

Ibn Sina is often credited as the originator or codifier of Unani medicine, a system he expounded upon in his medical encyclopedia *Al-Qanun fi al-Tibb*, or *Canon of Medicine* (1025). Interweaving Galenic theories with Islamic medicine and aspects of Ayurvedic medicine, Ibn Sina incorporated astrology and the Muslim faith into the practice of medicine. He held that both patients and the medicinal plants prescribed to them were subject to astrological influence, and that Allah (God) provided medicines for all human ailments.

The most significant contribution to Western medicine made by Ibn Sina and other leading Arab physicians of his era was in the field of pharmaceutical processing. They developed new botanical preparations, such as ointments, elixirs, pills, suppositories, inhalations and essential oil distillations, and introduced hundreds of medicinal plants from Arabia, Persia and India to the European pharmacy, classified and sorted according to Galenic categories. Through their work, Ibn Sina and his contemporaries solidified Galen's supreme authority as a revolutionary medical figure, not to be challenged until after Europe was ravaged by the Black Plague and syphilis.

The Doctrine of Signatures

In many pre-modern cultures, the look, shape, feel, sound or taste of a plant was used as a means of understanding its medicinal use. For example, the bright yellow latex of the greater celandine plant was seen to be an excellent signifier of its therapeutic role as a cholagogue, in supporting the production and release of bile — which many associate with a bright yellow fluid — from the liver and gallbladder. The root of ginseng (*Panax ginseng*) resembles a human figure, indicating its use as a general tonic for the entire body. Within European traditions, this concept came to be known as the Doctrine of Signatures, and these examples and countless others have since been confirmed through practical use and scientific research.

Paracelsus

Born Philippus Theophrastus Bombastus von Hohenheim, Paracelsus (1493–1542) is regarded as a key figure in the history of both botanical and homeopathic medicine. As a young boy, he developed a keen interest in medicine, learning about plants and alchemy from his father, who taught him to trust in observation and experience over books and dogmas. He graduated from medical school in northern Italy and quickly started an unconventional practice using surgery (a method that was at that time forbidden by the Hippocratic Oath and relegated to barber-surgeons) as well as medicines. He traveled extensively throughout Europe and the Middle East, learning all he could from folk healers and shamans. In 1527, he was granted the position of municipal doctor in Basel, where he was best known for burning a copy of Ibn Sina's *Canon of Medicine* to show his contempt for medical dogma. He was subsequently forced to flee Basel and spent much of his later years working out his own system of medicine.

Many of the concepts familiar to naturopathic medicine can be traced back to Paracelsus's writings. He defined the *archeus*, or life force, in much the same way that the *vis medicatrix naturae* (the healing power of nature) is understood by naturopathic philosophy: as a dynamic, intelligent force with powers of repair and restoration. He described the Doctrine of Signatures as the physical manifestation of the energetic template or essence of a plant, the outward sign of each plant's inner virtue. This virtue, or *arcana*, could be isolated through alchemical refinement (foreshadowing the modern extraction of active constituents) and through minimal doses (similar to homeopathic dilutions). Paracelsus coined the phrase "*similia similibus curantur*," or "like treats like," a principle he applied to the Doctrine of Signatures, just as homeopathic practitioners would later apply it to symptoms.

Paracelsus presented a system that was holistic in nature, unifying chemistry and spirit. His work represents the intertwining of biomedical science and magical or intuitive medicine, the balance of traditional wisdom with phytochemical science.

Did You Know?

Not a Quack, After All

Although Paracelsus was considered a quack by many of his contemporaries and was run out of several towns because of his theories, his ideas would later form the basis of modern science and conventional, or allopathic, medicine. His doctrines also shaped the development of Western herbalism, homeopathy and flower essence therapy, making him the father of alternative medicine.

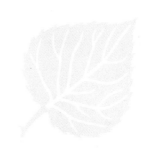

The Herbal Code

The herbal code is a legendary list of herbs disguised by other names. Throughout the ages, herbal practitioners guarded their herbal lore carefully, knowing it could be dangerous in the wrong hands. They created a code to keep their recipes secret and to discourage their use by the uninitiated. The following list is part of the herbal code common to several traditions.

- Adder's tongue: plantain
- Bat's wing: holly leaf
- Bear's foot: lady's mantle
- Blood: elder sap
- Blood of Hestia: chamomile
- Brains: congealed gum from a cherry tree
- Capon's tail: valerian
- Corpse candles: mullein
- Crow foot: wild geranium
- Dragon's scales: bistort leaves
- Ears of a goat: St. John's wort
- Eyes: eyebright or daisy
- Fingers: cinquefoil
- Hair: maidenhair fern
- Hand: the unexpanded frond from a male fern
- Heart: walnut
- Lion's tooth: dandelion
- Skin of a man: fern
- Skull: skullcap
- Tongue of a dog: hound's tongue
- Urine: dandelion
- Unicorn horn: true unicorn root

These animals indicated the following herbs:

- Blue jay: bay laurel
- Cat: catnip
- Cuckoo: orchid, plantain
- Eagle: wild garlic or fenugreek
- Hawk: hawkweed
- Lamb: lamb's lettuce
- Linnet: eyebright
- Lizard: calamint
- Nightingale: hops
- Rat: valerian
- Sheep: dandelion
- Snake: fennel or bistort
- Toad: sage
- Weasel: rue
- Woodpecker: peony
- Worms: thin roots

Native North American Traditions and Early Colonists

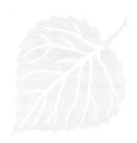

When the first colonists arrived in North America, they encountered many different indigenous groups with extensive herbal materia medica and a long history of medical practice. Some plants had different applications, being used by one group to treat one disease while another group would use the same plant to treat an entirely different health condition. Other plants were used in much the same way across the continent. Acute diseases were frequently addressed through the use of emetics (herbs to induce vomiting), cathartics (medicines that cause the bowels to purge) and various techniques to induce sweating, the most familiar of which is the sweat lodge. Chronic diseases were treated holistically and often involved the whole community in prayer and group healing rituals.

The colonists, struck by a myriad of epidemics and lacking both physicians and apothecaries, should naturally have turned to the expertise of indigenous medicine men and women. Some settlers did, in fact, study under aboriginal mentors and came to be called "Indian doctors." Unfortunately, the majority were so unwilling to recognize the legitimacy and value of aboriginal knowledge that barely any attempt was made by professional and semi-professional physicians, or "book doctors," to learn herbal lore from indigenous peoples. Medical practices and pharmacies in the early colonies continued to be stocked with herbs and remedies imported from Europe, and research into the medicinal properties of herbs reflected this rejection of native plants and traditional aboriginal medicine.

Physiomedicalism

As the boundaries of the colonies expanded westward, frontier settlers increasingly came to rely on indigenous plant medicines. Because professional doctors were scarce in frontier settlements, folk doctors, or "root doctors," increased in popularity, borrowing primarily from aboriginal medicine. One of the most famous of these folk doctors was Samuel Thomson (1769–1843). Thomson developed a theory that disease was brought about by cold, or loss of vital energy, which then resulted in an obstruction, or canker. His treatments consisted mainly of hot steam baths with lobelia (*Lobelia inflata*), cayenne pepper (*Capsicum frutescens*) and other herbs, and a cold friction rub, all used to purge the system and restore body heat. Through his use of herbs, in stark contrast to the bleeding advocated by most physicians of his time, he revived the concept of the *vis medicatrix naturae*. In 1813, he patented his system and sold rights to its use via agents.

Alva Curtis (1797–1881) drew from Thomson's ideas, started the Botanico-Medical School and Infirmary and gave the system a new name: physiomedicalism. Like Ayurvedic medicine, physiomedicalism recognized three basic tissue changes: relaxation, stimulation and contraction. Physio-medicalists believed it was important to ensure free flow of elimination through the skin, lungs, large intestine and kidneys. The liver, blood and lymph nodes were also considered significant for their ability to ensure clean metabolism and free movement of fluids. Alteratives — herbs that maintain the cleanliness and detoxification of the major organ systems — constituted the core of their treatments.

Homeopathy

Although they are distinct medical modalities, homeopathy and botanical medicine share both the common historical figure of Paracelsus as a governing influence and belief in the *vis medicatrix naturae* (the healing power of nature) as a guiding principle. Developed by Samuel Hahnemann (1755–1843), homeopathy employs dilutions of plants, animal products and other natural elements using the theory of *similis similibus curentur* ("like cures like") to create an artificial illness in the body similar to the one experienced by the patient, in order to stimulate the body's own healing powers. Hahnemann primarily used remedies made from toxic plants, in infinitesimal dilutions selected according to the individual's range of symptoms, taking into account the person's mental, emotional, spiritual and physical states, as in the naturopathic principle of *tolle totum* ("heal the whole person"). Later homeopaths greatly expanded on symptom pictures and proven remedies.

Rajan Sankaran, a contemporary homeopath in India, has explored and identified specific symptomatological themes that emerge among plants in the same family, such as Ranunculaceae (which includes delphiniums and clematis) or Solanaceae (the nightshades, such as tomatoes, potatoes and peppers). Sankaran teaches that plants within

the same family share common characteristics or sensations. For example, the Asteraceae family (also known as the Compositae family), which includes asters, daisies and sunflowers, carries the sensations of being "injured, hurt or insulted, shocked, burnt or scalded, fear to be touched, hurt, approached," and the active reaction is "touching, hurting others, cruel, violent strikes, insulting."

We can see glimpses of this school of thought in the way eclectics and flower essence therapists use some Asteraceae plants. For example, *Echinacea* species are used for physical, mental and spiritual abuse where one's sense of identity has disintegrated. Chamomile (*Matricaria chamomilla*) is prescribed for nervous irritability, peevishness and sudden fits of temper and irascibility during menstruation. Sankaran's theory of plant family sensations has not yet been explored within the context of botanical medicine. This area shows great promise for deepening our understanding of both individual and related groups of plant medicines, both the unique and the familial energetic essences of medicinal herbs.

Bach Flower Essences

Flower essence therapy grew out of Edward Bach's (1886–1936) experience with bacteriology and homeopathy. He found that medicinal plants had a special healing virtue that could be transmitted to water, as when dew collected on flowers. He grouped these virtues into seven basic types related to human personality types or spiritual typology. Almost fifty years after his death, other practitioners began to add new flower essences to Bach's original thirty-eight.

Bach presented a view of the relationship between the *vis* of plants and the *vis* of humans that differed from that of homeopathy or other vitalistic traditions. He believed that flower essences cured "by flooding our bodies with the beautiful vibrations of our Higher Nature." In other words, flower essences hold a specific positive virtue until the recipients can hold the same virtue for themselves. These remedies are yet another example of how botanical medicines heal at the spiritual and psychological levels as well as at the physiological level.

Eclecticism

Did You Know?

An Eastern Foundation

The eclectics' methods of reaching a diagnosis by assessing bodily functions, in particular assimilation and metabolism, temperature regulation, the functionality of the nervous system, excretion, and the qualities of blood and circulation, are reminiscent of the teachings of traditional Chinese, Ayurvedic and Tibetan medicine.

Wooster Beach (1794–1868) is often cited as the founder of the Eclectic movement. Before attending medical college in New York, he apprenticed under Jacob Tidd, a German doctor who exclusively used local medicinal plants. Beach sought to reform the profession from within, "combining what was useful in the old practice with what was best in the new." He advocated the use of safe botanical remedies, moderation in the use of drugs and surgery, and the exclusion of chemical poisons. Beach called his movement "reform medicine" when he started teaching it in the 1820s; his followers renamed it "eclectic medicine" in the 1840s. The early years of the movement lacked focus and philosophical foundations beyond mere substitution — instead of mercury or bloodletting, they promoted the use of milder herbs. The basic doctrine underlying their approach was not discernibly different from that of the conventional medical system.

Recognizing the need for a distinctive philosophy, John Scudder (1829–94) incorporated allopathic, homeopathic and Native medicine concepts and remedy pictures into one system. Scudder's understanding of the vital force, which extended to the relationship between the vitality of the doctor and the vitality of the patient, was integral to both diagnosis and treatment. He believed that, through this relationship, the doctor could perceive the presence of a "wrong" or disturbance to the vitality of the patient, which could be sensed both instinctively and physically, by assessing patterns in the pulse, tongue and complexion. The doctor then treated the diagnosed disturbance with specific medicines, which he chose based on an analysis of the experience of eclectic doctors, botanic empirics and folk doctors alike.

Eclectic pharmacists, such as John King (1813–93) and John Uri Lloyd (1849–1936), became increasingly interested in phytopharmacy, investigating the possibility of using concentrated extracts instead of tinctures, decoctions or syrups. They soon isolated podophyllin, the active ingredient in mayapple (*Podophyllum peltatum*), as well as many other organic compounds, and created high-quality botanical preparations. Often, however, isolated compounds were found to be completely inert. Ultimately, the eclectic pharmacists' focus on phytochemistry and extracting chemical constituents became a source of conflict within the movement.

The Flexner Report

The Flexner Report was commissioned by the Council on Medical Education (CME), which was created by the American Medical Association to promote medical education reform. Prior to the report, medical schools varied widely in their quality and content of instruction. The CME's goals were to create stringent standards for admission and training and to reduce the number of students seeking admission, and thus the number of practicing doctors. After visiting 168 medical schools in North America, Abraham Flexner recommended reducing the number to just thirty-one. He also suggested increasing the prerequisites for entry to medical school, increasing scientific research and evidence-based practice, and increasing state regulations regarding licensure.

One of the unfortunate results of the Flexner Report was the closure of schools that taught "alternative" medicine, such as naturopathic, homeopathic, osteopathic, eclectic and chiropractic medicine. Medical schools that offered education in these fields were told they needed to stop teaching these subjects or lose accreditation. Even more problematic were Flexner's recommendations to close all women-only medical schools and five of the seven schools that admitted black students. The ultimate result was a reversion to almost exclusively white, male-only admittance policies, and the near elimination of women and black physicians, that persisted well into the latter half of the twentieth century.

Divisions within the profession, the inability to establish and maintain medical schools and the 1910 Flexner Report on medical education all contributed to the downfall of the movement. Conventional medical schools flourished and the pharmaceutical industry gained ground through the discovery of patentable synthetic drugs. In North America, laboratory and clinical trials became the accepted standard and, as Alex Berman and Michel Flannery state in *America's Botanico-Medical Movements: Vox Populi*, medical culture came to view "vegetable materia medica as the product of a bygone era." But while the eclectic movement itself died off, herbalists and naturopathic doctors in North America carried on its traditions and approach to botanical medicine, publishing *Naturae Medicina* (1953), a compendium of over 300 herbs, many of which were mainstays in eclectic practice.

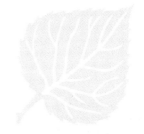

Pharmacognosy

In recent years, a renewed interest in herbal medicine has emerged in developed countries that once shunned traditional plant knowledge for modern pharmaceutical drugs (the irony being that many pharmaceuticals are derived from plant constituents). Over the past several decades, there has been an explosion of scientific research on the phytochemistry of herbal medicines, on the standardization of plant extracts and on creating a modern, evidence-based herbal pharmacopoeia.

Social interest in ensuring safe and effective medicines in Great Britain brought together previously disparate herbal organizations to create the British Herbal Medicine Association and write the *British Herbal Pharmacopoeia* (first published in 1971). In other European countries, where herbal medicine was already incorporated into conventional medical practice, research into phyto-medicinals has proliferated. Germany, ranked today as the leader in methodologically sound pharmacognostic research, created legal requirements for all drugs, including botanical medicines, culminating in the Commission E Monographs (published between 1983 and 1995).

Energetics

At the same time that pharmacognostic research has proliferated, there has been a revival of appreciation for the energetics of medicinal herbs, which goes beyond their phytochemical properties to recognize their healing spirit. Research has cast new light on old herbal remedies. For example, crude extracts based on traditional formulations have often proven more effective than isolated "active" constituents in clinical studies. Reductionistic or mechanistic models had pushed this kind of knowledge to the background and denied its relevance in modern therapeutics. This point of view is regrettable, as it neglects the salient contributions of vitalism, energetics and traditional herbalism.

Herbalists such as Matthew Wood, Peter Holmes, Michael Tierra, David Frawley and Vasant Lad have all explored the energetics of European and North American herbs, integrating flower remedies, homeopathy, traditional Chinese medicine and Ayurveda. Political and cultural movements, such as deep ecology and feminism, have also informed and inspired this herbal renaissance, as

can be seen in the works of David Hoffmann, Stephen Harrod Buhner, Mary Bove and Susun Weed. Schools of herbal energetics and traditional herbalism are enjoying unprecedented popularity, rejuvenating vitalism through their underlying belief in the transcendent power of plants. Unifying these approaches is a view that goes beyond the mechanistic phytochemical actions of plants to encompass a holistic philosophy recognizing plant intelligence, or consciousness, and ecological integration between plants and humans.

Naturopathic Integration

On the surface, there may appear to be a conflict between traditional herbal energetics and evidence-based pharmacognosy, one view of botanical medicine being vitalistic, the other being mechanistic. Naturopathic botanical medicine is particularly well suited to bridge these apparent gaps between vitalistic and mechanistic botanical medicine philosophies.

Cultures around the globe have developed distinct and seemingly disparate systems of healing, such as traditional Chinese medicine, Ayurvedic medicine, Unani medicine, curanderismo, North American Native medicine, homeopathy, Western botanical medicine and more. Naturopathic botanical medicine is able to incorporate these traditions by recognizing the commonalities in the philosophy and practice of healing, and by gaining a fuller, more holistic understanding of the essence — or *arcana*, as Paracelsus described it — of each plant used in naturopathic medical practice.

Balance is the cornerstone of health in all of these traditions, where disease is seen as a disturbance to the body's intrinsic state of homeostasis. The healer's or physician's duty is to restore balance, and thus health, by supporting the patient's own innate powers of recuperation. Different herbal traditions use different names — qi, *prana*, spirit, *dynamis*, vital force, *archeus* or *vis*, for example — but all describe an intrinsic and intelligent energy that connects individual vitality to universal energy. In naturopathic medicine, we refer to this energy as the *vis medicatrix naturae*, the healing power of nature. In this context, plants are seen as our allies and teachers, assisting us in our return to health and a state of balance through their inner vitality, energetic qualities, phytochemical structure and relationship with humans.

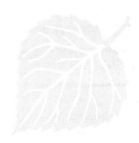

Did You Know?

Synthesis and Synergy

In both philosophy and practice, naturopathic botanical medicine is inclusive. It successfully synthesizes the art and the science of herbalism, seamlessly merging traditional and empirical knowledge with pharmacognosy and evidence-based approaches. Encompassing the whole of botanical history, naturopathic botanical medicine employs the best practices of these influences in case management.

Did You Know?

Environmental Stewardship

It is important to stress the need for environmental stewardship within botanical medicine traditions. Some of the plants presented in Part 3 of this book are endangered in their native habitats because of overharvesting, human encroachment or invasion by non-native species. Naturopathic doctors and herbalists are at the forefront of nurturing the special reciprocal relationship humans have with their plant allies, taking care of and with them to support the balance of the planet as much as that of patients. Continuing to pursue a deeper and more holistic understanding of plants, both scientifically and energetically, is essential to support the future of botanical medicine and the *vis medicatrix naturae* called upon in clinical practice.

Bioindividualism

An understanding of the value of both art and science is required in order to treat the whole person as a unique individual, matching our method of dispensing herbs to the needs of the patient. For example, an evidence-based or phytopharmacological approach to botanical prescribing might be more appropriate for a patient who is a mechanistic thinker, whereas an energetic approach may be better suited for a spiritually oriented person. Where the root cause of a physical ailment is mental, emotional or spiritual in nature, consideration of the energetics of the potential treatments is of the utmost importance in the choice of appropriate herbs. Where the cause is determined to be primarily physiological in nature, or the treatment of a proximate material cause is desired before treatment of the root cause, the pharmacological actions of a particular plant may be given priority over its energetic themes.

The Healing Power of Nature

The *vis medicatrix naturae*, or healing power of nature, is an essential template of health inherent in all living things. At the individual level, it is the biological process that enables humans and other animals to heal wounds and respond to infections, and that allows plants to change their chemical constituents to avoid being eaten or to communicate with neighboring plants.

The healing power of nature also refers to a plant's essence, or spirit, which is captured in different ways by traditional Chinese medicine, Native American medicine, Ayurvedic medicine, flower essence therapy, homeopathy and other herbal medicine systems. A medicinal herb, respectfully prepared as food, an infusion, a tincture or some other whole plant preparation, conveys not only the plant's pharmacology but also its energetic essence. Thus, plants may be used to heal not only at the physical level but also at the emotional, mental and spiritual levels.

Herbal medicine is the acknowledgment of a deep, harmonious relationship between humans and plants that moves beyond the pharmacological action of individual plant constituents to an understanding of the whole plant and its connection to the people working with it. It is a reflection of the mutual healing relationship best depicted by the basics of breathing: humans and other animals breathe in oxygen and breathe out carbon dioxide; plants breathe in carbon dioxide and breathe out oxygen. The more you work with medicinal plants, the more this relationship develops. Making an infusion, decoction, compress or salve at home allows for a greater opportunity to get to know medicinal plants than by simply taking an herbal pill.

Botanical Preparations

Herbs are prepared in a number of forms, ranging from teas to concentrated extracts to salves. In general, people are most familiar with drinking a cup of herbal tea for pleasure every once in a while. Fewer people regularly use herbal teas as medicine. Fewer still have used botanical medicines in the form of decoctions, tinctures, supplemental extracts or topical preparations.

Regardless of what form the medicine comes in, the whole plant is usually used (with the exception of some standardized or enhanced extracts, which isolate a particular plant chemical). This means that you are consuming a variety of plant constituents, or chemicals. Not only is the medicine complex, but its interaction with your body is complex. This meeting of one complex system (you) with another complex system (the plant) is one reason that herbal medicine is holistic. But it can also make it difficult to understand and evaluate how herbal medicines work.

Whole Fresh Plant

In this form of preparation, the plant is simply eaten or applied to the surface of the skin, either freshly picked or ripened in some way. For example, dandelion (*Taraxacum officinale*) greens, which contain bitter compounds, are used in salads to stimulate the appetite and digestive processes for the remainder of the meal. The gel of the *Aloe vera* plant is readily available by cutting open one of the spikes, and is well known for its topical use on sunburns and other minor skin irritations.

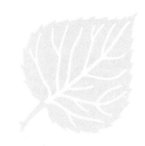

Infusion (Tea)

An infusion is better known as a tea. In most cases, hot water is poured over or mixed with the fresh or dried herb and then steeped, covered, for several minutes. Infusions are most appropriate when the parts of the plant used are leaves or flowers, which break down easily through steeping. The water draws out certain plant chemicals, especially volatile oils (the chemicals that give plants their smell) and starches. Infusions are often used for herbs that have an effect on the respiratory, digestive and nervous systems. They are best for conditions such as colds, flus and coughs, where steam can help open sinus passages and drinking lots of fluid is a good idea anyway.

Decoction

A decoction is an extract of a plant that has been simmered in hot water for 15 minutes to an hour. Decoctions are usually used for harder parts of the plant: roots, bark and seeds. This produces a more concentrated extract. Many botanicals used in traditional Chinese medicine, such as ginseng and dang gui, are made into decoctions.

Tincture

Herbal medicines can also be extracted with a solvent, usually ethanol. The resulting liquid is called a tincture. The herb, either fresh or dried, is added to a concentrated hydro-alcohol solution (25% to 90%, depending on the herb and plant constituents) and allowed to sit for days or weeks. The alcohol draws out certain constituents that cannot be extracted through water-based methods. Apéritifs and digestifs are essentially herbal tinctures that are drunk before or after meals to stimulate digestion.

Vinegar or glycerin is sometimes used instead of alcohol to extract botanical constituents. Glycerin tinctures are sweet and alcohol-free, so they are often used for children. However, vinegar and glycerin tinctures are less common, may not extract all the plant constituents desired and have shorter shelf lives than alcohol-based tinctures.

Naturopathic doctors, following the historical precedent of the eclectic physicians, use tinctures quite frequently, as it is easy for them to make customized medicinal formulas. (Although dried herbs can also be easily combined into custom formulas, they may not be appropriate in all cases,

Did You Know?

Help for Anxiety

Teas are also helpful for conditions such as anxiety, when the ritual of making tea can be an opportunity to breathe, connect to the present moment and feel more grounded and relaxed.

Did You Know?

Concentration

Tinctures are usually made with a 1:5 concentration, which means that 1 gram of the herb is mixed with 5 grams of alcohol (or vinegar or glycerin), but other concentrations are possible. Stronger liquid extracts can be made in 1:2 or 1:1 concentrations, using specialized equipment to distill or percolate the herbs. This type of concentration may require heat, pressure or other chemical solvents to achieve.

or for all herbs.) Another advantage of tinctures is their long shelf life. Alcohol-based tinctures can last many years, retaining their medicinal qualities and strength throughout. Tinctures are also convenient, as very little liquid is needed to achieve an effective dose, and they are easily absorbed.

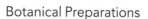

Solid Extract

In the case of a solid extract, a solvent such as ethanol is used to extract compounds from the plant. The solvent is then partially or completely evaporated or otherwise removed. This leaves a very thick solid or near-solid material that can be redissolved in water for use. Solid extracts are less commonly available.

Standardized Extract

A relatively new form of botanical preparation, standardized extracts have become increasingly popular. A standardized extract provides a very precise amount of a given constituent extracted from the plant. Although some standardized extracts are made from the whole plant, more often one or more plant chemicals are concentrated, resulting in an extract that contains constituents in ratios that are different from those found in nature.

Standardized extracts are typically patented and are the most common form of herbal medicine used in clinical trials. Produced in pill form, they are convenient, familiar to users of pharmaceutical drugs, patentable and highly portable. Turmeric is frequently found as a standardized extract, concentrated to a specific level of curcumin, the main active plant constituent responsible for turmeric's medicinal qualities.

Topical Preparations

Topical herbal medicines are applied to the surface of the skin rather than ingested orally. They come in various preparations, each of which is useful for different purposes.

Compress

To make a compress (also known as a fomentation), a clean cloth is dipped into an infusion, decoction or tincture and then placed directly on the skin. Compresses are often used on skin conditions or lesions.

Treatment on the Go

Since poultices are often made with fresh herbs, they are perfect for on-the-spot harvesting and application when you are out for a hike in the woods or otherwise enjoying nature. Plantain leaves, for example, can be chewed and applied over a mosquito bite for instant relief, while yarrow leaves and flowers can be used to stop bleeding from small cuts.

Poultice

A poultice is made by chopping, chewing or pounding plant material (usually leaves, flowers and/or powdered roots) and mixing it with water to make a paste. Flour is sometimes added, as with mustard or cayenne poultices. The paste is then applied to the skin. Poultices are traditionally used for skin lesions or infections. They may be covered by a wet cloth or herbal compress to further enhance their effects.

Infused Oil

Many different oils can be used as a base for topical delivery of herbs. Olive oil is a common choice, though other options, such as coconut, sesame or jojoba oil, may be used for their own medicinal qualities. Herbs are infused in the oil over time (anywhere from days to weeks) to extract the phytochemical constituents. The oil is then strained and applied to the skin, imparting medicine from the herbs and oil as well as moisture from the oil. Infused oils are best used on large areas of the body, where they are massaged into the skin, and on the scalp, where hair can make it difficult to apply other preparations. Infused oils can also be used vaginally in cases of atrophic vaginitis, or released in drops into the ear for ear infections.

Salve or Cream

A salve is an ointment traditionally made by mixing an infused oil with beeswax to create a semisolid product that can be applied topically to a specific area of the skin. The beeswax also seals in moisture and creates a barrier that protects the skin from infection.

Creams are similar to salves but are created by emulsifying the infused oil into a water-based cream. As a result, they are less likely to stain clothes.

Suppository

Herbal oil infusions can be made with oils that are solid at room temperature, such as coconut oil, and then formed into small ovoid shapes to be inserted into the rectum or vagina. Alternatively, tinctures may be mixed with coconut oil and then shaped as described. Suppositories are commonly used for health conditions such as hemorrhoids, anal fissures, cervical dysplasia and vaginitis. A panty liner is worn to prevent the oil from saturating or staining underclothes.

Botanical Preparations: Advantages and Disadvantages

Preparation	Advantages	Disadvantages
Whole fresh plant	• Can be incorporated into regular diet • Simple to prepare • Minimal processing	• Might not be strong enough in certain cases • Strength of medicine can vary greatly between individual plants
Infusion/tea (hot or cold)	• Easy to prepare • Alcohol-free • Good form for tasty herbs such as mint, chamomile, lemon balm	• Concentration may not be strong enough • Some plant constituents do not extract well in water • May be inconvenient for some people • Some herbs taste very bitter or pungent, which may not appeal to some people
Decoction	• Can be made relatively quickly • Alcohol-free • Stronger concentration than infusion	• Concentration may not be strong enough, or may not be suitable for certain plant constituents • May be inconvenient for some people • Some herbs taste very bitter or pungent, which may not appeal to some people
Tincture	• Alcohol extracts have a long shelf life • Can be easily mixed into combinations • More concentrated than infusions and decoctions • Easily absorbed • Liquid form is convenient; less liquid is needed to achieve therapeutic doses	• Contains alcohol (not appropriate for some people, very young children) • Taste cannot be hidden very easily
Solid extract	• Concentrated form without the alcohol found in tinctures	• Reduced shelf life • Not readily available commercially
Standardized extract	• Dose is very specific and consistent • Can deliver a specific amount of a plant substance • Can isolate a certain plant constituent • Form of herbal medicine most often used in clinical trials • Pill form is convenient	• Not necessarily a whole plant extract • Not consistent with traditional use of plants • Cannot mix and combine easily (need to take additional pills) • Not available for all herbal medicines • More expensive

Preparation	Advantages	Disadvantages
Compress	• Easy to prepare at home	• Messy
Poultice	• Easy to prepare at home • Good for on-the-spot application	• Cost-effective • Messy
Infused oil	• Easy to massage onto large areas of skin or into the scalp • Basis for other preparations, such as salves and creams	• Messy • Can become rancid if exposed to air or light • May stain clothes
Salve or cream	• Convenient format • Less messy than other topical preparations	• Messy • May stain clothes
Suppository	• Easy to insert into vagina or rectum for local applications	• Need to wear a panty liner or pad to avoid staining undergarments

Dosage

Dosage can be an issue in botanical medicine because of problems in gauging potency, ensuring purity and standardizing doses. However, many herbal manufacturers are now testing their batches in laboratories to ensure consistent purity and potency, and government agencies, such as the Food and Drug Administration in the United States and the National Health Products Directorate in Canada, are establishing dosage standards and regulations. In the U.S. and Canada, health claims on a label must be supported by evidence. Nevertheless, the nature of the botanical medicine marketplace still allows for a wide variation in quality, and it is important to source botanicals from suppliers who accurately define their products and are known to be compliant with federal agencies.

Unlike pharmaceuticals, for which dosage is more clearly defined and studied, in herbal medicine the dose is usually less precise. Tinctures and solid extracts are usually prescribed by the teaspoon (5 mL) and infusions by the cup (250 mL). A dose might be taken once a day or repeated two or more times per day. Botanicals in capsule or tablet form, for example, might be taken several times a day.

Although dosage precision is not always possible, neither is it always necessary: certain commonly used botanicals have been observed, over decades or centuries, to bring about a clinical improvement at a wide range of doses, and they are considered to have a high margin of safety. However, for some botanicals with very low safety margins, the dose must be much more specific. Kava, for example, has been linked to liver toxicity, so in countries where it is legally available for use, maximum doses may be set to ensure safety. Although herbs are all natural, not all herbs are safe at any dose.

The introduction of standardized extracts is changing the picture. It is now possible for doctors to prescribe a precise quantity of a given botanical compound. This is useful when the doctor's rationale for the prescription is based on scientific studies that used a standardized extract of the botanical, or where there are dosage-related safety concerns.

Purity Issues

Substandard quality control and processing methods can make it difficult to know what, exactly, you're getting when you purchase an herbal medicine. In some historical cases, certain herbs have been replaced with cheaper, similar-looking herbs with different medicinal actions. Contamination (when other substances, such as pharmaceutical drugs, are unintentionally added to an herbal product) and adulteration (when the addition of other substances is intentional) are both illegal but unfortunately still occur. Substitutions, contamination and adulterations have been implicated in unexpected drug–herb interactions and serious adverse effects.

Contaminants may include mold, dust, pollen, insects, microbes, fungi and even heavy metals. Fluffy leafy herbs, such as raspberry leaf, are more susceptible to mold growth during the drying process. Herbs that draw minerals from deep in the earth into their roots and leaves, such as nettle, red clover and dandelion (also known as dynamic accumulators), are more likely to be contiminated with heavy metals.

Drug–Herb Interactions

Botanicals can alter the effect of drugs in many ways. Herbs can increase the actions of drugs, decrease the actions of drugs, oppose the actions of drugs or change how drugs are metabolized in the body. Some herbs can enhance the action of certain drugs, as devil's claw, ginger and willow bark do when taken with non-steroidal anti-inflammatory drugs (NSAIDs). In other cases, the interaction may have unwanted consequences. For example, St. John's wort can be helpful for depression but has effects on drug metabolism that may make oral contraceptive pills ineffective, potentially resulting in an unplanned pregnancy.

There are now excellent databases for checking drug–herb and herb–herb interactions, but doctor discretion is always needed, along with a thorough patient history that includes herb, drug and over-the-counter product use. Before starting any herbal medicine, it is always best to consult with a regulated health professional who is knowledgeable in the area of herb–drug interactions.

Plant Classifications

Herbs can be classified by botany/taxonomy or by therapeutic uses. Throughout history, many authors have compiled extensive classification systems for plants according to their medicinal properties. To a certain degree, such classification is arbitrary, because most herbs have more than one action, act on more than one body system and/or have different actions depending on the part used or the preparation used. Many of the classifications are ancient and are based on culturally specific language and medical philosophies, rather than on the modern scientific classifications used for pharmaceutical drugs. Nonetheless, these classifications can be useful in terms of reflecting how herbs are used in actual practice.

Botanical Classification

Latin binomials are used to name plants, following the same genus and species classification applied to all organisms. For example, *Echinacea angustifolia* tells you the specific species — *angustifolia* — within the genus *Echinacea*. On a pragmatic level, this system is essential to avoid confusing species and perhaps using the wrong herb. The genus *Echinacea* has three species — *angustifolia*, *purpurea* and *pallida* — each with a somewhat different chemical composition. *Symphytum officinale* (comfrey), used therapeutically to promote wound healing, has been confused with another species of comfrey, *Symphytum uplandicum*, which is linked to liver cancer.

Common names used for herbs, such as "comfrey," can result in confusion, too. "Echinacea" is both the genus name (when uppercase and in italics) and the common name, but echinacea is also known by the common names "purple coneflower" and "snakeroot." When a plant has several common names, mix-ups can occur if those names are used interchangeably.

Therapeutic Classification

Therapeutic classifications are a time-honored way to organize botanicals for study and clinical use. Herbs are commonly classified by health condition, by body system or organ, by constituent or by action. Some herbs function in several different categories within a therapeutic classification.

Classification by Health Condition

The classification of herbal medicines by specific symptoms (or indications) is based on case observations from a wealth of collective experience in which a particular herb has consistently acted best for patients with that symptom or set of symptoms. Most herbal medicine traditions include very specific information about plants and their effects on people, to simplify the process of choosing herbs. Further classification may be based on pulse, the appearance of the tongue, spiritual or mental symptoms, or other factors.

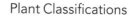

Classification by Body System or Organ

Medicinal herbs are now commonly classified by the body system or organ they affect. For example, a "hepatic" herb affects the hepatic system, which includes the liver, while a "cardiac" herb affects the cardiovascular system, which includes the heart. The herbs discussed in this book are classified within a variety of body systems, including the gynecological, gastrointestinal, musculoskeletal and nervous systems.

Classification by Constituent

Scientists and pharmacologists often group herbs by their chemical constituents (phytochemicals) to better understand how herbs affect specific body systems and physiological pathways. This system can also help us to better understand herb–drug interactions. Classification by constituent sometimes produces a list similar to the one created when herbs are classified by therapeutic action.

Classification by Action

Herbs can also be grouped by therapeutic action: their healing effect on the body. For example, many herbs are cholagogues — they increase the expulsion of bile from the gallbladder — though each may elicit this reaction in a slightly different way. Sometimes the chemical constituent responsible for producing an action is known; in other cases, it is unknown which plant chemicals are responsible for the action, or how exactly they work in the body.

Therapeutic Actions

Herbal medicine uses some archaic or non-English action-related terms. Here are definitions of some of the terms used in this book. See the Glossary (page 363) for more terms.

Term	Definition
Adaptogen	Helps the body adapt to new or stressful situations by building resistance to stress, reducing stress response and increasing endurance
Alterative	Restores overall function, detoxifies and eliminates waste
Analgesic	Relieves pain
Antihemorrhagic	Stops bleeding
Anti-inflammatory	Reduces inflammation locally and/or systemically
Antimicrobial	Supports innate immune responses; is active against bacteria, viruses, fungi and protozoa
Antispasmodic	Reduces pain caused by smooth and/or skeletal muscle spasm
Aphrodisiac	Increases sexual arousal
Astringent	Constricts and tones tissues and mucous membranes; stops bleeding
Bitter	Increases digestive secretions, increases appetite, awakens metabolism and consciousness
Cardioactive	Stimulates or regulates the heart
Cardiotonic	Tonifies the heart and cardiovascular system
Carminative	Soothes and relaxes the digestive tract; relieves gas in the intestines
Cholagogue	Encourages release of bile from the gallbladder into the intestines to help digest food, especially fats
Counterirritant	Activates nerve cells in the skin to alter the perception of pain
Demulcent	Coats, soothes and protects mucous membranes
Diuretic	Increases urinary excretion
Galactagogue	Increases breast milk production
Hepatic	Promotes better liver and gallbladder function and/or detoxification through the liver
Hypnotic	Promotes sleep
Hypotensive	Decreases blood pressure
Laxative	Promotes bowel activity and movement
Nervine	Affects the nervous system by relaxing, stimulating, tonifying, combating depression or sedating
Tonic	Strengthens an organ or a person's overall vitality

Part 2

Women's Health Conditions

Acne

Acne is probably the most common and most visible skin condition experienced by women. About 85% of women experience at least some degree of acne at some point in their lives, most likely during their teen years. Even though acne is so prevalent, it is quite common for women (and men) to become self-conscious about how they look or how they are perceived when they have acne, a worry that has negative psychological and social effects. The trouble is that acne is so visible, usually affecting the very part of our bodies that people look at the most: the face. Acne can have an impact on self-esteem, body image, social life and sexuality. Studies show that adolescent girls tend to be more vulnerable than boys to these psychosocial effects.

Changes in hormone levels during puberty can lead to inflammation of oil-producing glands in the skin, resulting in acne. Acne can show up as whiteheads, blackheads or, less frequently, cysts. It is most often seen on the face, chest and back, where oil-producing glands are most common. For some women, it can persist into adulthood, particularly when hormone levels are irregular or excessive. Acne can also show up at other times of great hormone changes, such as birth and menopause. Over time, acne can lead to enlargement of the oil glands, scarring and changes in skin tone or color.

Signs and Symptoms
- Oily skin
- Blackheads
- Whiteheads
- Nodules or cysts

Associated Conditions
- Congenital adrenal hyperplasia
- Depression and/or anxiety
- Insulin resistance (theorized)
- Polycystic ovarian syndrome (PCOS)

First-Line Herbal Care: TEA TREE OIL

Tea tree oil (*Melaleuca alternifolia*) is an extract from a tree native to Australia that has strong antibacterial and antifungal properties. Although it is not safe to take orally because of its highly concentrated essential oils, tea tree oil is an excellent topical treatment for acne, especially in cases that respond to topical antibiotic treatment.

In a double-blind study, a 5% tea tree oil gel applied twice daily significantly decreased the number and severity of acne lesions when compared to a placebo. A previous single-blind study found no difference in treatment effects between 5% tea tree oil gel and benzoyl peroxide, the first-line pharmaceutical therapy for acne. In that study, the positive effects took longer to become apparent with the use of the tea tree oil gel, but it was better tolerated and had fewer reported side effects.

Other Herbal Treatments

Anti-inflammatory herbs, such as calendula, can be applied topically. Herbs that help support healthy liver function and hormone metabolism, such as barberry, can be taken orally. Antianxiety or mood-stabilizing herbs, such as St. John's wort, may be used to treat significant psychosocial effects.

Did You Know?

Barberry and PCOS

Recent research on barberry has centered on its use in the treatment of polycystic ovarian syndrome (PCOS). Barberry has been shown to be comparable to metformin, a common pharmaceutical treatment.

Barberry

The skin, as one of the means through which the body naturally rids itself of toxins, can become overburdened if another organ of metabolism and detoxification, such as the liver, is not working well. One of the goals of herbal therapy in the treatment of skin conditions is to ensure that other detoxification organs are functioning at optimal levels. Barberry (*Berberis vulgaris*), as a hepatic, promotes the function of the liver and gallbladder.

A 2012 study on the use of barberry to treat moderate to severe acne in teenagers showed promising results. Compared to a placebo, 600 milligrams of barberry extract, taken daily, significantly decreased the number of acne lesions and the severity of lesions after four weeks of use. No side effects were noted in the study.

Calendula

Calendula (*Calendula officinalis*) is one of the best herbs for skin conditions of all kinds. It is a gentle but excellent anti-inflammatory, soothing and cleansing the skin. Calendula is also mildly antimicrobial, perfect for helping to balance skin bacterial flora. A simple infusion of calendula can be applied as a compress after cleansing the skin, or it can be put into a misting bottle and sprayed onto the face like a toner. Calendula is also available as a cream, to be used as an herbal moisturizer. No matter which application is used, calendula is best applied after washing the face, in the morning and again before bed.

Green Tea

Among its many medicinal uses, green tea (*Camellia sinensis*) can be used as a topical treatment for acne. In one study, a 2% green tea extract applied to skin twice a day for six weeks significantly decreased both the number of acne lesions (also known as "zits") and the overall severity of the acne.

CASE STUDY
Acne

Courtney, a twelve-year-old girl with acne covering her cheeks and chin, came to see me because she thought she looked ugly. She was deeply affected by sociocultural expectations of beauty and body image. As a result, she was suffering moderate social anxiety and depression and was avoiding socializing with her friends and peers.

Courtney had had her first period around the same time that the acne became bothersome, less than six months before. Since then, her periods had been irregular.

I recommended a tincture of barberry, black cohosh, dang gui and dandelion, along with herbal skin-care compresses. I also suggested that Courtney apply castor oil to her face before bed each night.

Over the next few visits, Courtney explored her feelings about puberty, her changing body and ideas of attractiveness and identity. After six weeks, the acne was mostly resolved, and she was no longer quite so bothered when she did have an occasional breakout.

Common Combinations

- A compress of calendula and green tea, with a couple of drops of tea tree oil and castor oil, applied overnight
- Barberry, burdock and dandelion for stubborn acne plus slow bowel function or mild constipation
- Chaste tree, peony and barberry for acne due to PCOS

Conventional Medical Treatments

- **Topical:** Benzoyl peroxide; antibiotics; retinoid creams
- **Systemic:** Antibiotics; oral contraceptives; isotretinoin in severe cases

Further Reading

Elsaie ML, Abdelhamid MF, Elsaaiee LT, Emam HM. The efficacy of topical 2% green tea lotion in mild-to-moderate acne vulgaris. *Journal of Drugs in Dermatology*, 2009 Apr; 8 (4): 358–64.

Enshaieh S, Jooya A, Siadat AH, Iraji F. The efficacy of 5% topical tea tree oil gel in mild to moderate acne vulgaris: A randomized, double-blind placebo-controlled study. *Indian Journal of Dermatology, Venereology and Leprology*, 2007 Jan–Feb; 73 (1): 22–25.

Fouladi RF. Aqueous extract of dried fruit of *Berberis vulgaris* L. in acne vulgaris: A clinical trial. *Journal of Dietary Supplements*, 2012 Dec; 9 (4): 253–61.

Anemia

Among the various forms of anemia, iron-deficiency anemia is the most common. In order to treat the anemia, the cause of the iron deficiency has to be determined. In adults, iron-deficiency anemia is most often seen in conjunction with heavy menses or during pregnancy. In cases of heavy menses, blood, and thus iron, is lost each month, making women vulnerable to iron-deficiency anemia. In pregnancy, more blood is created, and therefore greater amounts of iron are required. Other reasons for iron deficiency include insufficient iron from dietary sources, inadequate absorption, and blood loss from causes other than menses, such as a bleeding stomach ulcer.

Iron-deficiency anemia is often asymptomatic and found by routine blood tests. Common mild symptoms include fatigue, dizziness and shortness of breath with exercise. More severe symptoms include pagophagia (eating ice), pica (eating non-foods), anorexia, glossitis (soreness or inflammation of the tongue), angular stomatitis (inflammation of the corners of the lips) and pallor.

Signs and Symptoms

- Fatigue
- Dizziness
- Shortness of breath with exercise
- Pagophagia
- Pica
- Anorexia
- Glossitis
- Angular stomatitis
- Pallor

Associated Conditions

- Colon cancer
- Menorrhagia
- Peptic ulcer disease
- Pregnancy
- Uterine cancer

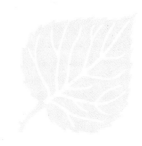

First-Line Herbal Care: NETTLE

Nettles (*Urtica dioica*) have a long history of use in treating anemia because they are a rich source of minerals. They draw up whatever minerals are present in the soil, concentrating them in their roots and leaves. Their nutritive qualities make them an excellent herb at any age, and especially during puberty, pregnancy, breastfeeding or menopause.

Traditionally, nettles have been used in soups and stews as spring and fall tonics, nourishing people during times of seasonal transition. They are an excellent source of vegetarian iron and also contain vitamin C, which increases iron's absorption. According to the United States Department of Agriculture (USDA), 100 grams of cooked nettles contain 1.6 milligrams of iron.

Caution

Because nettles pull minerals — and heavy metals — out of the soil, care should be taken when sourcing them. Whether you are buying nettles or wildcrafting them (harvesting them from the wild), be cautious about their soil quality and growing conditions. Don't pick nettles from land that is known to be toxic or that was previously used for industrial purposes.

Kitchen Lore

Nettle Tea

My favorite way to prepare nettles is as a strong infusion, or tea. I use a 1-quart (1 L) mason jar, but any glass container with a sealable lid will do.

> 4 cups (1 L) water
> 1 cup (250 mL) nettles (about 1 oz/30 g)
> 1 tbsp (15 mL) cider vinegar

1. Bring the water to a boil. Place the nettles in the jar and cover almost to the top with the boiled water. Add cider vinegar to improve mineral absorption.
2. Close the lid tightly and steep overnight.
3. Strain.
4. Drink the contents over the course of two days, keeping the infusion refrigerated after straining.

Tip
Add 1 tablespoon (15 mL) of molasses to increase the iron content of the drink even more.

Other Herbal Treatments

Herbal treatment of iron deficiency is typically twofold: increase intake of iron-rich herbs and blood tonics, and decrease blood loss, if necessary.

Dandelion

Like nettles, dandelion (*Taraxacum officinale*) concentrates minerals from the soil in its roots and leaves. One hundred grams of cooked dandelion leaves contains 1.8 milligrams of iron.

A study in which a water-and-alcohol-based extract of dandelion was injected into mice found that it significantly improved red blood cell markers compared to a placebo, increasing both total red blood cell count and hemoglobin levels. This study supports the traditional use of dandelion to treat anemia.

Dang Gui

Dang gui, also known as dong quai or by its Latin name, *Angelica sinensis*, is considered a blood tonic — traditionally used to treat anemia — within traditional Chinese herbal medicine. It is an archetypal example of an herb used to increase the production of blood. As a blood tonic, it is useful in cases of anemia, amenorrhea, irregular menstrual cycles, infertility and even menopause.

Recent clinical trials have supported the use of dang gui in the treatment of anemia. Several studies on iron-deficient animals have shown that the polysaccharides in dang gui improve the animals' hemoglobin, red blood cell and hematocrit levels. The same blood marker improvements were found in studies that used dang gui for anemia caused by drugs used to treat autoimmune disease and as chemotherapy for cancer.

Traditionally, dang gui is prepared as a decoction of the root. In traditional Chinese medicine, the typical daily dosage can be anywhere from 3 to 15 grams of the whole root when it is made into a decoction, depending on how the herb is used in combination with other herbs. Dang gui is also available as a tincture, an encapsulated extract or an herbal tablet.

Caution

Although dang gui may be useful for regulating an abnormal menstrual cycle over time, it should be used cautiously during menses itself, as it may increase bleeding.

Common Combinations

- Nettles, dandelion and burdock to increase mineral intake and absorption
- Dang gui, cooked rehmannia and white peony to address blood deficiency

Conventional Medical Treatments

- Iron supplementation, whether orally, by injection or, in severe cases, intravenously

Further Reading

Liu PJ, Hsieh WT, Huang SH, et al. Hematopoietic effect of water-soluble polysaccharides from *Angelica sinensis* on mice with acute blood loss. *Experimental Hematology*, 2010 Jun; 38 (6): 437–45.

Modaresi M, Resalatpour N. The effect of *Taraxacum officinale* hydroalcoholic extract on blood cells in mice. *Advances in Hematology*, 2012; 2012: 653412.

Wang PP, Zhang Y, Dai LQ, Wang KP. Effect of *Angelica sinensis* polysaccharide-iron complex on iron deficiency anemia in rats. *Chinese Journal of Integrative Medicine*, 2007 Dec; 13 (4): 297–300.

Anxiety

Anxiety disorders are a collection of common health conditions characterized by excessive and/or chronic feelings of anxiety, worry and/or fear. The umbrella term includes such conditions as panic disorder, generalized anxiety disorder, social phobia, obsessive-compulsive disorder (OCD) and post-traumatic stress disorder (PTSD).

Anxiety is one of the most common complaints I see in my naturopathic practice. It manifests emotionally, behaviorally and physically in different ways in different women. Some women with anxiety also experience depression; some women's anxiety is related to irritable bowel syndrome or a skin rash. Some women use substances like alcohol, cigarettes or other drugs to cope with their anxiety; some women redirect their anxiety toward other health issues or their body image.

No matter how anxiety manifests, it is more often than not a major health concern for the women (and men) who experience it. Yet social stigma, access to care and associated health conditions can all pose significant challenges to people seeking help for anxiety.

Signs and Symptoms

Symptoms of anxiety are often described as being either somatic (of the body) or psychological (of the mind).

Somatic Symptoms
- Shortness of breath
- Heart palpitations
- Excessive sweating
- Restlessness
- Insomnia
- Dizziness
- Nausea
- Diarrhea
- Headache

Psychological Symptoms
- Anxiety
- Worry
- Fear
- Difficulty concentrating
- Feeling on edge
- Irritability

Associated Conditions

- Chronic pain
- Depression
- Disordered eating
- Irritable bowel syndrome
- Other anxiety disorders
- Personality disorders
- Substance abuse

First-Line Herbal Care: LAVENDER

Most of us already think of lavender as a relaxing scent, in part because it is commonly stuffed into eye pillows to encourage a good night's sleep. Lavender (*Lavandula angustifolia*) is traditionally administered through aromatherapy or in the form of tea, but lavender oil capsules are becoming more common.

Clinical studies have shown that lavender essential oil, used as aromatherapy, is effective in reducing anxiety before tests, surgery and dental work. One small pilot study investigated the use of lavender essential oil as aromatherapy in high-risk postpartum women. Compared to a control group, the group that used lavender showed significant improvements in both depression and anxiety symptoms.

Between 2010 and 2014, a slew of clinical trials explored the therapeutic use of lavender oil capsules for a wide range of anxiety disorders. In a large double-blind, placebo-controlled study of people diagnosed with generalized anxiety disorder, anxiety symptoms were significantly reduced after the participants took lavender oil capsules for ten weeks. Their scores on an anxiety questionnaire decreased by up to 50%. These results were shown to be better than those achieved with a placebo, and at least as good as those seen with the antidepressant drug paroxetine.

A review of the use of lavender oil capsules for anxiety concluded that lavender reduced anxiety symptoms substantially more than a placebo in subsyndromal anxiety (anxiety that is present but doesn't meet the threshold for diagnosis) and generalized anxiety disorder. Antianxiety effects were evident in some trials after as little as two weeks, and were comparable to the effects of lorazepam, a benzodiazepine. Other trials have shown significant improvements in the symptoms of post-traumatic stress disorder and somatization disorder.

Lavender oil capsules have fewer side effects than either antidepressant drugs or benzodiazepines and do not appear to lead to dependency. Lavender is non-drowsy, unlike many other nervine herbs. Dosage ranges from 80 to 160 milligrams daily.

Other Herbal Treatments

Nervines and antianxiety herbs are typically used to treat anxiety. I highlight some of them below, but there are many more that I use in clinical practice, including skullcap, blue vervain and milky oats. Where anxiety is strongly associated with chronic stress and fatigue, adaptogens such as ashwagandha may be helpful. For severe anxiety and insomnia, stronger herbs that are considered hypnotics, such as valerian or hops, may be indicated. Stronger herbs may induce drowsiness, affecting the ability to work, drive a car or operate heavy machinery. Hypnotic herbs should be taken only in consultation with a health-care professional.

Chamomile

Chamomile (*Matricaria recutita* or *Chamaemelum nobile*) is well known as a gentle digestive and de-stressing herb. But despite its long history of use as a mild antianxiety herb, only a handful of clinical studies have looked at chamomile for anxiety. The studies that have been conducted, however, are positive and support its use in mild anxiety. One study comparing chamomile extract to a placebo found that the people who took chamomile reported significantly less anxiety. Another study found that, in addition to its anxiety-reducing effects, chamomile also reduced symptoms of depression when they occurred in tandem with anxiety.

In these studies, chamomile was given in capsules containing 220 milligrams of herb, standardized to 1.2% apigenin. Participants took two to four capsules daily. Traditionally, chamomile is used as a tea.

Kava

Kava (*Piper methysticum*) has been traditionally used in South Pacific cultures for medicinal, spiritual, cultural and social purposes. It is valued for its ability to produce a hypnotic effect and euphoria while maintaining, or even enhancing, thought processes. The traditional method of preparing kava varies, but it can be an elaborate and ritualized process that often includes chewing the root.

Caution

At this time, caution is strongly advised when it comes to taking kava. Consultation with and monitoring by a health-care professional is highly recommended.

Kava's antianxiety effects were demonstrated in clinical studies in the early 2000s, and it has been widely regarded as the most effective herb for anxiety. A large review published in 2003 concluded that kava was an effective treatment for anxiety when compared to a placebo. A 2006 review came to a similar conclusion but raised concerns about the safety of kava. Two of the three studies reviewed were stopped early and never published because of concerns about liver damage. Case reports on the use of kava have documented liver damage, cirrhosis, hepatitis, liver failure and even death. In light of the links between liver damage and kava, many countries have restricted the use of kava or removed it from the commercial market altogether.

Kava's potential toxicity highlights the importance of several issues in the preparation of herbal medicines, as well as ethnographic and cultural considerations in botanical

The Kava Debate

Kava remains available for sale in both the United States and Canada. In 2002, the U.S. Food and Drug Administration (FDA) issued a consumer advisory and a letter to health-care professionals outlining the potential risk of severe liver toxicity associated with using kava, and encouraging consumers to consult with a physician before using any supplements that contain kava. In Canada, kava-containing products are approved for sale only if they are whole-root or water-based extracts containing no more than 125 milligrams of kavalactones (the active medicinal component) per dosage unit and no more than 250 milligrams of kavalactones per recommended daily dosage.

Recent studies have attempted to allay fears about liver toxicity by preparing kava supplements as whole-root or water-based extracts as outlined above. One study noted significant antidepressant and antianxiety effects when kava was compared to a placebo in adults diagnosed with generalized anxiety disorder. A six-week double-blind, placebo-controlled trial recorded similarly positive results. Neither trial found any significant adverse effects, nor any significant difference in liver function tests between the kava and placebo groups.

research and treatment. Questions have been raised about whether acetone- and alcohol-based extraction methods are the cause of liver toxicity or whether traditional water-based preparations may also be of concern. More long-term, high-quality studies of standardized water-based extracts are needed. It is also not clear whether the reported liver toxicity has been due to dosage, herb–drug interactions, allergic reactions, mislabeling, contamination or adulteration (not actually kava in the product but another substance that is toxic to the liver).

As highlighted by a report from the World Health Organization, kava is an excellent example of the need for better understanding of the principles behind the traditional uses of herbal medicines.

Lemon Balm

Lemon balm (*Melissa officinalis*) is a member of the mint family and is both delicious and calming. I use it often to treat anxiety, in part because it tastes so good. The lemony flavor is refreshing, and the herb is particularly effective for releasing nervous tension. Herbalists consider lemon balm to have a specific use for anxiety accompanied by heart palpitations, hyperactivity and frenetic sensations. Non-human animal studies and a pilot trial in human volunteers support the traditional use of lemon balm as an herb for anxiety.

Did You Know?

Hyperthyroidism
Herbalists have recently been using lemon balm to treat hyperthyroidism, a use supported by in vitro research. Although there is no clinical evidence that lemon balm may worsen hypothyroidism, caution is advised.

Passionflower

Passionflower (*Passiflora incarnata*) has historically been used for anxiety and insomnia due to a racing mind or circular thinking. The flower's concentric shapes and colors are reminiscent of a kaleidoscope or a mandala, a design that provides a clue to the plant's traditional use: it is perfectly suited for treating cases of anxiety in which a person's thoughts are stuck in a loop of negative self-talk or worry.

Clinical studies haven't yet caught up with traditions. Many of the studies that do exist have been poorly designed or are missing vital information about the preparation of the herbal extracts. There are, however, a limited number of studies that support herbalists' empirical knowledge that passionflower is a great herb for anxiety. One small study demonstrated that passionflower improved sleep quality and reduced anxiety in healthy adults when compared to a placebo. Another study found that passionflower reduced anxiety symptoms in adults with general anxiety disorder, with effects comparable to oxazepam, a benzodiazepine drug. Additional research shows that passionflower may effectively reduce the anxiety that commonly arises before surgery and dental work.

More studies are needed before any clear scientific conclusions can be drawn.

Common Combinations

- Lemon balm, passionflower and lavender for generalized anxiety
- Lavender and chamomile essential oil inhaled for postpartum anxiety
- St. John's wort and passionflower for anxiety mixed with depression
- Ashwagandha and lavender for anxiety, stress and fatigue

Conventional Medical Treatments

- *Acute:* Benzodiazepines
- *Chronic:* Various antidepressants; antipsychotics in severe cases

Further Reading

Conrad P, Adams C. The effects of clinical aromatherapy for anxiety and depression in the high risk postpartum woman — A pilot study. *Complementary Therapies in Clinical Practice*, 2012 Aug; 18 (3): 164–68.

CASE STUDY
Anxiety

Sarah came to me looking for help with managing her moderately severe anxiety disorder. At fifty-five, she had struggled with anxiety and panic disorder for most of her adult life. She had been taking benzodiazepines on and off since her early twenties, but she didn't like how they made her feel. Her anxiety was generalized and sometimes appeared to come out of nowhere, but it was also triggered by interpersonal relationships. She often felt uncertain, unloved and afraid of being abandoned by friends and lovers, even when those relationships were stable. Her anxiety resulted in a lot of negative self-talk and obsessive, intrusive thoughts. She was restless and could not even sit still in my office chair. Several nights a week, her internal dialogue kept her awake, unable to find the sense of calmness that would allow her to fall asleep. At times her anxiety had been so severe that she had been hospitalized for a week or two at a time.

Together, we formulated a plan to bring stability and calmness back into Sarah's life. In the office, we used acupuncture, visualization and cognitive behavioral therapy techniques to model a state of relaxation and give Sarah some tools and skills she could use to break the cycle of anxiety and panic. In between visits, Sarah continued with the mind–body techniques I had taught her. She also drank a tea throughout the day that included lavender, passionflower, lemon balm, skullcap and oat straw.

Although it took several months and she occasionally had setbacks, overall her anxiety became less severe. She was able to fall asleep easily most nights of the week and was able to identify and manage her symptoms of anxiety before they turned into panic or interfered with her social life.

Kasper S. An orally administered lavandula oil preparation (Silexan) for anxiety disorder and related conditions: An evidence based review. *International Journal of Psychiatry in Clinical Practice*, 2013 Nov; 17 Suppl 1: 15–22.

Kasper S, Gastpar M, Müller WE, et al. Lavender oil preparation Silexan is effective in generalized anxiety disorder — A randomized, double-blind comparison to placebo and paroxetine. *International Journal of Neuropsychopharmacology*, 2014 Jun; 17 (6): 859–69.

Sarris J, Stough C, Bousman CA, et al. Kava in the treatment of generalized anxiety disorder: A double-blind, randomized, placebo-controlled study. *Journal of Clinical Psychopharmacology*, 2013 Oct; 33 (5): 643–48.

Uehleke B, Schaper S, Dienel A, et al. Phase II trial on the effects of Silexan in patients with neurasthenia, post-traumatic stress disorder or somatization disorder. *Phytomedicine*, 2012 Jun 15; 19 (8–9): 665–71.

World Health Organization. *Assessment of the Risk of Hepatotoxicity with Kava Products*. Geneva: WHO Document Production Services, 2007.

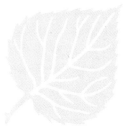

Arthritis (Osteoarthritis)

Osteoarthritis is the most common form of arthritis, with rheumatoid arthritis (see page 63) second in line. Osteoarthritis is considered benign, but many people are severely affected and may have difficulty with even basic daily activities because of the intense pain and discomfort that is typical of the condition.

Osteoarthritis is a chronic degenerative disease of the joints, caused by normal wear and tear. Degeneration and inflammation cause a loss of cartilage in the joints. As bone rubs against bone, new bone is often formed, creating outgrowths or spurs (osteophytes) and leading to further deformity and pain. The joints most often affected are the hips, knees, neck and lower back.

Signs and Symptoms

- Aches and pain in joints, especially after use
- Stiffness on waking or after periods of inactivity
- Limited movement in joints
- Cracking, popping or other sounds or sensations in joints as they move
- Bony growths and swelling of the joint

Associated Conditions

- Diabetes
- Heart disease
- High cholesterol
- Hypothyroidism
- Obesity

First-Line Herbal Care: CAYENNE PEPPER

Cayenne pepper (*Capsicum frutescens*) is frequently used in cooking to add heat. Many people have first-hand experience of its ability to increase circulation through a local sensation of heat in the mouth and stomach, as well as the runny nose that sometimes occurs when you eat food cooked with cayenne. Most people wouldn't dream

Cayenne Pain-Relief Balm

With just a few ingredients you can make your own pain-relieving balm at home.

> ½ cup (125 mL) virgin coconut oil
> 3 tbsp (45 mL) cayenne pepper
> 1 tsp (5 mL) cornstarch or arrowroot powder
> 1½ cups (375 mL) grated cocoa butter (about 2 oz/60 g)
> 10 drops peppermint essential oil

1. In a double boiler or a nonreactive bowl placed over a pot, melt coconut oil over gently simmering water. Stir in cayenne, being careful not to inhale the fumes, and set aside to cool. Stir in cornstarch.
2. Place infused oil in the refrigerator or freezer until it is semisolid on top.
3. In a large bowl, using an electric mixer, whip together infused oil, cocoa butter and peppermint oil until peaks begin to form.
4. Transfer balm to a glass jar with a tight-fitting lid. Store it in a cool, dark place and use within six months.

How to Use the Balm

1. Use a spoon or cotton swab to apply the healing balm, or wash your hands thoroughly after application with the fingers.
2. Cover the applied balm with gauze or cloth to avoid staining clothing or furniture.

Caution

Be careful not to touch your eyes or other mucous membranes after handling cayenne pepper or balm, as it can burn. Wash your skin with soap and water immediately if a burning sensation occurs. Do not use balm on broken skin. Do not apply heat on top of balm, as this will increase the likelihood that a burning sensation will occur.

Quick Fix

In a pinch, you can just mix ½ teaspoon (2 mL) of cayenne pepper and 2 drops of peppermint essential oil in 1 tablespoon (15 mL) of coconut or castor oil and apply directly to painful joints. The cornstarch and cocoa butter are included to solidify the balm and make it less oily.

of putting cayenne on their skin, but the same increase in circulation works to reduce pain when it is applied topically over an arthritic joint. Mustard powder has been used traditionally in much the same way. Herbalists traditionally make a paste with flour, water and a little cayenne and apply it as a poultice over inflamed joints.

Studies on topical capsaicin, the active constituent in cayenne, support cayenne's traditional use in arthritis. Since topical cayenne produces a slight burning sensation on the skin, it is relatively easy for people to tell whether they've been given a placebo in clinical trials, which is less than ideal from a study design perspective. Nonetheless, topical cayenne cream (0.025% to 0.075% weight per volume) applied four times daily has been shown to reduce pain in people with osteoarthritis.

Other Herbal Treatments

Herbal treatments for osteoarthritis focus on decreasing inflammation and swelling as well as on reducing pain. Treatments can be either topical or ingested. Some commonly used anti-inflammatory herbs, such as willow, meadowsweet and wintergreen, contain salicylates, which are related to Aspirin but do not have the unfortunate side effect of causing stomach ulcers. Other herbs, such as ginger and cayenne, work by increasing circulation and clearing irritating by-products of inflammation that build up in the joints. Dandelion leaf and celery seed act as diuretics, removing fluid that has built up in the joints.

Turmeric, nettles, boswellia, ginger and devil's claw are all believed to work by inhibiting the physiochemical process of inflammation. Whereas most pharmaceutical anti-inflammatory drugs simply block the enzyme cyclooxygenase-2 (COX-2), many anti-inflammatory herbs have been shown to inhibit inflammation caused by both COX-2 and the enzyme 5-lipoxygenase (5-LOX).

Herbs used topically are frequently counterirritants; that is, they alter the perception of pain by activating certain nerve cells in the skin. Cayenne and menthol are well-known counterirritants.

Combinations of herbs that work to decrease inflammation and pain through several different mechanisms at the same time have proven to be particularly effective.

Did You Know?

Salicylates
Herbs that contain salicylates have long been used for their anti-inflammatory and pain-relieving properties. Willow bark, which contains significant concentrations of salicylates, has an extensive history of use in chronic musculoskeletal pain.

Boswellia

Scientific research backs up the traditional use of boswellia (*Boswellia serrata*), also known as Indian frankincense, as an anti-inflammatory and pain-relieving herb. A recent systematic review found that boswellia extract significantly improved pain scores in adults with osteoarthritis. Another study investigating the use of an Ayurvedic formula containing boswellia, ginger, amla and guduchi showed that the formula was just as effective in the treatment of osteoarthritis of the knee as either glucosamine or celecoxib, a common COX-2 inhibitor.

Devil's Claw

Devil's claw (*Harpagophytum procumbens*) is a traditional herbal remedy native to the Kalahari savannah in southern Africa. The San and Khoi peoples used it for muscle and joint pain, indigestion, fever, malaria, postpartum pains, sprains and other maladies. Knowledge of its use as a powerful pain reliever and anti-inflammatory was first introduced to Europe in the early 1900's by a German farmer who learned about the plant from the indigenous peoples of Namibia. It has since become a popular treatment for arthritic pain throughout Europe and North America.

A review of the clinical research on the use of devil's claw for osteoarthritis found that it reduced pain more effectively than a placebo and appeared to have fewer side effects than non-steroidal anti-inflammatory drugs (NSAIDs), although it may cause gastrointestinal distress. Other studies have shown that devil's claw is as effective as diacerein in its ability to reduce pain. In one study, participants taking devil's claw took fewer NSAIDs and other pain-relieving medications than the group taking diacerein.

Dosage of devil's claw is typically 2 to 3 grams per day of dried root, in a decoction or as a powdered capsule. Extracts used in clinical trials are standardized to contain approximately 50 to 100 milligrams of harpagoside (the active ingredient in devil's claw) as a daily dosage.

Nettle

Traditionally, fresh nettles (*Urtica dioica*) have been used much like other counterirritants. Small hairs on the leaves and stems of nettle contain formic acid, histamine and other compounds that increase blood circulation locally, helping to relieve swelling and inflammation — and giving the plant its longer name: stinging nettle. The practice

of urtication, or flogging oneself with nettles, is at least 2,000 years old. Beating a swollen, painful joint with nettles relieves pain and decreases inflammation. During the First World War, soldiers were said to have intentionally stung their hands or feet as treatment for frostbite.

Few studies exist that look at urtication for osteoarthritis, and results are mixed: one study reported positive results, while another found no change in pain levels. More research is needed to confirm nettle's traditional use as a counter-irritant and its efficacy in treating joint pain and arthritis. In the meantime, nettles may be considered cost-effective pain-relieving treatment, as they can be found growing wild in many parts of the world.

Common Combination

- Boswellia, turmeric and ginger for inflammation and pain relief

Conventional Medical Treatments

- Acetaminophen
- Non-steroidal anti-inflammatory drugs (NSAIDs)
- Cyclooxygenase-2 (COX-2) inhibitors
- Narcotics
- Injections of cortisone or hyaluronic acid (in severe cases)

Further Reading

Brien S, Lewith GT, McGregor G. Devil's claw (*Harpagophytum procumbens*) as a treatment for osteoarthritis: A review of efficacy and safety. *Journal of Alternative and Complementary Medicine*, 2006 Dec; 12 (10): 981–93.

Cameron M, Chrubasik S. Oral herbal therapies for treating osteoarthritis. *Cochrane Database of Systematic Reviews*, 2014 May 22; 5: CD002947.

Cameron M, Chrubasik S. Topical herbal therapies for treating osteoarthritis. *Cochrane Database of Systematic Reviews*, 2013 May 31; 5: CD010538.

Cameron M, Gagnier JJ, Little CV, et al. Evidence of effectiveness of herbal medicinal products in the treatment of arthritis. Part I: Osteoarthritis. *Phytotherapy Research*, 2009 Nov; 23 (11): 1497–515.

Laslett LL, Jones G. Capsaicin for osteoarthritis pain. *Progress in Drug Research*, 2014; 68: 277–91.

Arthritis (Rheumatoid)

Rheumatoid arthritis is a chronic inflammatory disease that primarily affects the small joints in the hands, wrists and feet. Unlike osteoarthritis, it affects the lining of the joints rather than the cartilage, causing swelling, pain and, potentially, bone erosion and joint deformity.

Although the precise causes of rheumatoid arthritis are unknown, it is an autoimmune condition in which the body's own immune system attacks the lining of the joints. Theories suggest that a combination of environmental and genetic factors may trigger this immune system response. In some cases, rheumatoid arthritis can also affect other parts of the body, including the lungs, heart, skin and eyes.

Rheumatoid arthritis affects women three times more often than men.

Signs and Symptoms

- Red, hot, swollen and/or painful joints
- Affected joints on both sides of the body (bilateral)
- Stiffness on waking or after periods of inactivity
- Fatigue
- Nodules or bony growths under the skin

Associated Conditions

- Anemia
- Anxiety
- Depression
- Heart disease
- Osteoporosis

First-Line Herbal Care: EVENING PRIMROSE

Evening primrose oil (*Oenothera biennis*) — like other plant-derived oils, such as borage oil and blackcurrant seed oil — contains high amounts of gamma-linolenic acid (GLA), an omega-6 fatty acid that is known to reduce inflammation. GLA is important in treating rheumatoid arthritis because it can help the body move away from producing inflammatory fatty acids, such as arachidonic

Folklore

Cure-All

During the early 1600s, evening primrose was called "king's cure-all." An extract of the whole plant was believed to cure asthma, whooping cough and gastrointestinal disorders, and to reduce pain. Many traditional herbalists still use the whole plant for these conditions today.

Personalized Formulas

Most herbal traditions worldwide focus on creating personalized combinations of herbs rather than a single-herb preparation to treat a particular health condition. Herbs that act to increase circulation are particularly likely to be added to formulas, for this purpose alone.

acid, and thereby transition from a pro-inflammatory response to a non-inflammatory response. Adequate B vitamins, vitamin C, magnesium and zinc are needed to help support this anti-inflammatory pathway.

Several clinical studies using GLA from evening primrose and other plant sources have consistently shown significant decreases in overall pain, joint tenderness, swelling and duration of morning stiffness in people diagnosed with rheumatoid arthritis. At least six months of treatment with evening primrose oil may be needed before positive effects can be seen.

Other Herbal Treatments

There is a lot of crossover between the herbs used for rheumatoid arthritis and those used for osteoarthritis, because relieving pain and reducing inflammation are usually the primary goals for people with either disease. Typically, pain-relieving herbs containing salicylates, anti-inflammatory herbs and antirheumatic herbs are used. (Even pharmacologically, the day-to-day medications that are recommended are often non-steroidal anti-inflammatory drugs, regardless of which kind of arthritis has been diagnosed.)

Ginger

Ginger (*Zingiber officinale*) is a great herb for increasing circulation in painful, inflamed joints. It is traditionally used in Ayurvedic medicine to reduce nausea and other gastrointestinal complaints, treat colds and flus, and decrease pain in muscles and joints.

Ginger alone is likely not enough to reduce the pain and inflammation of rheumatoid arthritis, so it is typically included as one component of a larger formula. I often include it in combination formulas to improve the action of other herbs through its ability to increase circulation.

Certain constituents in ginger are known to act as anti-inflammatories. In animal studies, ginger has been shown to reduce prostaglandins and leukotrienes — types of inflammatory markers that are associated with rheumatoid arthritis. A combination Ayurvedic formula with ginger and guduchi was shown in a clinical study to be as effective as a disease-modifying antirheumatic drug (DMARD) in reducing pain. Unfortunately, the study was poorly designed and more research is needed.

Turmeric

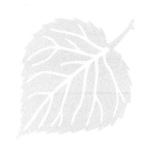

Turmeric (*Curcuma longa*), an herb native to India, has a lot of potential as an anti-inflammatory in the treatment of rheumatoid arthritis. In traditional Chinese medicine, turmeric is used for its ability to move qi (vital energy) and blood. In rheumatoid arthritis, increased blood circulation is important for reducing swelling and pain.

Turmeric's medicinal qualities are attributed to the curcuminoids present in the plant. Curcumin, one of those curcuminoids, has been the major focus of research. Most clinical trials use standardized extracts that have very high concentrations of curcuminoids.

Preclinical in vitro and animal studies support the use of turmeric in the management of rheumatoid arthritis. One small human study showed that turmeric was just as effective as diclofenac sodium in reducing tenderness and swelling of involved joints. More clinical trials are needed to confirm the specific use of turmeric in rheumatoid arthritis.

Kitchen Lore

Golden Milk

Try mixing turmeric into warm milk or coconut oil instead of taking a capsule.

> 2 tsp (10 mL) ground turmeric
> 1 tsp (5 mL) ground ginger
> ⅛ tsp (0.5 mL) freshly ground black pepper
> 2 tbsp (30 mL) water or melted virgin coconut oil
> 1 cup (250 mL) milk or unflavored nondairy milk
>   (such as almond, coconut or soy)
> Raw honey or other sweetener (optional)

1. In a bowl, combine the turmeric, ginger and pepper. Add the water or coconut oil and stir to make a paste.
2. In a small saucepan, combine milk and herbal paste until well blended. Heat over low heat until warmed through.
3. If desired, add raw honey to taste.

Variation

If you prefer a cool beverage, use a blender to combine the ingredients and serve over ice.

Willow

Plant-derived salicylates, from herbs such as willow, meadowsweet and aspen, were the inspiration for the development of acetylsalicylic acid (ASA), known better by its brand name, Aspirin. However, researchers and herbalists caution against focusing exclusively on salicylate extracts rather than whole-plant extracts.

Several studies have investigated the use of willow bark (*Salix nigra* or *Salix alba*) in different arthritic conditions. A double-blind trial with over 200 participants found that willow bark standardized to 240 milligrams of salicin relieved back pain (including back pain caused by rheumatoid arthritis) significantly better than a placebo, and that people using willow bark used pharmaceutical drugs less frequently. Other studies have found that willow bark extract is comparable to NSAIDs in its ability to relieve pain. However, several studies have failed to show pain relief greater than that achieved by a placebo. More research is needed.

Common Combination

- Willow bark, ginger, turmeric and boswellia to address pain and inflammation

Conventional Medical Treatments

- Non-steroidal anti-inflammatory drugs (NSAIDs)
- Corticosteroids
- Disease-modifying antirheumatic drugs (DMARDs)
- Biologics

Perspectives on Willow

Willow branches were historically used to make rounded structures, skirts and baskets because they bend easily and can be formed into arches or woven into fabrics. In Taoism, willow represents the concept of strength in weakness. Energetically, willow bark helps us increase our emotional pliability and adaptability without losing our sense of authentic identity.

My children often refer to willow trees as "monkey trees" because they always hope to see a monkey swinging from one branch to the next. Whenever they get the chance, they too swing from a willow's branches. I find the flower essence of willow most useful for restoring the optimism, playfulness and resilience of spirit embodied so well by children. It is also helpful when someone is stuck in self-pity, feeling bitter and resentful.

Willow in any form is an excellent herbal treatment when physical pain is accompanied by, or is a manifestation of, difficulty finding flexibility and optimism in life. Willow works best when someone's thinking is as rigid and stiff as their muscles and joints.

CASE STUDY
Rheumatoid Arthritis

Rheumatoid arthritis is often diagnosed in people between the ages of thirty and sixty, a time when many women find themselves busy with families, hobbies and careers. Gabrielle was no exception. She was thirty-four years old at the time of diagnosis, with two children under the age of two who kept her on her toes. She had just gone back to work after taking parental leave, returning to a busy job with a lot of pressure to perform.

Her symptoms began with severe pain and swelling in her wrists and fingers while she was typing, writing or knitting. Her hand joints were stiff and achy even after a good night's sleep — sometimes they actually seemed worse when she first got out of bed in the morning.

Gabrielle initially thought carpal tunnel syndrome was the culprit, but after imaging and blood tests, she was diagnosed with rheumatoid arthritis. She wanted to avoid the known negative side effects of DMARDs, and her rheumatologist agreed to a trial of complementary therapies before starting more aggressive pharmaceutical treatment.

Gabrielle's diet was already quite healthy, but she started consciously choosing anti-inflammatory foods while avoiding alcohol and coffee. I prescribed a tincture for her: an alcohol-based herbal extract containing boswellia, turmeric, devil's claw and ginger. I also recommended that she take evening primrose oil capsules containing 2 grams of oil every day. Together, we also created a plan for her to set aside some quiet time during the week for self-care, including meditation and baths. She took breaks at work to just breathe for a few minutes.

After two weeks, she was able to starting knitting again. She felt more inspired, energetic and patient with her kids. She remained on the tincture for some time as her pain and inflammation slowly decreased, but after several months, she was able to decrease the dosage of the herbs to a maintenance level.

Further Reading

Cameron M, Gagnier JJ, Chrubasik S. Herbal therapy for treating rheumatoid arthritis. *Cochrane Database of Systematic Reviews*, 2011 Feb 16; (2): CD002948.

Chandran B, Goel A. A randomized, pilot study to assess the efficacy and safety of curcumin in patients with active rheumatoid arthritis. *Phytotherapy Research*, 2012 Nov; 26 (11): 1719–25.

Chopra A, Saluja M, Tillu G, et al. Comparable efficacy of standardized Ayurveda formulation and hydroxychloroquine sulfate (HCQS) in the treatment of rheumatoid arthritis (RA): A randomized investigator-blind controlled study. *Clinical Rheumatology*, 2012 Feb; 31 (2): 259–69.

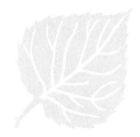

Breast Cancer

Breast cancer is the most commonly diagnosed cancer in women worldwide. In 2012, nearly 1.7 million women were diagnosed with breast cancer, and more than 500,000 women lost their lives to it. Breast cancer incidence rates are highest in North America, Western Europe, Australia and New Zealand. In some countries, there are over 100 new cases of breast cancer per 100,000 women annually.

Signs and Symptoms

- A hard, immovable lump, bumps, indentation, erosion, shape/size changes, dimpling
- Nipple discharge or growing veins
- Swelling, redness, heat or thickening of the skin

Associated Conditions

- Depression
- Fibrocystic breast disease
- Menopause
- Obesity
- Ovarian cancer

First-Line Herbal Care: SOY

Soy (*Glycine max*) has had a tumultuous history with breast cancer. Early epidemiological studies noted that the incidence of breast cancer was lower among Asian women. Some theories pointed to green tea consumption, while others suggested that soy's isoflavones were protective against the development of breast cancer.

As breast cancer researchers began to better understand estrogen-receptor-positive (ER-positive) breast cancer, controversy arose around whether soy was protective or potentially harmful. Researchers wondered whether soy's phytoestrogenic isoflavones might increase estrogen in the body and thus increase the risk of recurrence or death in women with ER-positive breast cancer.

In vitro and animal studies provided conflicting results. However, human cohort studies show that dietary soy intake is not only safe but may also be preventive. A 2012 systematic review on soy and breast cancer concluded that high daily soy intake (two to three servings daily) may protect against the development of breast cancer and its recurrence. Two other reviews published in the same year similarly concluded that soy intake may be associated with a lower risk of breast cancer, as well as lower mortality in women already diagnosed with breast cancer.

Other Herbal Treatments

Herbal treatment usually focuses on enhancing the effects of, or reducing the side effects of, biomedical cancer treatment. Herbs can also be used to reduce the occurrence and recurrence of breast cancer. Since conventional medical treatment for cancer varies widely and there are many potential herb–drug interactions, it is difficult to specify herbs that may be appropriate in general terms, especially for women undergoing radiation or chemotherapy. As always, it is critical to consult with a regulated health-care provider before starting herbal treatment.

Ashwagandha

Fatigue, exhaustion and low white blood cell counts are common side effects of chemotherapy. In vitro and animal studies have demonstrated that ashwagandha may reduce some of these side effects without interfering with the desired tumor-reducing actions of the drugs. Other in vitro studies have shown that ashwagandha may enhance the effectiveness of radiation as well.

A recent open-label, non-randomized trial on ashwagandha in women undergoing chemotherapy for breast cancer showed that 2 grams of ashwagandha taken every eight hours during chemotherapy significantly reduced fatigue compared to chemotherapy alone. The women who took ashwagandha reported significant improvements in fatigue, physical functioning, insomnia and emotional and social functioning.

More studies are needed to confirm the potential benefits of using ashwagandha as adjunctive care with chemotherapy and/or radiation in breast cancer.

Did You Know?

Soy Safety
Earlier concerns about phyto-estrogens have been set aside, as research shows no increase in circulating estrogen in women who consume larger amounts of soy.

Did You Know?

Insomnia Cure
Ashwagandha's Latin species name, *somnifera*, means "sleep-inducing," an indication of its use in promoting healthy sleep patterns and relieving insomnia.

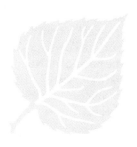

Barberry

Barberry (*Berberis vulgaris*) and other berberine-containing herbs, such as coptis and Oregon grape root, have attracted research attention for their potential anticancer effects. Berberine has been found to promote apoptosis (the death of cancer cells) in vitro. In other studies, it has been shown to enhance the effects of common chemotherapy drugs and estrogen receptor antagonist drugs in ER-positive breast cancer cells. Human trials haven't yet been conducted, but this early research supports barberry's inclusion in many traditional anticancer herbal formulas.

Ginger

Nausea and vomiting is one of the most common complaints of patients undergoing chemotherapy as part of cancer treatment. As a traditional herbal remedy for nausea, ginger (*Zingiber officinale*) is a seemingly safe, cost-effective and convenient herb for chemotherapy-induced nausea and vomiting.

Several studies have attempted to measure the benefits of ginger for this use. In a 2013 review, the authors found mixed results in the studies they looked at. Out of seven good-quality studies, two reported that ginger was just as effective as metoclopramide, three showed some decrease in nausea, and two claimed no benefit. An earlier review also found mixed results.

Although conclusive results are lacking, ginger is considered a relatively safe herb with few side effects.

Green Tea

Epidemiological research has shown that the risk of breast cancer is significantly lower in Asian-American women who regularly consume green tea (*Camellia sinensis*). However, studies on Japanese women have not found an association between green tea consumption and decreased risk of breast cancer, regardless of hormone-receptor subtype or menopausal status. Nonetheless, in vitro and animal studies suggest that epigallocatechin gallate (EGCG), the most abundant catechin in green tea, alters cancer cell regulation, inducing apoptosis and decreasing the proliferation of cancer cells. Some of these studies also suggest that EGCG may enhance the effects of tamoxifen, a drug commonly used in the treatment and prevention of ER-positive breast cancer.

How to Brew Green Tea

Green tea comes in many varieties. The most common are sencha, gunpowder and matcha.

Whatever type of green tree you are brewing, the temperature of the water is the most important detail. The water should have just begun to simmer but not yet begun to boil. This stage is sometimes called "first boil." If the water is too hot, the resulting tea will taste bitter. The ideal temperature for steeping most green teas ranges from 160°F to 180°F (71°C to 82°C), depending on the variety.

Traditionally, hot water is poured into the teapot and cups before steeping, to cleanse and heat them, ensuring an even temperature during steeping. This step is also an important part of the tea ritual. Once the pot and cups are warm, the water is poured out.

Most green tea is steeped using about 1 teaspoon (5 mL) of loose tea leaves per 1 cup (250 mL) of water. The tea leaves can be placed either directly in a teacup or pot (ideally made of glass, ceramic, china, clay or stainless steel) or in an infuser or tea ball in the cup or pot. Pour hot water over the tea, cover the cup or pot and steep for 1 to 3 minutes, depending on the variety of tea. Strain the tea, pour it into a heated cup and enjoy!

Red Clover

Clover, both red and white, is grown in many places in the world as a forage crop for livestock, because of its high mineral content. A nitrogen-fixer, it enriches the soil and improves future crop yields and has long been used in crop rotation systems of agriculture. The human body likewise makes good use of the minerals red clover provides.

Like soy, red clover (*Trifolium pratense*) contains a class of phytoestrogens known as isoflavones, which have been isolated and extracted primarily for research into their effects on menopausal symptoms (see page 124). Theoretical concerns have been raised about the possibility that phytoestrogens may help ER-positive breast cancers grow faster. However, a recent systematic review found that the existing studies fail to show that red clover had any breast cancer–promoting effects in menopausal women. In the studies reviewed, red clover extracts did not adversely affect breast density, bone strength, endometrial thickness or cardiovascular health. On the contrary, one in vitro study found that formononetin, a constituent in red clover, induced the death of ER-positive breast cancer cells.

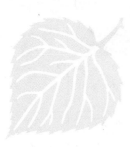

Turmeric

Most people think of turmeric (*Curcuma longa*) as a kitchen spice — the ingredient that gives curry powder its golden hue and dyes our hands and cutting boards. But turmeric also has a long history of use in the religious and medical practices of South Asia. In India, turmeric is used in a variety of ceremonies as a marker of protection from evil, and it is frequently applied as a paste over the third eye for this purpose. In Ayurvedic medicine, turmeric is considered a balancing herb. It has been used historically as an anti-inflammatory for joint pain and to treat parasites, ringworm, jaundice and ulcers.

Modern scientific research has focused on curcumin, turmeric's active constituent, for its anti-inflammatory and anticancer effects. Curcumin has been found in several in vitro studies to inhibit ER-positive cancer cells. Other studies have noted that curcumin may inhibit breast cancer cell growth and metastasis and may improve the efficacy of certain chemotherapy drugs. One study found that high-dose curcumin (2 grams, three times daily) significantly decreased radiation-induced dermatitis (skin inflammation) compared to a placebo in women being treated for breast cancer. Research into the many potential benefits of turmeric for cancer patients continues to build.

Common Combination

- Soy and red clover for the prevention of breast cancer and to reduce recurrence and mortality

Conventional Medical Treatments

Pharmaceutical treatment varies depending on the stage and type of breast cancer but commonly includes radiation, chemotherapy, hormonal therapy (such as tamoxifen) and/or bisphosphonates.

Further Reading

Biswal BM, Sulaiman SA, Ismail HC, et al. Effect of *Withania somnifera* (ashwagandha) on the development of chemotherapy-induced fatigue and quality of life in breast cancer patients. *Integrative Cancer Therapies*, 2013 Jul; 12 (4): 312–22.

Chen M, Rao Y, Zheng Y, et al. Association between soy isoflavone intake and breast cancer risk for pre- and post-menopausal women: A meta-analysis of epidemiological studies. *PLoS One*, 2014 Feb 20; 9 (2): e89288.

Fritz H, Seely D, Flower G, et al. Soy, red clover, and isoflavones and breast cancer: A systematic review. *PLoS One*, 2013 Nov 28; 8 (11): e81968.

Marx WM, Teleni L, McCarthy AL, et al. Ginger (*Zingiber officinale*) and chemotherapy-induced nausea and vomiting: A systematic literature review. *Nutrition Reviews*, 2013 Apr; 71 (4): 245–54.

Ryan JL, Heckler CE, Ling M, et al. Curcumin for radiation dermatitis: A randomized, double-blind, placebo-controlled clinical trial of thirty breast cancer patients. *Radiation Research*, 2013 Jul; 180 (1): 34–43.

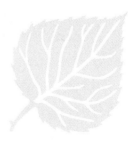

Cervical Dysplasia

Cervical dysplasia describes an abnormal change in the cells of the cervix. In time, the majority of slightly to moderately abnormal cells spontaneously revert back to being healthy cells on their own. However, these types of changes in cells may be precancerous, so early diagnosis is important to avoid a progression to invasive cervical cancer. Cervical cancer is the second most common cancer in women worldwide, but it is also easily prevented. Regular Pap smears and HPV testing are recommended to detect any potential abnormalities. Vaccines that protect against the strains of HPV most commonly associated with cervical cancer and anogenital warts are also available.

Cervical dysplasia is most common in women between the ages of twenty-five and thirty-five, although it can affect women of any age. Eighty to ninety percent of women with cervical dysplasia have a human papilloma virus (HPV) infection.

Signs and Symptoms

Typically, there are no symptoms. Cervical dysplasia is found through gynecological exams, Pap smears and HPV testing. Occasional symptoms may include:

- Genital warts
- Abnormal bleeding or spotting
- Vaginal discharge
- Low back pain

Associated Conditions

- Cervical cancer
- Genital warts
- Other sexually transmitted infections

First-Line Care: GREEN TEA

Green tea (*Camellia sinensis*) has been touted for its anti-cancer effects, with much research focused on polyphenols called catechins. In vitro studies have suggested that green tea may both stall the growth of cancer and encourage cancerous cells to die off. Since cervical dysplasia can be regarded as a precancerous condition, green tea may be an effective treatment.

Few studies have been done in humans to confirm these theories. In one study, topical and oral use of green tea extracts contributed to a reduction or elimination of HPV, cervical lesions and/or abnormal cervical cells found in Pap smears. Remarkably, 69% of women using some form of green tea improved, compared to 10% of women who received no treatment. Although promising, this study's methodology was poor. A higher-quality study found no difference in outcomes when comparing oral green tea extract to a placebo in the treatment of low-grade cervical dysplasia.

While green tea is safe and well tolerated, at this time it is not clear if it is an effective treatment for cervical dysplasia, despite promising in vitro research.

Other Herbal Treatments

Since cervical dysplasia is often caused by HPV, herbal treatment focuses on antiviral herbs, used both orally and vaginally, to stimulate the immune system and the patient's innate ability to resolve the infection.

Herbal escharotics — treatments that cause tissue to die and then slough off — have traditionally been used topically to treat cancers close to the surface of the skin. Cervical escharotic treatment may be used in severe dysplasia but requires a licensed practitioner to apply herbs directly to the cervix during a speculum exam, carefully avoiding healthy vaginal tissues. A licensed practitioner is crucial because the risk of scarring or other serious injury is significant with escharotic herbs.

Echinacea

Echinacea (*Echinacea purpurea* or *Echinacea angustifolia*) is traditionally included in formulas for cervical dysplasia. As a stimulant to the immune system with broad-spectrum antimicrobial properties, echinacea is believed to increase the body's innate response to HPV, helping the body rid itself of the virus. As an immunostimulant, echinacea may also support the clearance of cancerous cells through proper functioning of the immune system.

To date, there are no clinical studies looking at the use of echinacea in the treatment or prevention of cervical dysplasia. However, research on using echinacea to prevent genital warts caused by HPV is promising (see page 101 for details).

Folklore

A Floral Hedgehog

The word "echinacea" comes from the Greek word *echinos*, meaning spiny or pointed, in reference to the seed head, which resembles a sea urchin or hedgehog. Native to the Great Plains of North America, echinacea stands tall and strong in the wind and open sky. Its bright purple-pink flower petals stand out among the other wildflowers of the prairies, while its rigid stem holds fast when the wind blows.

Licorice

In Ayurvedic medicine, licorice (*Glycyrrhiza glabra* or *Glycyrrhiza uralensis*) is often paired with shatavari and other herbs to address the imbalances that create the conditions for cervical dysplasia. Ayurvedic doctors have used ghee infused with licorice as a topical application directly to the cervix, alongside other herbal and dietary treatments.

Phytopharmacology and in vitro studies have shown that licorice has strong antiviral properties, including against some strains of HPV. An open-label, poorly reported trial noted resolution of cervical dysplasia in 74% of women after twelve weeks using an oral and topical licorice extract. More research is needed to confirm these results and determine whether these cases would have resolved on their own, without treatment.

> ## Caution
>
> Licorice is known to raise blood pressure. Anyone taking licorice should routinely monitor their blood pressure. People with high blood pressure should avoid taking licorice.

Common Combination

- Licorice, shatavari and turmeric orally to support clearance of HPV and cervical dysplasia

Conventional Medical Treatments

Medications are not used to treat cervical dysplasia. Depending on severity, treatment varies. "Watch and wait" is usually recommended for low-grade lesions, with repeat Pap smears scheduled six to twelve months later. Persistent or higher-grade lesions may be treated with cryosurgery to freeze the abnormal cells, laser therapy, loop electrosurgical excision procedure (LEEP) or cone biopsy. Vaccines are available to prevent infection from the types of HPV most commonly associated with cervical cancer.

Further Reading

Ahn WS, Yoo J, Huh SW, et al. Protective effects of green tea extracts (polyphenon E and EGCG) on human cervical lesions. *European Journal of Cancer Prevention*, 2003 Oct; 12 (5): 383–90.

Garcia FA, Cornelison T, Nuño T, et al. Results of a phase II randomized, double-blind, placebo-controlled trial of polyphenon E in women with persistent high-risk HPV infection and low-grade cervical intraepithelial neoplasia. *Gynecologic Oncology*, 2014 Feb; 132 (2): 377–82.

Valencia MH, Pacheco AC, Quijano TH, et al. Clinical response to glycyrrhizinic acid in genital infection due to human papillomavirus and low-grade squamous intraepithelial lesion. *Clinics and Practice*, 2011 Nov 8; 1 (4): e93.

Depression

Depression is one of the most common mental health conditions and the leading cause of disability worldwide. The World Health Organization (WHO) estimates that more than 350 million people of all ages suffer from depression. Rates of depression are higher in women than in men, and it is estimated that 10% of women experience depressive symptoms after giving birth (postpartum depression). Other stressful life events, such as divorce, the death of a loved one, a change in employment, or physical or sexual abuse, may also precipitate depressive episodes.

It is important to note that women (and men) have been socialized to restrain their emotions and apologize for their feelings, especially in certain cultures. At the same time, it is this very emotionality that enables the intuition, sensitivity and empathy that is socially expected of women, especially mothers. The need to appear even-keeled rather than "moody" creates tension and stress for many people. Crying, and what looks like overwhelming sadness, may actually be an expression of frustration or anger or vulnerability or empathy.

When sadness is debilitating, however, it becomes a health problem. Recognizing the difference between normal variations in mood and depression (or anxiety or PMS, for that matter) can sometimes be challenging, and the social stigma associated with mental health disorders is frequently a barrier to treatment. When in doubt, talk to your health-care provider.

Signs and Symptoms

- Low or flat mood, overwhelming sadness
- Loss of interest and pleasure in activities
- Change in appetite
- Disturbed sleep
- Fatigue or lack of energy
- Decreased libido
- Feelings of worthlessness or guilt
- Poor concentration or memory
- Suicidal thoughts

Associated Conditions

- Addiction
- Anxiety
- Cancer
- Diabetes
- Hypertension

First-Line Herbal Care: ST. JOHN'S WORT

St. John's wort (*Hypericum perforatum*) is the most thoroughly studied herb for depression, and one of the most effective non-pharmaceutical treatments known to date. It has been shown to be effective at treating all forms of depression, from mild to severe. In the majority of studies conducted, it has been proven to work better than a placebo and as well as standard antidepressant drugs.

I use St. John's wort often in my practice, though caution must be taken, as it has powerful effects on drug metabolism: when taken in combination with St. John's wort, certain pharmaceuticals become less active, with potentially drastic consequences. For example, St. John's wort may decrease the effectiveness of oral contraceptives, leading to breakthrough bleeding or pregnancy.

A small number of in vitro and animal studies suggest that antidepressant effects may be possible at lower doses of St. John's wort when it is combined with passionflower and valerian. Further research is needed to confirm these potential synergistic effects.

Herbal Sunshine

St. John's wort is one of those seminal herbs that I remember from my teenage years, when I first began learning about the medicinal properties of plants. I had read about the use of St. John's wort in treating depression and was looking for a seedling to grow in my backyard, as my younger brother suffered from depression. My mother graciously drove me around to different nurseries, looking for the seemingly elusive plant. Not finding it anywhere, I gave up, planning to buy seeds the following year. A month or so later, a single St. John's wort plant showed up in our garden, with none of us knowing exactly how it had got there but very grateful for its presence nonetheless.

Just looking at the bright yellow flowers of St. John's wort brightens the spirit. Taking a closer look at the leaves, you can better understand how this herb got its Latin name, *Hypericum perforatum*, referring to perforation. Each leaf of St. John's wort has many translucent spots. Both literally and figuratively, St. John's wort allows the sun to shine through, bringing clarity of mind and spirit to the person taking it.

Other Herbal Treatments

Bitter herbs, such as mugwort and dandelion, have traditionally been used alongside nervine tonics to treat depression. Bitters serve to regulate digestion and overall metabolism. They stimulate appetite, increase stomach acid, help the release of digestive enzymes and pancreatic hormones and aid the liver in detoxification. Many herbalists also emphasize the ability of bitters to bring about a shift in consciousness or a change in perspective in those suffering from depression. The use of bitters to treat depression is being reaffirmed by recent scientific theories, which posit that depression may be related to inflammatory processes and an imbalance of bacteria in the gut.

As many people with depression also experience anxiety and sleep disturbances, herbal treatment may also include herbs used primarily for their ability to reduce anxious tension, such as passionflower and valerian.

Lavender

Research has confirmed lavender's traditional use in alleviating anxiety. Given that depression is often mixed with anxiety, researchers have started to investigate lavender's potential use in treating depression as well. In an open-label study on depressed patients taking the drug citalopram, a lavender infusion significantly decreased symptoms of depression compared to the control group. A series of case studies also reported that the concurrent use of lavender oil capsules with antidepressant medication resulted in improvements in depression symptoms, anxiety, agitation and insomnia. More placebo-controlled research on the use of lavender for depression is needed.

Rhodiola

Rhodiola (*Rhodiola rosea*) has been investigated for use in mild to moderate depression. In one study, it showed improvements in depressive symptoms and insomnia when compared to a placebo. More research is needed to confirm these results.

Saffron

Saffron (*Crocus sativa*) may also be effective in the treatment of depression. Several studies on saffron petals and stigmas have shown the herb to be more effective than a placebo and comparable to certain selective serotonin reuptake inhibitors (SSRIs). One small study showed a reduction of fluoxetine-induced sexual dysfunction in women, a common side effect of SSRIs.

Did You Know?

A Valuable Remedy

By weight, saffron is one of the most expensive spices in the world. It takes about 75,000 saffron flowers to yield just 1 pound (500 g) of saffron stigmas.

CASE STUDY
Depression

Depression can range from mild to severe and can be caused or affected by various life events and major transitions, including adolescence, pregnancy and menopause. I have had patients at every age and stage of life who were experiencing depression. As evidenced by health statistics, depression and anxiety are increasing in prevalence among children and teenagers.

Keisha, a fifteen-year-old girl, came to see me to help her address her feelings of extreme sadness and lack of motivation at school and at home. Her parents had noticed changes in her mood over the past several years. Her grades had dropped. She was going to bed quite late and having a lot of difficulty getting up in the morning. Most days of the week, she was late for school and skipped classes.

Keisha told me she felt overwhelmingly depressed and spoke of being "worthless" and "unlovable." She wasn't having suicidal thoughts per se, but she did feel hopeless and sometimes wished she were dead. She felt socially isolated and cried herself to sleep most nights thinking about how she didn't fit in.

Keisha had friends but felt that they didn't really understand her. Her parents were loving and supportive but she felt uncomfortable talking to them about many things, especially issues concerning sex and sexuality. She knew she was more attracted to girls than to boys, but she hadn't shared that with anyone, and she wasn't sure how to handle all her jumbled feelings about telling her friends or parents, or how to navigate dating. Keeping all these feelings inside without any support was eating her up.

We spent a lot of time talking. I suggested that Keisha join a peer support group for LGBT teens and referred her for more counseling with a psychotherapist. She started using meditation podcasts to help her fall asleep earlier, and joined a pick-up soccer team to get active (exercise is also great for alleviating depression).

While we worked on the big picture and long-term healing, Keisha started taking a combination of St. John's wort, rhodiola and mugwort, as well as fish oil, to help stabilize her mood. She felt an immediate sense of relief from sharing her experiences and continued to improve over the next several months.

Common Combinations

- St. John's wort, rhodiola and passionflower for depression with difficulty sleeping
- St. John's wort and dandelion root for depression with low appetite
- St. John's wort, passionflower and lavender for mixed anxiety and depression

Conventional Medical Treatments

- Monoamine oxidase inhibitors (MAOIs)
- Selective serotonin reuptake inhibitors (SSRIs)
- Serotonin-norepinephrine reuptake inhibitors (SNRIs)
- Tricyclic antidepressants (TCAs)

Further Reading

Akhondzadeh Basti A, Moshiri E, Noorbala AA, et al. Comparison of petal of *Crocus sativus* L. and fluoxetine in the treatment of depressed outpatients: A pilot double-blind randomized trial. *Progress in Neuro-Psychopharmacology & Biological Psychiatry*, 2007 Mar 30; 31 (2): 439–42.

Darbinyan V, Aslanyan G, Amroyan E, et al. Clinical trial of *Rhodiola rosea* L. extract SHR-5 in the treatment of mild to moderate depression. *Nordic Journal of Psychiatry*, 2007; 61 (5): 343–48.

Dwyer AV, Whitten DL, Hawrelak JA. Herbal medicines, other than St. John's wort, in the treatment of depression: A systematic review. *Alternative Medicine Review*, 2011 Mar; 16 (1): 40–49.

Fiebich BL, Knörle R, Appel K, et al. Pharmacological studies in an herbal drug combination of St. John's wort (*Hypericum perforatum*) and passion flower (*Passiflora incarnata*): In vitro and in vivo evidence of synergy between *Hypericum* and *Passiflora* in antidepressant pharmacological models. *Fitoterapia*, 2011 Apr; 82 (3): 474–80.

Kashani L, Raisi F, Saroukhani S, et al. Saffron for treatment of fluoxetine-induced sexual dysfunction in women: Randomized double-blind placebo-controlled study. *Human Psychopharmacology*, 2013 Jan; 28 (1): 54–60.

Linde K, Berner MM, Kriston L. St. John's wort for major depression. *Cochrane Database of Systematic Reviews*, 2008 Oct 8; (4): CD000448.

Moshiri E, Basti AA, Noorbala AA, et al. *Crocus sativus* L. (petal) in the treatment of mild-to-moderate depression: A double-blind, randomized and placebo-controlled trial. *Phytomedicine*, 2006 Nov; 13 (9–10): 607–11.

Nikfarjam M, Parvin N, Assarzadegan N, Asghari S. The effects of *Lavandula angustifolia* Mill. infusion on depression in patients using citalopram: A comparison study. *Iranian Red Crescent Medical Journal*, 2013 Aug; 15 (8): 734–39.

Sarris J, Panossian A, Schweitzer I, et al. Herbal medicine for depression, anxiety and insomnia: A review of psychopharmacology and clinical evidence. *European Neuropsychopharmacology*, 2011 Dec; 21 (12): 841–60.

Diabetes Mellitus

Diabetes mellitus is a condition in which a person's blood sugar, or blood glucose, is too high. Sometimes this is because the pancreas does not make insulin, which is needed to move sugar from the blood into cells, where it can be used for energy. This type of diabetes is often called type 1 diabetes, or insulin-dependent diabetes. More often, the body makes insulin but the cells don't respond to it; they are said to be insulin-resistant. This type of diabetes is often called type 2 diabetes, or non-insulin-dependent diabetes. About 90% of people with diabetes have type 2 diabetes.

The causes of type 2 diabetes are primarily lifestyle-related. High intake of refined carbohydrates and added sugars, obesity and lack of exercise all promote insulin resistance. Herbal treatment of diabetes is best used to augment and support dietary and lifestyle changes in people who are not dependent on insulin. Increasing the consumption of whole foods, such as non-starchy fruits and vegetables, high-fiber complex carbohydrates and healthy fats and proteins, is the first step to managing blood sugar. Health authorities also generally recommend avoiding sugars and foods with a high glycemic index, as well as losing weight if indicated. Once lifestyle changes have been implemented, herbs can help to blunt spikes in blood sugar and decrease insulin resistance.

Did You Know?

Diabetes Demographics

Diabetes affects approximately 250 million people worldwide, half of whom are women. In North America, diabetes is more prevalent among black, Latina, Native and Asian women than among Caucasian women. Elderly women and low-income women are also at greater risk of developing diabetes. Women with diabetes are more likely to have a heart attack, and at a younger age than women without diabetes. Diabetes is especially problematic during pregnancy, when it can be harmful to both mother and child.

Signs and Symptoms

- Excessive thirst or hunger
- Excessive urination
- Fatigue
- Frequent urinary tract infections or vaginal yeast infections
- Sexual dysfunction (vaginal dryness, inability to orgasm, pain during intercourse)
- Weight loss (type 1 only)

Associated Conditions

- Arthritis
- Depression
- Eating disorders
- Gestational diabetes
- Heart disease
- High cholesterol
- Hypertension
- Metabolic syndrome
- Obesity
- Polycystic ovarian syndrome (PCOS)
- Stroke

First-Line Herbal Care: CINNAMON

Cinnamon (*Cinnamomum verum* or *Cinnamomum cassia*) not only adds delicious flavor to baked goods and smoothies but also curbs blood sugar spikes. This effect is possibly why people added cinnamon to sweets to begin with, to balance out the impact of high-sugar meals.

There is plenty of research to support the use of cinnamon in type 2 diabetes. Several meta-analyses and systematic reviews have summarized the findings of clinical trials. These studies overwhelmingly show that cinnamon significantly reduces fasting blood sugar, hemoglobin A1c, total cholesterol, low-density lipoprotein (LDL), or "bad," cholesterol and triglycerides. Cinnamon also increases high-density lipoprotein (HDL), or "good," cholesterol.

Dosage in the studies ranged drastically, from 1 to 6 grams daily. The density of ground cinnamon varies, with 1 teaspoon (5 mL) weighing anywhere from about 2.5 to 5 grams. Adding 1 teaspoon of ground cinnamon to food daily is a great way to make use of this powerful herb.

Folklore

Historical Uses of Cinnamon

Cinnamon is mentioned in the Bible for its use in incense and as an anointing oil. It was used during funerals in ancient Rome and for embalming mummies in ancient Egypt.

Other Herbal Treatments

In general, herbal treatment for diabetes falls into two overlapping categories: herbs that alter the taste of and response to sugar, and herbs that regulate blood sugar by stimulating proper digestion. Herbs such as cinnamon and gymnema are understood to affect the taste of sugar and the body's response to it. Bitter herbs, such as milk thistle, barberry and dandelion, are thought to improve blood sugar levels by increasing pancreatic secretions and optimizing digestion and liver metabolism. Milk thistle, bilberry and grape seed are used in diabetes as antioxidants, to protect blood vessels from the potential damage of uncontrolled blood sugar. Green tea may be useful in cases of metabolic syndrome, where blood sugar, blood pressure and cholesterol are all abnormal.

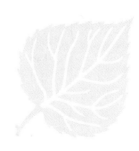

Barberry

Although barberry (*Berberis vulgaris*) and its main constituent berberine do not have a history of traditional use for diabetes specifically, barberry has long been used to optimize liver and gallbladder function. Through its work in the liver, barberry has beneficial impacts on blood sugar by reducing the production of glucose and improving insulin sensitivity. In preclinical trials, berberine has been shown to act similarly to sulfonylureas or metformin.

A recent but small double-blind, randomized clinical trial found that barberry significantly decreased blood sugar, insulin, insulin resistance and cholesterol compared to a placebo in people with type 2 diabetes. The dosage used in this study was 1 gram of whole barberry extract, three times a day.

CASE STUDY
Diabetes

Margaret needed help regulating her blood sugar. Now sixty, she had been diagnosed with type 2 diabetes in her forties and had been struggling for several years to keep her blood sugar within the normal range. Her fasting blood sugar hovered around 9 mmol/L (normal is under 7) first thing in the morning, and her hemoglobin A1c was also too high. She felt things had gotten worse after menopause as she found herself being less and less active. Her blood pressure had also started to increase. Although she had been prescribed metformin, she took it irregularly. Her medical doctor had advised her to see a nutritionist and start exercising.

Margaret told me that, on her birthday that year, she had taken stock of her life and realized she was ready to make some major changes. She knew her diet and lack of exercise were part of the problem. "I can't say no to cookies," she confessed. Overall, her digestion was good, and she didn't have any signs of complications due to long-standing blood sugar dysregulation.

I recommended that she avoid all added sugars and increase her intake of fruits and vegetables. She agreed to go for a brisk walk for twenty minutes, five days a week. She started taking a liquid botanical formula that included hawthorn, bilberry, cinnamon, fenugreek and gymnema. Within three months, Margaret's fasting blood sugar was around 7. After six months, it was consistently in the normal range.

Fenugreek

Fenugreek (*Trigonella foenum-graecum* L.), an herb native to Asia, has been traditionally included in cooking to reduce blood sugar. In clinical trials, it has been shown to acutely lower blood sugar after meals and to significantly reduce fasting blood sugar and hemoglobin A1c compared to controls.

Fenugreek seeds are very high in fiber, being made up of approximately 45% dietary fiber. Since the seeds are easily ground, fenugreek flour is often incorporated into bread flour mixes to boost fiber content and improve blood sugar control. Fenugreek should not be used by people with allergies to peanuts or chickpeas, as it is from the same family of plants.

Gymnema

Gymnema (*Gymnema sylvestre*) is an herb from the Ayurvedic medicine tradition that is commonly used by herbalists in the management of diabetes. In Hindi, gymnema is known as *gurmar*, meaning "sugar destroyer." Chewing gymnema suppresses the taste of sweet on the tongue. This property led researchers to investigate the use of gymnema in diabetes. In vitro animal studies and human cell studies support gymnema's ability to delay the absorption of glucose into the blood. In addition, two small open-label trials noted decreases in fasting blood sugar and hemoglobin A1c. Randomized clinical trials are needed to confirm these results.

Milk Thistle

Milk thistle seeds (*Silybum marianum*) are best known for protecting the liver from damage from drugs or diseases like hepatitis. Because of its protective effect against a variety of toxins, milk thistle is also used to support general detoxification and cleansing.

Although less well known for its hypoglycemic qualities, milk thistle is another great herb for helping to control blood sugar. As an antioxidant, it protects fragile blood vessels in the kidneys and eyes that can be damaged by persistent uncontrolled blood sugar. Milk thistle also protects the liver from high cholesterol, which contributes to an increased risk of heart attack or death in women with diabetes.

Clinical research supports the traditional use of milk thistle for diabetes. One high-quality randomized, controlled trial found that a milk thistle extract significantly reduced

fasting blood sugar, hemoglobin A1c, total cholesterol, low-density lipoprotein (LDL) and triglycerides in people with type 2 diabetes when compared to a placebo. In this study, milk thistle was given as 200 milligrams of silymarin extract, three times daily.

In another study, milk thistle, when given alongside a drug commonly used to treat kidney problems in diabetes, significantly reduced the amount of protein in the urine (a sign of kidney damage) compared to the drug alone. More studies are needed to confirm these results.

Common Combinations

- Cinnamon, fenugreek and gymnema to control blood sugar and reduce cholesterol
- Barberry and milk thistle to control blood sugar in advanced cases of diabetes, and with PCOS

Conventional Medical Treatments

- Insulin
- Meglitinides
- Metformin
- Sulfonylureas
- Thiazolidinediones

Further Reading

Akilen R, Tsiami A, Devendra D, Robinson N. Cinnamon in glycaemic control: Systematic review and meta-analysis. *Clinical Nutrition*, 2012 Oct; 31 (5): 609–15.

Allen RW, Schwartzman E, Baker WL, et al. Cinnamon use in type 2 diabetes: An updated systematic review and meta-analysis. *Annals of Family Medicine*, 2013 Sep–Oct; 11 (5): 452–59.

Nahas R, Moher M. Complementary and alternative medicine for the treatment of type 2 diabetes. *Canadian Family Physician*, 2009 Jun; 55 (6): 591–96.

Neelakantan N, Narayanan M, de Souza RJ, van Dam RM. Effect of fenugreek (*Trigonella foenum-graecum* L.) intake on glycemia: A meta-analysis of clinical trials. *Nutrition Journal*, 2014 Jan 18; 13: 7.

Shidfar F, Ebrahimi SS, Hosseini S, et al. The effects of *Berberis vulgaris* fruit extract on serum lipoproteins, apoB, apoA-1, homocysteine, glycemic control and total antioxidant capacity in type 2 diabetic patients. *Iranian Journal of Pharmaceutical Research*, 2012 Spring; 11 (2): 643–52.

Suksomboon N, Poolsup N, Boonkaew S, Suthisisang CC. Meta-analysis of the effect of herbal supplement on glycemic control in type 2 diabetes. *Journal of Ethnopharmacology*, 2011 Oct 11; 137 (3): 1328–33.

Endometriosis

In endometriosis, tissue that normally grows inside the uterus is also located outside of it. Endometriosis most often occurs in the pelvis, but in some cases lesions can also be found outside the pelvis. Approximately 6% to 10% of women have pelvic endometriosis. Somewhere between 35% and 50% women who complain of pelvic pain or infertility are eventually diagnosed with endometriosis.

Signs and Symptoms

- Pelvic pain occurring with menstruation, bowel movements or sexual intercourse
- Spotting or bleeding between periods
- Chronic pain in the lower back or pelvis
- Infertility

Associated Conditions

- Dysmenorrhea
- Infertility

First-Line Herbal Care: TURMERIC

Turmeric (*Curcuma longa*) has a long-standing use in traditional Ayurvedic and Chinese medicine formulas for endometriosis. In Ayurveda, turmeric is considered one of the most important herbs for medicinal and spiritual purposes and is referred to in the Vedas as *aushadhi*, meaning simply "herb." It has almost as many names in Ayurveda as it has uses. In terms of women's health, it has been traditionally used to regulate female reproductive functions and purify the uterus by increasing circulation.

In traditional Chinese medicine, turmeric is known as *jiang huang*, or yellow ginger, an accurate name given that turmeric is a member of the ginger family. Turmeric has been used in China to promote the movement of blood and qi, improve menstrual flow and alleviate pain.

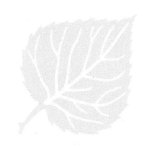

Traditional Chinese medicine (TCM) considers most cases of endometriosis to be a pattern of blood stasis, where blood in the pelvis cannot move freely and thus congeals into endometrial lesions. Herbal treatment is centered on promoting the free-flowing circulation of blood. Herbs such as dang gui, red peony, turmeric and cinnamon are included in TCM herbal formulas for endometriosis. Studies and case reports on traditional formulas, such as *xuefu zhuyu tang* and *guizhi fuling*, have shown promising results in relieving dysmenorrhea and shrinking lesions in women with endometriosis. High-quality placebo-controlled trials are needed to confirm these results.

The traditional Persian system of medicine, Unani, used turmeric to purify, stimulate and build blood.

Human studies on turmeric for other conditions have shown that it stimulates the production and release of bile from the liver and gallbladder. In this way, turmeric also supports the proper metabolism and excretion of hormones, as estrogen needs to be bound to bile before it can be excreted in stool.

A small number of in vitro and animal studies show preliminary evidence-based support for the use of turmeric in endometriosis.

Other Herbal Treatments

The focus of herbal treatment for endometriosis can be either acute or chronic, palliative or curative in nature. A symptom-relieving approach often focuses on decreasing pain and abnormal bleeding patterns. Antispasmodic, pain-relieving and astringent herbs, such as cramp bark, trillium, lady's mantle and yarrow, are used. See the sections on dysmenorrhea (page 135) and menorrhagia (page 139) for details.

An approach designed to address the cause of endometriosis will stress hormonal balance and optimal liver function. Long-term goals focus on decreasing production of estrogen and increasing the metabolism of excess estrogen, which is often a factor in the development and recurrence of endometriosis. This is especially true when women with endometriosis also show signs of hormonal excess, such as breast tenderness, acne, premenstrual syndrome (PMS), bloating and constipation.

Green Tea

A few recent in vitro and animal studies have demonstrated the ability of the green tea (*Camellia sinensis*) extract epigallocatechin gallate (EGCG) to slow, and even reverse, the growth of endometrial lesions. More studies are needed.

Yarrow

Yarrow (*Achillea millefolium*) is an astringent herb with a long history of use for both breaking up congealed blood and staunching bleeding where it shouldn't occur. It is an excellent herb for endometriosis because it can both address excessive and abnormal uterine bleeding and promote the healthy circulation of blood through the uterus, breaking up the congealed blood usually associated with endometriosis.

CASE STUDY
Endometriosis

Sonja came to my clinic looking for help in preventing a recurrence of her endometriosis. Now twenty-eight years old, she had recently had laparoscopic surgery and was hoping to get pregnant in a few years. She wanted to avoid needing to have surgery again before she started trying to conceive, but she wasn't yet ready to become a parent. Historically, her menses had been extremely painful, with heavy bleeding during the first two days. Vaginal penetration during sex was often uncomfortable for her. She considered her premenstrual symptoms to be pretty mild, but she had infrequent bowel movements and had struggled with constipation most of her life.

I recommended a tincture of dandelion root, burdock, dang gui and yarrow throughout the month to increase liver and gallbladder function and improve blood circulation. During her menstrual flow, Sonja switched to a formula that included yarrow, cinnamon, trillium, cramp bark and valerian. She also traded coffee for green tea and added 1 teaspoon (5 mL) of ground turmeric to a smoothie every morning.

After a week, Sonja's bowel movements became regular. Within two months, her menstrual flow was less heavy and her cramps no longer interfered with her daily activities.

A single placebo-controlled animal study found that an alcohol-based extract of *Achillea biebersteinii*, a related species native to Turkey and Iran, reduced the size of endometrial lesions, adhesions and immunological growth factors associated with endometriosis. As this is the only study of its kind, more research is needed to confirm its results.

Common Combinations

- Yarrow, trillium and lady's mantle for abnormal uterine bleeding
- Yarrow, dang gui, red peony and cinnamon for pain and abnormal bleeding
- Burdock, dandelion root and milk thistle to optimize liver function and hormone balance in the long term

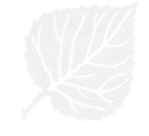

Conventional Medical Treatments

- Danazol
- Gonadotropin-releasing hormone (GnRH) analogs
- Laparoscopic surgery
- Non-steroidal anti-inflammatory drugs (NSAIDS)
- Oral contraceptive pills

Further Reading

Flower A, Liu JP, Lewith G, et al. Chinese herbal medicine for endometriosis. *Cochrane Database of Systematic Reviews*, 2012 May 16; 5: CD006568.

Kong S, Zhang YH, Liu CF, et al. The complementary and alternative medicine for endometriosis: A review of utilization and mechanism. *Evidence-Based Complementary and Alternative Medicine*, 2014; 2014: 146383.

Wieser F, Cohen M, Gaeddert A, et al. Evolution of medical treatment for endometriosis: Back to the roots? *Human Reproduction Update*, 2007 Sep–Oct; 13 (5): 487–99.

Fibrocystic Breast Changes

Fibrocystic changes in breast tissue are one of the top reasons women visit a doctor or gynecologist. Fifty percent of women have fibrocystic changes during their lifetime, usually sometime between menarche and menopause. These noncancerous alterations in breast tissue most often manifest in the form of premenstrual breast tenderness, pain and/or lumps. They are usually caused by normal changes in hormones during the menstrual cycle and are generally not a health concern. Symptoms are often cyclical or change over the course of a menstrual cycle.

Signs and Symptoms

- Breast swelling, tenderness or pain
- Lumps of various sizes and textures, including fibrous, ropey tissue and fluid-filled cysts

Associated Conditions

- Hormonal imbalances, primarily with excess estrogen or progesterone deficiency
- Menstrual irregularities

First-Line Herbal Care: CHASTE TREE

Chaste tree (*Vitex agnus-castus*) is often regarded as one of the best herbal hormonal regulators for a multitude of women's health conditions and at many stages of a woman's life. It has been used to treat premenstrual syndrome (PMS), mastalgia, irregular menses, dysmenorrhea, infertility, hyperprolactinemia, insufficient lactation, menopause and acne.

In clinical studies, chaste tree has been proven more effective than a placebo in treating PMS, especially where breast tenderness and swelling (cyclic mastalgia) is one of the major complaints. Other studies have found that chaste tree reduces premenstrual symptoms better than vitamin B_6 (pyridoxine) or magnesium oxide.

Chaste tree is best suited to cases where fibrocystic changes and mastalgia are associated with a short luteal phase (the part of the menstrual cycle between ovulation and menses) or latent hyperprolactinemia (too much prolactin in the blood).

Other Herbal Treatments

Herbal treatment focuses on correcting hormonal imbalances and reducing inflammation and pain in the breasts. Where fibrocystic breast changes are related to hyperprolactinemia or polycystic ovarian syndrome (PCOS), chaste tree is often recommended. When mastalgia is primarily premenstrual but without other hormonal changes, evening primrose oil, borage oil or blackcurrant oil, all high in gamma-linolenic acid, are used to reduce inflammation and pain.

Evening Primrose

Evening primrose oil (*Oenothera biennis*) is high in gamma-linolenic acid, which acts as an anti-inflammatory when consumed in high doses. Research has shown that evening primrose oil may be more effective at reducing premenstrual breast pain, or cyclic mastalgia, than either a placebo or non-steroidal anti-inflammatory drugs (NSAIDs). A recent study found that evening primrose oil, both on its own and when taken with vitamin E, significantly reduced pain scores for women with cyclic mastalgia when compared to a placebo.

A placebo-controlled trial of a proprietary formula containing evening primrose oil, vitamin B$_6$ and vitamin E found significant changes in premenstrual symptom scores in the areas of mood, behavior and physical symptoms. Other studies, however, have not consistently shown positive results, although negative findings may be related to the length of the studies or other methodological limitations. Evening primrose oil needs to be taken for long periods of time (at least four to six months) for beneficial results to be seen.

The dose of evening primrose oil used in the studies ranged from 1 to 3 grams daily, approximately equivalent to 100 to 300 milligrams of gamma-linolenic acid. Borage oil, which is even higher in gamma-linolenic acid than evening primrose oil, may also be a good choice.

Folklore

Moon Plant
Frequently included in moon gardens — gardens that highlight plants that bloom or look aesthetically pleasing at night — evening primrose's flowers bloom at night and appear to glow in the dark. Evening primrose is associated with the yin/feminine aspects and is said to stimulate the solar plexus and heart.

Common Combination

- Evening primrose oil, vitamin B_6 and vitamin E for premenstrual mastalgia

Conventional Medical Treatments

Pharmaceutical treatment is not usually necessary. If pain relief is needed, NSAIDs may be prescribed. In more severe cases, oral contraceptive pills, spironolactone and/or bromocriptine may be useful.

Further Reading

Carmichael AR. Can *Vitex agnus-castus* be used for the treatment of mastalgia? What is the current evidence? *Evidence-Based Complementary and Alternative Medicine*, 2008 Sep; 5 (3): 247–50.

Pruthi S, Wahner-Roedler DL, Torkelson CJ, et al. Vitamin E and evening primrose oil for management of cyclical mastalgia: A randomized pilot study. *Alternative Medicine Review*, 2010 Apr; 15 (1): 59–67.

Sharma N, Gupta A, Jha PK, Rajput P. Mastalgia cured! Randomized trial comparing centchroman to evening primrose oil. *Breast Journal*, 2012 Sep; 18 (5): 509–10.

van Die MD, Burger HG, Teede HJ, Bone KM. *Vitex agnus-castus* extracts for female reproductive disorders: A systematic review of clinical trials. *Planta Medica*, 2013 May; 79 (7): 562–75.

Did You Know?

Lifestyle Changes

Dietary treatment can be quite helpful in reducing the pain of fibrocystic breast changes. Health authorities often recommend avoiding or limiting caffeine in coffee, tea and chocolate. Wearing a supportive bra without underwire can also reduce pain.

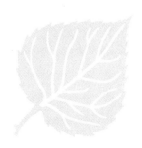

Fibroids

Fibroids are benign smooth muscle tumors of the uterus. They are also called leiomyomas (*lie-o-my-O-muhs*). Fibroids are classified based on their location within the uterus, but all are growths within the walls of the uterus. Since fibroids are dependent on estrogen to help them grow, they are most common between menarche and menopause. Fibroids also tend to grow during pregnancy, when estrogen levels are particularly high. Many fibroids shrink or disappear after pregnancy or after menopause. Fibroids are not associated with an increased risk of uterine cancer.

Many women don't even know they have fibroids, because they don't experience any symptoms. One common symptom is heavy and/or prolonged menstrual bleeding, which is usually caused by fibroids that are growing in the internal wall of the uterus or those that are pedunculated. Constipation or urinary symptoms may occur if a large fibroid presses against the bowel or bladder. It is rare for fibroids to cause difficulties with embryo implantation leading to infertility.

Signs and Symptoms
- Heavy and/or prolonged menstrual bleeding
- Sensations of pelvic fullness
- Pain during intercourse or noncyclic pelvic pain
- Constipation
- Urinary frequency, nocturia or urinary incontinence
- Infertility (rare)

Associated Conditions
- Anemia
- Diabetes
- Hypertension
- Infertility (rare)
- Menorrhagia
- Obesity
- Polycystic ovarian syndrome (PCOS)

First-Line Herbal Care: CASTOR OIL

Although most people don't have castor oil (*Ricinus communis*) in their kitchen cupboards anymore, just a generation or two ago it was a well-known herbal treatment for use at home. Some people might remember the thick, bitter taste of the oil from their childhood, as it was a popular folk remedy for constipation and was often given to children to prevent and treat intestinal worms.

Castor oil can be quite strong, causing intense cramping and spasmodic diarrhea. In fact, it has been traditionally used in China and other places to induce labor and expel the placenta by encouraging spasms in smooth muscles, which include both the intestines and uterus.

As a treatment for fibroids, castor oil is (thankfully) not used orally but topically, typically as a pack placed over the abdomen and pelvis, where it is believed to improve the circulation of blood and lymph in the underlying tissues.

Castor Oil Packs

Very few studies have looked at the health impacts of regular use of castor oil packs for any specific condition. None have been conducted on fibroids specifically. Nonetheless, studies do support Edgar Cayce's rationale for using castor oil topically (see sidebar). One study showed that castor oil packs increase the production of white blood cells in the day following the treatment. This stimulation of the immune system improves both blood and lymph circulation, as white blood cells travel through these systems, boosting the body's natural defenses.

Whatever the direct physiological benefits of castor oil packs, there are other benefits as well. By lying down for thirty to sixty minutes, you encourage rest and relaxation through the parasympathetic nervous system. This increases blood circulation through the organs and promotes proper functioning of the immune system. Given the stresses of modern life, the importance of self-care and relaxation cannot be overlooked.

Other Herbal Treatments

Traditional approaches to the treatment of fibroids are very similar to those for endometriosis (see page 87). From the perspective of traditional Chinese medicine, fibroids and endometriosis have a lot in common. Both are often

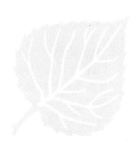

How to Prepare a Castor Oil Pack

A castor oil pack can be used for many conditions involving the pelvic organs, including fibroids, endometriosis and polycystic ovaries, and even for general hormone imbalance leading to irregular menstrual cycles. Castor oil packs increase circulation in the area covered, release local tension, reduce inflammation, clear congestion, stimulate bowel function and support healthy immune system responses. They also help to connect you with your body, set a healing intention through daily ritual and encourage relaxation.

Before your first castor oil pack, do a patch test of castor oil on a small area of skin to make sure you don't have an allergic reaction.

> 1 piece of cotton flannel large enough to cover
>   the area from bra line to pubic bone
> Cold-pressed organic castor oil
> Plastic wrap (optional)
> Hot water bottle or heating pad
> Old towel

1. Soak the cotton flannel in castor oil so that it is saturated but not dripping.
2. Lying down in a comfortable position, place the flannel over your abdomen so that it covers the entire area from bra line to pubic bone.
3. If desired, cover the flannel with plastic wrap to prevent castor oil from leaking onto your clothes or furniture.
4. Place the heating pad or hot water bottle on top and cover with the towel to keep in the heat.
5. Relax for thirty to sixty minutes. This is a great time to read a book, write in a journal, meditate, breathe deeply, visualize or nap.
6. After removing the pack, cleanse the skin with a mixture of baking soda and water. The castor oil pack can be stored in a closed container in the refrigerator and reused for up to two weeks.
7. Repeat the castor oil pack treatment three to five days a week.

Caution

Do not use a castor oil pack over broken skin or during pregnancy. Exercise caution when using castor oil packs during menses. In some cases they may help to alleviate pain associated with dysmenorrhea, but they may also increase blood flow, worsening menorrhagia.

Note

Castor oil will stain clothing and can be difficult to remove. Use a mixture of baking soda and water to wash any fabrics that come in contact with castor oil. Lying down on an old towel will protect furniture.

understood as decreased circulation of blood in the uterus, which then stagnates and congeals into benign masses.

Fibroids are estrogen-dependent — that is, they depend on a relative excess of circulating estrogen. Although time and menopause often resolve fibroids on their own, herbs that act as hormonal regulators can also be helpful. Herbs are also used to resolve heavy bleeding and encourage the metabolism of estrogen through the liver.

Black Cohosh

Black cohosh has traditionally been used for almost every female reproductive or menstrual condition imaginable, and at every stage of life. Native Americans and herbalists have long used black cohosh to normalize hormones such as estrogen, progesterone, luteinizing hormone and follicle-stimulating hormone in conditions as varied as fibroids, amenorrhea, dysmenorrhea, premenstrual syndrome and menopause.

As with many herbs that contain phytoestrogens, concerns were once raised about the use of black cohosh when the patient also has an estrogen-dependent tumor (such as fibroids or estrogen-receptor-positive breast cancer). These speculations, however, have been refuted through in vitro and human clinical trials. In one large controlled study, black cohosh was shown to have protective effects against breast cancer development. In terms of its effects on estrogen in the uterus, in vitro studies have shown that black cohosh may actually halt the growth of fibroid cells.

A randomized, controlled trial comparing black cohosh to the drug tibolone for menopausal symptoms conducted a subgroup analysis of women who had uterine fibroids at the start of the trial. Fibroid size was measured before and after the three-month treatment. In the group taking Remifemin, a standardized extract of black cohosh, 70% of the women experienced a decrease in fibroid size and volume, with the largest fibroid in each woman shrinking significantly. For those taking tibolone, fibroids actually increased in size on average, and only 36% showed decreases in fibroid size. Although these are the results of only one study, black cohosh may be helpful in reducing fibroid size, particularly in perimenopausal women.

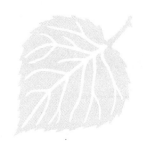

Cinnamon

Cinnamon (*Cinnamomum verum* or *Cinnamomum cassia*) is one of the main ingredients in a traditional Chinese medicine formula for fibroids called *guizhi fuling*, in which cinnamon is paired with poria, tree peony root and peach kernel to warm the menses and resolve blood stasis. The warming effects of cinnamon help to break up stagnation and move blood.

In a recent systematic review of nine clinical trials, researchers found that *guizhi fuling* used in conjunction with mifepristone, a commonly prescribed pharmaceutical, resulted in a greater reduction of fibroid volume and overall uterus size than when mifepristone was used alone.

Yarrow

Yarrow (*Achillea millefolium*) is often used in the treatment of fibroids for the same reason that it is used in endometriosis — it helps to regulate the circulation of blood through the uterus.

Yarrow has long been used to control the blood, either starting or stopping its flow as needed. Leaves rolled up and placed in the nostrils were traditionally used to induce a nosebleed — and thus relieve a headache — or to stop an existing nosebleed.

In women's health traditions, yarrow is used as both an emmenagogue and an antihemorrhagic. It can bring on menses when blood is congealed or stagnant, but it can also prevent excessive menstrual flow. Yarrow is thus considered a normalizing herb for the blood and for circulation. It relieves congestion and tones blood vessels, moves and stops blood, and strengthens and relaxes circulation.

This action is key in cases of fibroids, where heavy menses, or menorrhagia, is the most common physical symptom. Unfortunately, no scientific research has been conducted on yarrow specifically with respect to the treatment of fibroids.

Folklore

Achilles' Heal

Yarrow is said to get its Latin name, *Achillea*, from the Greek hero Achilles, who was taught by the great healer Chiron the centaur how to use the plant to heal wounds. According to myth, when Achilles asked Chiron for protection against the wounds he was sure to incur in his role as warrior, Chiron brewed up a large vat of yarrow tea, grabbed Achilles by the ankle and dunked him headfirst into the yarrow bath. This elixir made Achilles completely invulnerable to attack — except, of course, for his heel.

Common Combinations

- Yarrow, geranium and lady's mantle for heavy menstrual flow due to fibroids
- Black cohosh, raspberry, dang gui and chaste tree to address hormonal imbalances
- Dandelion root, burdock root and milk thistle to promote optimal liver function
- Cinnamon and poria formula (*guizhi fuling*) where there is a traditional Chinese medicine diagnosis of cold phlegm and blood stagnation

Conventional Medical Treatments

Often, a "watch and wait" approach or no treatment is recommended. If fibroids are very large or very bothersome, oral contraceptives, hormonal intrauterine devices or gonadotropin-releasing hormone analogs may be prescribed. Other treatment options include uterine artery embolization, surgical removal and, in some cases, hysterectomy.

Further Reading

Liu JP, Yang H, Xia Y, Cardini F. Herbal preparations for uterine fibroids. *Cochrane Database of Systematic Reviews*, 2013 Apr 30; 4: CD005292.

Mehl-Madrona L. Complementary medicine treatment of uterine fibroids: A pilot study. *Alternative Therapies in Health and Medicine*, 2002 Mar–Apr; 8 (2): 34–36, 38–40, 42, 44–46.

Xi S, Liske E, Wang S, et al. Effect of isopropanolic *Cimicifuga racemosa* extract on uterine fibroids in comparison with tibolone among patients of a recent randomized, double blind, parallel-controlled study in Chinese women with menopausal symptoms. *Evidence-Based Complementary and Alternative Medicine*, 2014; 2014: 717686.

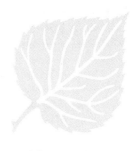

Genital Warts

Did You Know?

Social Stigma

As with many sexually transmitted infections, genital warts often have a social stigma applied to them and may impact psychosocial aspects of health. Telling sexual partners that you have, or have had, genital warts can be stressful and anxiety-inducing for some people. Fear of being judged and rejected is common.

Genital warts are one of the most common sexually transmitted infections. Like cervical dysplasia (see page 74), genital warts are caused by specific strains of human papilloma virus (HPV). HPV is transmitted through sexual contact. It is estimated that over half of all sexually active people are exposed to HPV at some point in their lifetime. Not everyone who is exposed will get genital warts, but some people do. Those who are immunocompromised are more likely to develop warts after contact with the virus.

Vaccines exist to help protect against certain strains of HPV. In the United States, before the introduction of HPV vaccines, the rate of genital warts in sexually active young women was estimated to be 6% overall, and up to 10% in women aged twenty-five to thirty-four. In Canada, it was estimated to be 2% among sexually active young women. Preliminary studies show that these rates have already decreased significantly through national vaccination programs directed at young women. In Australia, where approximately 70% of women under twenty-eight have received the HPV vaccine, the treatment rates for genital warts in private hospitals declined by 85% post-vaccine in women aged fifteen to twenty-four, according to a recent study.

Signs and Symptoms

- Growths on or near the vagina or anus that appear as small, moist, flesh-colored bumps or may resemble cauliflower
- Warts in the mouth or throat (if the virus was contracted through oral sexual contact)

Associated Conditions

- Cervical dysplasia
- Cervical cancer
- Other sexually transmitted infections

First-Line Herbal Care: GREEN TEA

Catechins in green tea (*Camellia sinensis*) have been well studied as a topical treatment for genital warts. Most studies have involved a proprietary cream called Polyphenon E, which contains 10% to 15% catechins by weight. Several well-designed clinical trials have found that Polyphenon E applied three times daily is an effective treatment for genital warts. A recent review showed that over 50% of people using Polyphenon E had complete resolution of the warts within sixteen weeks of use, and more than 75% showed partial resolution.

Side effects from topical green tea extracts are similar to those seen with a placebo, and local skin reactions are generally mild to moderate. Studies also consistently show low rates of recurrence after treatment has ended.

In 2006, the United States Food and Drug Administration (FDA) officially approved Polyphenon E ointment as a treatment for genital and perianal warts caused by HPV. Polyphenon E is sold as Veregen in the United States, Canada and many European countries.

Other Herbal Treatments

Herbal treatment for genital warts is similar in many ways to the treatment of cervical dysplasia, since both are caused by HPV. Antiviral and anticancer herbs are used both topically and internally to stop the growth of new warts and to stimulate the immune system to resolve the virus. For those people who experience anxiety and stress about the possibility of recurrence, antianxiety herbs, such as lavender and lemon balm, may be appropriate.

Echinacea

Echinacea (*Echinacea purpurea* or *Echinacea angustifolia*) may be used in the treatment and prevention of genital warts, as it may help to improve immune responses to HPV. As an immunostimulant, echinacea is traditionally used anytime the immune system isn't able to respond effectively to clear viruses (or bacteria) on its own.

Little research has been conducted on echinacea specifically for the treatment of genital warts. One study compared the use of a combination herbal product to no treatment after surgical removal of genital warts, to see if herbs were effective in preventing the recurrence of warts

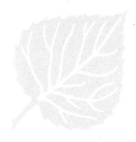

(which is common even after treatment). For patients who used the herbal formula for one month after surgery, recurrence rates six months later were significantly lower than for those who had no treatment. The herbal product used in this study contains echinacea, cat's claw, pau d'arco, andrographis, grapefruit seed extract and papaya.

Lemon Balm

Lemon balm (*Melissa officinalis*) is traditionally used for both its calming and its antiviral effects. Although it has not been studied for use in the treatment of HPV, lemon balm gently stimulates the immune system by easing anxiety and stress.

St. John's Wort

Well known for its effective use in depression, St. John's wort (*Hypericum perforatum*) has also been shown through in vitro studies to have antiviral effects against many different viruses. In cases where genital warts appear alongside feelings of depression, hopelessness or overwhelming sadness, St. John's wort may be a good choice.

Common Combinations

- Echinacea, andrographis and St. John's wort to prevent recurrence of genital warts
- Echinacea, lemon balm and lavender to prevent recurrence and reduce anxiety
- Topical green tea extract with 15% catechins to treat warts

Conventional Medical Treatments

- *Topical Creams:* Imiquimod, podophyllin (a drug developed from plants) or trichloroacetic acid
- Liquid nitrogen to freeze off warts

Further Reading

Mistrangelo M, Cornaglia S, Pizzio M, et al. Immunostimulation to reduce recurrence after surgery for anal condyloma acuminata: A prospective randomized controlled trial. *Colorectal Disease*, 2010 Aug; 12 (8): 799–803.

Tzellos TG, Sardeli C, Lallas A, et al. Efficacy, safety and tolerability of green tea catechins in the treatment of external anogenital warts: A systematic review and meta-analysis. *Journal of the European Academy of Dermatology and Venereology*. 2011 Mar; 25 (3): 345–53.

Caution

St. John's wort has been shown to speed up the metabolism and decrease the effectiveness of many commonly used pharmaceutical drugs, including oral contraceptives. Consult with a healthcare provider who is familiar with drug–herb interactions before taking St. John's wort. The use of St. John's wort may lead to photosensitivity; be cautious when exposing your skin to the sun while taking this herb.

Herpes

Herpes simplex virus (HSV) is a very common viral infection that affects the mucous membranes around the mouth and/or genitals. Typically, HSV-1 is associated with oral herpes (commonly known as a cold sore or fever blister) and HSV-2 is associated with genital herpes, although this is not always the case.

Herpes can affect people of any age, and once someone has herpes, they have it for life. The virus can go into a hibernation of sorts, hiding in the nervous system and reappearing during times of stress, menses, skin trauma or illness. Some people go for years without the virus manifesting, while others may struggle with recurrent herpes breakouts. Unfortunately, the herpes virus can sometimes be spread through skin contact even when there is no visible sore, making transmission more widespread.

Herpes can be triggered by stress and can be a source of stress in itself. Many women are concerned about the effect herpes will have on their sexual practices, and are worried about transmitting the virus to their sexual partners or children. Having sores around the mouth or genitals can also lead to body-image issues and a sense of being stigmatized.

Signs and Symptoms

- Tingling, itching or burning before the appearance of blisters around the mouth or genitals
- Small fluid-filled blisters that break open into painful sores, ooze fluid and crust over
- Flu-like symptoms
- Painful or difficult urination as urine passes over genital sores
- Less frequently, herpes lesions on the hands or eyes

Associated Condition

- Increased risk of transmission of other sexually transmitted infections, most notably human immuno-deficiency virus (HIV)

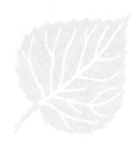

First-Line Herbal Care: LEMON BALM

Lemon balm (*Melissa officinalis*) and other well-known mint family plants, including peppermint and rosemary, have been studied for their use in treating herpes lesions. Three separate randomized, controlled trials looked at the topical use of 1% lemon balm cream for the treatment of oral herpes sores. Applied four times daily, the cream significantly reduced the size and severity of the sores after forty-eight hours compared to a placebo. One of these trials even demonstrated that prolonged use of lemon balm cream increased the time span between outbreaks.

In vitro studies show that water-based extracts of lemon balm have strong antiviral activity against HSV-1 and HSV-2, even in cases where the virus has become resistant to standard pharmaceutical drugs.

Other Herbal Treatments

Along with changes in diet and stress reduction, herbal treatment plays a central role in reducing symptoms and preventing outbreaks. Herbal treatment focuses on supporting the immune system to help decrease the severity and longevity of acute herpes lesions. Especially useful are those herbs with specific antiviral activity, such as lemon balm, St. John's wort, sage and propolis. Strengthening the immune system and improving the body's response to stress helps to prevent future outbreaks.

In my clinical practice, I frequently suggest that patients use schisandra, licorice, astragalus and rhodiola on a long-term basis to help tonify the immune system and improve the body's physiological response to daily stresses. Stress management techniques such as breathing exercises, mindful meditation and adequate rest are the cornerstone of any treatment plan for recurrent herpes outbreaks.

Echinacea

All parts of the echinacea plant (*Echinacea purpurea* or *Echinacea angustifolia*) are known to stimulate the immune system and protect against infections. In vitro and animal studies show that echinacea has strong antiviral activity against both HSV-1 and HSV-2. Since echinacea has been shown to act best as prophylactic immune support, it is also useful for supporting the healthy function of the immune system to prevent future outbreaks.

Propolis

Propolis is a resinous mixture that honey bees collect from various trees and use to seal small open spaces within their hives. The exact makeup of propolis varies depending on the season and the trees it is collected from, but it is usually harvested from conifers, poplars and willow trees in temperate climates. Bees in other regions may use other trees and even flowers to make propolis.

A randomized, single-blind study compared a 3% propolis ointment applied four times daily with topical 5% acyclovir (a pharmaceutical antiviral), also applied four times daily, in women and men with HSV-2. The group that used the propolis ointment reported fewer symptoms and healed faster. The propolis cream was also effective at resolving superinfections in women with intravaginal or cervical herpes lesions.

St. John's Wort

St. John's wort (*Hypericum perforatum*) is best known for its use in treating depression, but it has also been used topically to heal skin wounds and burns. Since herpes is, essentially, a skin wound, herbalists often include St. John's wort in formulas for herpes.

In vitro studies have shown that St. John's wort may suppress the ability of the herpes virus to replicate, which, in theory, could reduce the time it takes for herpes lesions to heal. One study on the use of St. John's wort for depression suggested that St. John's wort taken orally also helped prevent HSV-1 and HSV-2 outbreaks. Two studies demonstrated that oral St. John's wort significantly decreased pain, itching, number of blisters and other subjective symptoms compared to a placebo; unfortunately, these studies were never published.

Common Combinations

- Lemon balm, echinacea and St. John's wort topically and internally for acute herpes
- Propolis ointment (readily available as a commercial product) topically

Conventional Medical Treatments

- Oral antivirals such as acyclovir or valacyclovir
- Topical antiviral cream

Did You Know?

Honey Bee Protection

Originally, beekeepers thought propolis helped protect bees from wind, rain and cold. Recent research suggests otherwise. The currently accepted theory is that bees use propolis as an antimicrobial, to protect the hive from bacteria, disease and putrefaction. Early scientific studies support the idea that propolis contains strong antimicrobial components.

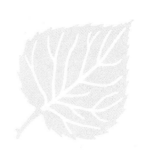

CASE STUDY
Genital Herpes

Thirty-one-year-old Kimberly came to see me during the first trimester of her pregnancy for advice on how to prevent an outbreak of genital herpes. There can be serious complications during labor and vaginal delivery if a woman has any active lesions within six weeks of delivery, and she wanted to avoid the possibility of a Caesarean section.

Kimberly already knew that stress and certain foods could trigger an outbreak. I recommended that she avoid foods high in arginine, an amino acid that is correlated to herpes outbreaks. I also suggested that she incorporate a variety of stress management techniques into her daily routine and take additional vitamin C and zinc to support optimal immune system function. During her second and third trimesters, whenever she felt she was at risk of getting an outbreak, she used an oral herbal formula that contained echinacea and St. John's wort for up to a week. At the first sign of tingling, she also applied a topical preparation of lemon balm and propolis to the area several times each day.

Kimberly had one outbreak in her second trimester that resolved within two days, and no further herpes lesions throughout the remainder of her pregnancy. She took acyclovir prophylactically during the last two weeks of pregnancy and gave birth vaginally to a healthy baby.

Further Reading

Koytchev R, Alken RG, Dundarov S. Balm mint extract (Lo-701) for topical treatment of recurring herpes labialis. *Phytomedicine*, 1999 Oct; 6 (4): 225–30.

Vynograd N, Vynograd I, Sosnowski Z. A comparative multi-centre study of the efficacy of propolis, acyclovir and placebo in the treatment of genital herpes (HSV). *Phytomedicine*, 2000 Mar; 7 (1): 1–6.

Wölfle U, Seelinger G, Schempp CM. Topical application of St. John's wort (*Hypericum perforatum*). *Planta Medica*, 2014 Feb; 80 (2–3): 109–20.

Yarnell E, Abascal K, Rountree R. Herbs for herpes simplex infections. *Alternative and Complementary Therapies*, 2009 April; 15 (2): 69–74.

High Blood Pressure and Heart Disease

High blood pressure (also known as hypertension) is exactly what it sounds like: the pressure of the blood moving through your blood vessels is higher than it should be. This can cause strain on the walls of the arteries, the heart (which is responsible for pumping blood) and the kidneys (which filter blood).

"Heart disease" is an umbrella term that refers to several conditions that affect the heart, including coronary artery disease, heart failure, abnormal heart rhythms (arrhythmia) and disorders involving the valves of the heart. For the most part, heart disease involves conditions where there is a narrowing of arteries in and around the heart, which increases the risk of having a heart attack or stroke.

Some people experience no obvious signs or symptoms preceding a cardiovascular event such as a heart attack or stroke. High blood pressure is often said to be a silent killer because it is usually discovered only incidentally during a visit to a health-care provider. Others may experience some or all of the symptoms listed in the box below. Symptoms may occur at rest or during physical activity, or they may be triggered by stressful situations.

Signs and Symptoms

- Dull, heavy, sharp or burning pain in the chest, neck, jaw, throat, upper abdomen or back
- Heart palpitations or a fluttering sensation in the chest
- Shortness of breath
- Fatigue, generalized weakness
- Swelling, weakness and/or numbness in the legs and feet

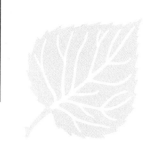

Associated Conditions

- Chronic kidney disease
- Diabetes
- Heart attack
- High cholesterol
- Obesity
- Stroke

Lifestyle Changes

In my experience, lifestyle is the single most important factor to address with high blood pressure or heart disease, well before the use of herbs.

Achieving and maintaining a healthy body weight is the first step, if indicated. Reducing daily intake of salt can also make a big difference, especially for people who add too much salt to their food or eat a lot of canned soups and other prepared foods, which typically contain way too much sodium. Another important step is increasing total daily servings of fruits and vegetables, which provide nutrients that help strengthen blood vessel walls and protect against heart disease and stroke.

Exercise is indispensable for controlling blood pressure over the long term. If there's anything most of us do too little of, it is exercise. A brisk walk for twenty to thirty minutes at least three times a week is my baseline recommendation for decreasing blood pressure and reducing the risk of complications.

First-Line Herbal Care: GARLIC

Garlic (*Allium sativum*) is an easy addition to any treatment plan for lowering blood pressure and cholesterol. As long as you don't mind the taste and smell, it is easy and accessible. For those who don't want to smell like garlic, odorless garlic is available in supplement form.

Two recent meta-analyses reported on the results of a small number of high-quality studies, which found that garlic reduces systolic blood pressure by 20 to 30 mmHg and diastolic blood pressure by 10 to 20 mmHg compared to a placebo. More research is needed to confirm how effective garlic is at preventing more serious heart disease or death.

The doses of garlic in these trials ranged from 480 to 960 milligrams of encapsulated garlic powder per day. Because the size and quality of garlic differ from clove to clove, it is difficult to determine how many cloves would be beneficial, but two to four cloves of garlic, weighing about 2 to 5 grams total, is recommended. If taking raw garlic, eat the cloves or oil with food, as garlic can cause stomach upset.

Other Herbal Treatments

Herbal treatment for high blood pressure typically consists of herbs that are traditionally known as cardiotonics; in other words, they tonify the cardiovascular system. Hawthorn, motherwort, hibiscus, garlic and linden are a few examples of cardiotonics.

Herbal diuretics are often used as well, and many are particularly useful because they do not decrease potassium in the blood, which is a well-known adverse effect of pharmaceutical diuretics. Examples of herbal diuretics include dandelion leaf, yarrow and celery seed.

Cardioactive herbs, such as foxglove, lily-of-the-valley and mistletoe, are sometimes used in more severe cases of high blood pressure or heart disease, but because these are also very toxic, they should not be used without the guidance of a licensed health-care practitioner.

Dandelion Leaf

Dandelion leaf (*Taraxacum officinale*) is traditionally used as a diuretic. In French, dandelion is known as *pissenlit*, which literally translates as "urine in bed." This name is a declaration of its excellent diuretic action, and perhaps also a caution against drinking dandelion leaf tea before bed.

One very small study showed that dandelion tincture increased urinary frequency compared to a baseline, confirming its diuretic action. An animal model found dandelion leaf to be comparable to furosemide, a pharmaceutical diuretic. However, since dandelion leaf is a source of minerals, it doesn't cause a loss of minerals through urine, unlike many pharmaceutical diuretics.

I frequently add dandelion leaf or another diuretic to formulas for high blood pressure and congestive heart failure, especially when the patient has edema or swelling or has responded to pharmaceutical diuretics in the past.

Green Tea

Green tea (*Camellia sinensis*) has gone from everyday beverage to panacea herb status in recent years. Much of this interest stems from the belief that green tea is an herb of longevity, an idea bolstered by epidemiological studies showing that people in cultures where green tea is regularly consumed live longer lives and have lower rates of certain diseases.

In this way, green tea and soy have much in common. They are both native to Asia, where they are an important part of the diet of many cultures. Both have inspired large-scale population studies that have triggered many other clinical trials. One could say that green tea is to heart disease and cancer as soy is to menopause.

At the root of green tea's health benefits are its antioxidant polyphenols, which are understood to be the main constituent responsible for prolonging life and preventing heart disease and cancer. Many studies have looked at the role of green tea in addressing hypertension and heart disease. Scientific trials have supported the population studies and preclinical studies. Two recent meta-analyses showed that green tea significantly lowers systolic blood pressure, total cholesterol and low-density lipoprotein (LDL), or "bad," cholesterol. (Similar results were found with black tea.)

Hawthorn

Hawthorn (*Crataegus laevigata* or *Crataegus monogyna*) is one of the first herbs I think of when a patient has a cardiovascular condition, because it has such a broad range of use. I often include hawthorn in formulas for high blood pressure to help prevent the development of more serious cardiovascular disease.

Historically, hawthorn, a member of the rose family, has been used to strengthen and tone the heart in a variety of diseases. The dark red berries are high in antioxidant proanthocyanidins and flavonoids, which are understood to be responsible for many of the plant's medicinal effects.

In traditional Chinese medicine, hawthorn is used for a variety of conditions ranging from food stagnation (a diagnosis with symptoms such as belching, acid reflux, indigestion and bloating after eating) to postpartum lochia (a medical term for bloody discharge after giving birth). Although seemingly disparate, all of the conditions for which hawthorn is used result from stagnation, according to Chinese medical theory. Hawthorn is believed to move

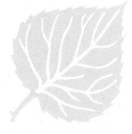

blood and resolve blood stasis. Its role in treating food stagnation is mirrored in its secondary effects of decreasing cholesterol and other blood lipids.

Hawthorn's potential as a treatment for heart disease is well documented by scientific research. For patients with heart disease that falls within the New York Heart Association functional classifications I to III (from mild heart disease with no limitations on activity to more severe heart disease with marked limitations on activity and comfort only during rest), hawthorn has been shown to significantly improve shortness of breath, fatigue, exercise tolerance and maximum workload compared to a placebo.

Most of the published studies have been performed on patients who were also using conventional pharmaceuticals, and have thus evaluated hawthorn's efficacy and safety as an adjunctive treatment. In a 2008 meta-analysis, the authors concluded that hawthorn is safe and effective for adjunctive use in patients with heart disease or chronic congestive heart failure. The dose used in most of the studies ranged from 450 to 900 milligrams twice daily.

More recently, a handful of studies have looked at the use of hawthorn in the treatment of high blood pressure. Although preliminary and very limited, these studies show a trend toward lowering blood pressure, even in people taking medications for hypertension and/or diabetes.

Kitchen Lore

Open Heart Tea
Drink 1 cup (250 mL) twice daily to gently tonify the cardiovascular system.

> 2 cups (500 mL) water
> ¼ tsp (1 mL) hawthorn berries, leaf and/or flower
> ¼ tsp (1 mL) dandelion leaf
> ¼ tsp (1 mL) yarrow leaf and flower
> ¼ tsp (1 mL) linden leaf and flower
> 1 green tea bag

1. Bring the water to a boil.
2. Mix together the hawthorn, dandelion, yarrow and linden and place them, along with the tea bag, in a tea infuser or loose in a teapot.
3. Cover the herbs with the boiled water and let steep for 5 minutes. Strain and enjoy.

Hawthorn's Doctrine of Signatures

Early one fall, I was walking with my family along an urban river valley, and we passed a large hawthorn tree. As I pointed out its characteristically long thorns to my kids, my eldest reached up to see for himself how pointy the thorns were. While I was trying to teach him to identify plants, with a side note of caution, he was pressing the thorn against his finger to determine if it was sharp enough to stab a vampire! As it turns out, we were both successful: the thorn easily drew a little blood, reminding me of hawthorn's ability to encourage the healthy flow of blood. Likewise, hawthorn's oval berries resemble drops of blood hanging from the tree.

Motherwort

Motherwort (*Leonurus cardiaca*) is often used for hypertension, especially in women who also experience anxiety or in cases where stress and/or worry lead to an increase in blood pressure.

"Wort" is another word for "herb," so motherwort is a mother's herb: an herb to mother mothers. Motherwort provides strength to women who spend most of their time taking care of other people, leaving them with little energy for themselves. It bolsters courage and confidence while calming an overactive mind. Its Latin name, *Leonurus cardiaca*, translates as "lion heart," referring to the strength and power it restores to the spirit.

Motherwort was first used by the Greeks to soothe anxiety in pregnant women. Although it is no longer recommended for use during pregnancy, motherwort is an important herb when your heartbeat is revved up by anxiety or stress. It has a long history of use in anxiety, palpitations, tachycardia (fast heart rate) and high blood pressure.

Overall, phytochemical and in vitro research confirms the hypotensive and sedative effects of motherwort. One small clinical trial investigating the use of motherwort oil extract showed significant improvement in symptoms of anxiety and depression, as well as blood pressure, in patients with stage 1 and 2 hypertension, affirming motherwort's traditional use.

Yarrow

Although my first thoughts about uses for yarrow (*Achillea millefolium*) tend to be related to menstrual cycles or wounds, it is also an excellent herb for improving blood flow in the heart and blood vessels overall. Because it both controls blood and is a diuretic, yarrow may be useful in addressing heart health and high blood pressure, especially where there is stagnation of blood (a traditional Chinese medicine diagnosis meaning that overall circulation is poor).

Preliminary preclinical studies support the use of yarrow for high blood pressure. The evidence suggests that the flavonoids in yarrow may act in a similar way to angiotensin-converting-enzyme inhibitor (ACE inhibitor) drugs and have vasodilating effects in vitro. More studies are needed.

CASE STUDY
High Blood Pressure

Veronica came to see me for help lowering her blood pressure. It had been climbing steadily for several years even though she exercised regularly and ate a whole-food diet with lots of fruits and vegetables. She had a family history of heart disease and stroke on both sides of her family. Now forty-nine, she often worried about her health and whether she would have a heart attack or stroke. She talked about all the sources of stress in her life: responsibilities at work, young adult children and aging parents in ill health.

When I measured Veronica's blood pressure, it was 154/102 mmHg, significantly higher than normal. I noticed that her breathing was shallow and that she fidgeted when she talked about her family, so I asked about anxiety and worry. She started to cry as she told me how concerned she was about her mother, who had recently been diagnosed with cancer. She was also worried about her youngest child, who was still living at home because of his struggle with bipolar disease.

During that first visit, I led Veronica through a breathing and visualization exercise for five minutes. When we were done, I retook her blood pressure: it was 146/94! I recommended that she do this exercise for ten minutes twice a day. I made her an herbal formula with motherwort, hawthorn, St. John's wort and lavender. She also started taking garlic and fish oil supplements. Slowly but surely, her blood pressure started to lower, settling around 130/90 within a few months.

Common Combinations

- Hawthorn, garlic and dandelion root for high blood pressure with high cholesterol
- Hawthorn, motherwort and linden for high blood pressure with anxiety
- Dandelion leaf, yarrow and celery seed for high blood pressure with edema or arthritis

Conventional Medical Treatments

- Angiotensin-converting-enzyme inhibitors (ACE inhibitors)
- Beta blockers
- Calcium channel blockers
- Thiazide diuretics

Further Reading

Clare BA, Conroy RS, Spelman K. The diuretic effect in human subjects of an extract of *Taraxacum officinale* folium over a single day. *Journal of Alternative and Complementary Medicine*, 2009 Aug; 15 (8): 929–34.

Hartley L, Flowers N, Holmes J, et al. Green and black tea for the primary prevention of cardiovascular disease. *Cochrane Database of Systematic Reviews*, 2013 Jun 18; 6: CD009934.

Onakpoya I, Spencer E, Heneghan C, Thompson M. The effect of green tea on blood pressure and lipid profile: A systematic review and meta-analysis of randomized clinical trials. *Nutrition, Metabolism and Cardiovascular Diseases*, 2014 Aug; 24 (8): 823–36.

Pittler MH, Guo R, Ernst E. Hawthorn extract for treating chronic heart failure. *Cochrane Database of Systematic Reviews*, 2008 Jan 23; (1): CD005312.

Rohner A, Ried K, Sobenin IA, et al. A systematic review and meta-analysis on the effects of garlic preparations on blood pressure in individuals with hypertension. *American Journal of Hypertension*, 2014 Sep 18. pii: hpu165. [Epub ahead of print.]

Shikov AN, Pozharitskaya ON, Makarov VG, et al. Effect of *Leonurus cardiaca* oil extract in patients with arterial hypertension accompanied by anxiety and sleep disorders. *Phytotherapy Research*, 2011 Apr; 25 (4): 540–43.

Stabler SN, Tejani AM, Huynh F, Fowkes C. Garlic for the prevention of cardiovascular morbidity and mortality in hypertensive patients. *Cochrane Database of Systematic Reviews*, 2012 Aug 15; 8: CD007653.

Wang J, Xiong X, Feng B. Effect of *Crataegus* usage in cardiovascular disease prevention: An evidence-based approach. *Evidence-Based Complementary and Alternative Medicine*, 2013; 2013: 149363.

Caution

For people who have been diagnosed with high blood pressure or heart disease, knowing which herbs to avoid is just as important as knowing which herbs to take. Of note, licorice is known to increase blood pressure, as is Korean ginseng when combined with caffeine. Always consult with a health-care practitioner before using any herbs to treat high blood pressure or heart disease, especially if you are taking any pharmaceutical medications.

Hypothyroidism

Hypothyroidism results from either a lack of thyroid hormone circulating in the blood or a lack of response to thyroid hormone in the body's cells. It can be caused by a problem in the thyroid gland, hypothalamus or pituitary gland. Adrenal gland dysfunction due to chronic stress can also feed back to the thyroid through the hypothalamic-pituitary-adrenal (HPA) axis, contributing to hypothyroid symptoms. Sometimes changes can be related to an autoimmune process, as in Hashimoto's thyroiditis. Other times, hypothyroidism is the result of an iodine deficiency in the diet, or even an iodine overload, in certain people.

Hypothyroidism is five to eight times more common in women than in men and can arise at any stage of life, perhaps leading to menstrual irregularities and early menopause. It becomes more prevalent with age and may be triggered in the postpartum period. Testing for hypothyroidism before pregnancy or during the first trimester is recommended to screen for potential disease. Left untreated, the consequences of hypothyroidism during pregnancy include spontaneous abortion, gestational hypertension, premature delivery and postpartum depression.

Did You Know?

A Challenge to Diagnose

Because the symptoms of hypothyroidism are vague and nonspecific, hypothyroidism is often missed or misdiagnosed. The American Association of Endocrinologists estimates that half of all cases are left undiagnosed.

Signs and Symptoms

Symptoms are often vague, nonspecific or even absent. When hypothyroidism manifests externally, women experience some or all of the following symptoms:

- Fatigue, generalized weakness
- Depression
- Poor memory and/or concentration
- Sleep disturbances
- Weight gain
- Dry, pale skin and hair, or hair loss
- Low body temperature
- Low diastolic blood pressure
- Heavy menstrual bleeding
- Constipation

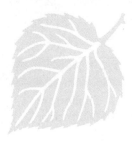

Associated Conditions

- Diabetes
- Dyslipidemia (abnormal cholesterol levels)
- Heart disease
- Infertility
- Menorrhagia

First-Line Herbal Care: ASHWAGANDHA

Ashwagandha (*Withania somnifera*) is a well-known adaptogen from the Ayurvedic tradition. Considered a general tonic, it has been called "Indian ginseng" because of the crossover in uses between the two herbs. Like ginseng, ashwagandha is touted for increasing longevity and maintaining youth in terms of physical health and mental capacity.

As an adaptogen, ashwagandha has been studied for a number of conditions, including hypothyroidism. Thyroid hormones, like most hormones, involve multiple organs and built-in feedback loops to ensure normal function. Adaptogens such as ashwagandha are used in hypothyroidism to promote optimal overall function and responses to stressful situations.

In animal studies, ashwagandha appears to increase the production of thyroid hormones. One case study reported a case of thyrotoxicosis (an overload of thyroid hormones, also known as hyperthyroidism) in a woman taking an ashwagandha supplement. No human clinical studies have yet been done to confirm these results.

Other Herbal Treatments

A common historical cause of hypothyroidism was a lack of iodine in the diet, so seaweeds high in iodine have an important place in traditional herbal treatment. Because of the widespread addition of iodine to table salt, iodine deficiency is now a less likely culprit; however, with recommendations to reduce salt intake to prevent high blood pressure, and food trends promoting non-iodized sea salt, we may see a resurgence of iodine deficiency.

If iodine deficiency is not a factor, adaptogenic herbs are the primary treatment, used to encourage optimal function of the thyroid and interrelated organs such as the adrenal glands, pituitary and hypothalamus.

Seaweed

Seaweed — and in particular bladderwrack and kelp — has long been used in cases of hypothyroidism caused by iodine deficiency. Seaweeds are naturally high in iodine, which is needed for the synthesis and activation of thyroid hormones. However, iodine overload may worsen existing hypothyroidism or even cause hypothyroidism where it didn't exist before. Be sure to consult with a licensed health-care provider before using seaweed.

Common Combination

- Ashwagandha, chaste tree and bacopa for hypothyroidism with menstrual irregularity and fatigue

Conventional Medical Treatments

- Cytomel
- Desiccated thyroid
- Levothyroxine

Further Reading

Di Matola T, Zeppa P, Gasperi M, Vitale M. Thyroid dysfunction following a kelp-containing marketed diet. *BMJ Case Reports*, 2014 October 29.

Jatwa R, Kar A. Amelioration of metformin-induced hypothyroidism by *Withania somnifera* and *Bauhinia purpurea* extracts in type 2 diabetic mice. *Phytotherapy Research*, 2009 Aug; 23 (8): 1140–45.

Panda S, Kar A. *Withania somnifera* and *Bauhinia purpurea* in the regulation of circulating thyroid hormone concentrations in female mice. *Journal of Ethnopharmacology*, 1999 Nov 1; 67 (2): 233–39.

Singh N, Bhalla M, de Jager P, Gilca M. An overview on ashwagandha: A rasayana (rejuvenator) of Ayurveda. *African Journal of Traditional, Complementary and Alternative Medicines*, 2011; 8 (5 Suppl): 208–13.

Infertility

Infertility describes any difficulty in conceiving, whether through assisted or non-assisted reproduction techniques. People struggle with infertility for a variety of reasons. Hypothyroidism, endometriosis and polycystic ovarian syndrome (PCOS) all commonly lead to fertility challenges. Primary ovarian insufficiency and structural abnormalities of the uterus or fallopian tubes can also lead to infertility.

In the United States, approximately 11% of women age fifteen to forty-four experience impaired fertility. It is estimated that approximately 10% to 15% of heterosexual couples trying to conceive through vaginal intercourse experience difficulties. Of those, approximately one-third are due to female fertility factors, one-third are due to male fertility factors and one-third are unexplained. Other contributing factors include age, substance use and being over- or underweight. Statistics on infertility in non-heterosexual families are lacking.

Trying to conceive but not succeeding puts tremendous stress on individuals and couples. Anxiety and depression are common side effects.

Signs and Symptoms

- Difficulty conceiving through assisted or non-assisted reproductive techniques

---

Associated Conditions

- Amenorrhea
- Anorexia nervosa
- Cancer
- Diabetes
- Endometriosis
- Hypothyroidism
- Obesity
- Pelvic infections
- Polycystic ovarian syndrome (PCOS)
- Primary ovarian insufficiency

First-Line Herbal Care: RASPBERRY

Raspberry (*Rubus idaeus*) is a classic tonic herb that has a strong association with women's health. As a gentle astringent and tonifier with an affinity for the female reproductive tract, raspberry has traditionally been included in formulas to improve fertility and the health of the uterus, but little research has been conducted on its traditional uses in menorrhagia, dysmenorrhea and infertility.

Raspberry is a biennial plant. The first year's growth produces only canes and leaves. The flowers, and thus berries, come only in the second year. Raspberry is a plant of patience, slowly building strength in its canes before bearing its fragile fruit. The same is true of how it is traditionally used: to build strength in the reproductive system slowly and gently over a long period of time.

As a uterine tonic, raspberry leaf has been used to prepare the uterus for both pregnancy and labor. Used before conception, it is said to support the growth of a healthy uterine lining and strengthen the muscles of the uterus, thanks to its nutritive qualities and gentle astringency. Midwives have also used it in the later stages of pregnancy to encourage more efficient contractions. Limited studies on raspberry leaf in pregnancy fail to show evidence of it shortening the first stage of labor. One study, however, found that raspberry leaf use was associated with a shorter second stage of labor and less frequent use of forceps during delivery. Another study noted an association between the use of raspberry leaf during pregnancy and increased rates of Caesarean delivery.

Folklore

Greek Myths

Raspberry's Latin name, *Rubus idaeus*, is derived from one of two Greek myths. One tells of the Olympian gods searching for, and presumably finding, raspberries on Mount Ida, on the island of Crete. In the other, raspberries were said to originally be white in color. One day, Zeus's nursemaid, Ida, pricked her finger on the thorns and bled over the berries, forever staining them bright red. Either way, the Greeks associated the whole plant with fertility and young infants.

Other Herbal Treatments

As with other medical approaches, herbal treatment of infertility is dependent on the cause. For discussions of specific conditions that may lead to infertility, such as hypothyroidism, endometriosis and PCOS, see the corresponding sections of this book. In general, an herbal approach focuses on correcting hormonal imbalances and normalizing the menstrual cycle through herbs such as raspberry, chaste tree and dang gui, to name a few.

Herbal support during assisted reproductive technologies, such as intrauterine insemination (IUI) and in vitro fertilization (IVF), can be helpful in minimizing side effects and maximizing positive outcomes. Emotional support and stress management using herbs and other strategies is important in many cases.

Berberine

Berberine is a constituent in certain plants, including barberry, Oregon grape root, goldenseal and coptis, that have been used to treat high blood sugar and insulin resistance in conditions such as diabetes and PCOS. Recently, research has also been conducted on the use of berberine for the treatment of infertility, with or without assisted reproductive technologies. In women with PCOS who were undergoing IVF, treatment with berberine was shown to increase pregnancy rates and reduce ovarian hyperstimulation. In one study, berberine was shown to be as effective in all parameters as metformin, a pharmaceutical commonly prescribed to women with PCOS who are attempting to conceive. In this study, berberine was associated with more live births and fewer side effects than metformin. This research is very promising, and more clinical trials are currently under way.

Black Cohosh

Black cohosh (*Actaea racemosa*) is one of the main herbs for women's health because of its ability to regulate menses at all stages. It has been used for dysmenorrhea, amenorrhea, menorrhagia, menopause, fertility and almost every reproductive health condition. It is no surprise, then, that it has also been studied in conjunction with assisted reproductive technologies.

In one small study, 120 milligrams per day of black cohosh was given to women with unexplained infertility, along with clomiphene citrate, a commonly used ovulatory stimulant drug. The group that received both clomiphene and black cohosh responded significantly better than those who were given clomiphene citrate alone. Women in the black cohosh group had shorter follicular cycle lengths, as well as higher estradiol, luteinizing hormone and progesterone levels. They also had significantly higher endometrial thickness and clinical pregnancy rates. Overall, black cohosh given in conjunction with clomiphene citrate resulted in better pregnancy outcomes. Another similar but larger study found similar effects, comparable to synthetic estrogen supplementation.

In a recent study that specifically focused on women with infertility and PCOS, clomiphene citrate plus black cohosh significantly improved hormone levels and overall clinical pregnancy rates compared to clomiphene citrate alone.

Common Combinations

- Chaste tree, fenugreek and berberine for infertility caused by PCOS
- Black cohosh for adjunctive care with ovarian stimulation drugs
- Raspberry and black cohosh to improve the uterine lining

Conventional Medical Treatments

Treatment is dependent on the cause identified. See the sections on hypothyroidism (page 115), endometriosis (page 87) and PCOS (page 148) for details. Assisted reproductive technologies may involve pharmaceutical ovarian stimulation, intrauterine insemination, in vitro fertilization, egg donor and embryo transfer, or surrogacy. Adoption is a non-medical option.

Further Reading

An Y, Sun Z, Zhang Y, et al. The use of berberine for women with polycystic ovary syndrome undergoing IVF treatment. *Clinical Endocrinology* (Oxford), 2014 Mar; 80 (3): 425–31.

Shahin AY, Ismail AM, Shaaban OM. Supplementation of clomiphene citrate cycles with *Cimicifuga racemosa* or ethinyl oestradiol — A randomized trial. *Reproductive BioMedicine Online*, 2009 Oct; 19 (4): 501–7.

Shahin AY, Ismail AM, Zahran KM, Makhlouf AM. Adding phytoestrogens to clomiphene induction in unexplained infertility patients — A randomized trial. *Reproductive BioMedicine Online*, 2008 Apr; 16 (4): 580–88.

Shahin AY, Mohammed SA. Adding the phytoestrogen *Cimicifugae racemosae* to clomiphene induction cycles with timed intercourse in polycystic ovary syndrome improves cycle outcomes and pregnancy rates — A randomized trial. *Gynecological Endocrinology*, 2014 Jul; 30 (7): 505–10.

Zheng J, Pistilli MJ, Holloway AC, Crankshaw DJ. The effects of commercial preparations of red raspberry leaf on the contractility of the rat's uterus in vitro. *Reproductive Sciences*, 2010 May; 17 (5): 494–501.

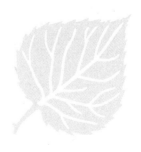

Menopause

Menopause means the end of menstrual cycles in a woman's life. It can be said to have taken place if menses hasn't occurred for twelve consecutive months. For most women, this happens some time between the ages of forty-four and fifty-five. The physiology of menopause is complex and varies considerably from one woman to another, not just in terms of when it happens but also in terms of how each woman experiences the transition.

Most women go through menopause at some point, but not everyone experiences symptoms. Cis-women, trans women and trans men starting or continuing hormone therapy are unlikely to experience any symptoms.

It is estimated that up to 45% of perimenopausal women experience vasomotor symptoms, such as hot flushes, while up to 50% have vaginal dryness or atrophy. Studies suggest that up to 50% of women worldwide use complementary and alternative medicines (CAM) for menopausal symptoms. Herbal medicine is cited as the most popular form of treatment in most studies. In North America and the United Kingdom, women's use of CAM therapies to address menopausal symptoms is even higher, closer to 60%.

Menopause can be challenging not just physically but also psychoemotionally and spiritually. All transitions are a time for self-reflection, but menopause often coincides with changing family dynamics: children are leaving the home, and some women may find themselves reassessing their roles in their family, career and relationships. In addition, menopause can bring to the forefront thoughts and feelings about beauty, aging, femininity and sexuality.

Signs and Symptoms

- Lack of menses for twelve months
- Hot flushes
- Night sweats and/or sleep disturbances
- Mood changes, irritability, anxiety and/or depression
- Vaginal dryness and/or atrophy
- Decreased libido and/or orgasm intensity

Associated Conditions

- Anorexia nervosa
- Breast cancer
- Depression
- Heart disease
- Insomnia
- Osteoporosis
- Uterine fibroids

First-Line Herbal Care: BLACK COHOSH

Black cohosh (*Actaea racemosa*) is one of the many herbs that Europeans learned about from the indigenous peoples of eastern North America, and is possibly the most important herb for women's health from this area. Many of the medicinal uses of black cohosh by Native peoples have been confirmed in modern clinical trials, in particular its uses in women's health.

In the energetic and homeopathic descriptions of this plant, the root, black in color, represents a dark, depressed or brooding mental state. As such, black cohosh is especially indicated for women whose menstrual or menopausal symptoms are accompanied by moping, gloominess or despondency.

Although many trials have shown promising results, a recent systematic review concluded that insufficient scientific evidence exists to support the clinical use of black cohosh for menopausal symptoms. The review cited poor trial quality, studies that were difficult to compare and inadequate reporting as some of the problems.

Another review, however, concluded that black cohosh was effective in treating hot flushes of mild to moderate severity. Since that review was published, several new positive studies have been conducted. The majority of these clinical trials demonstrated significant reductions in hot flushes, mood variability and other physical and sexual symptoms associated with menopause. Observational studies have produced similarly positive results.

European studies using the commercial preparation Remifemin have consistently shown black cohosh to be effective in treating menopausal symptoms. Several studies that used a combination of black cohosh with St. John's wort also found significant decreases in menopausal symptoms.

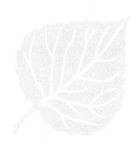

Other Herbal Treatments

Herbal treatment for menopause is as complex and varied as the symptoms experienced by women during their perimenopausal years. Phytoestrogenic herbs are commonly used, as are herbs that regulate hormones in general. Astringent herbs, such as sage, are used specifically for reducing hot flushes. Antidepressant herbs, such as St. John's wort, can be helpful for the emotional symptoms experienced by some women. Adaptogens (herbs used to help improve physiological responses to stress) have a long history of traditional use in Ayurvedic and Chinese herbal systems to increase energy, libido and vaginal lubrication in perimenopausal women. Traditional Chinese yin and blood tonics, such as dang gui, *he shou wu* and rehmannia, as well as nutritive tonics such as red clover, are also used.

Dang Gui

Dang gui (*Angelica sinensis*) is a quintessential herb for women's health. Most of the research on dang gui has been conducted on traditional Chinese medicine formulas containing many herbs. Researchers have noted that much of the therapeutic benefit of dang gui (and of many other herbs with a long history of use in Asia) is likely lost in translation. Extracting a single herb from the traditional Chinese medical model takes the herb out of context in several ways: traditional processing, traditional medicinal use and cultural milieu.

Mixed results have been found in studies evaluating the use of dang gui as part of a traditional Chinese medicine formula (*danggui buxue tang*) for hot flushes in postmenopausal women. Differences in preparation, dosage and research methodology make it difficult to assess the therapeutic benefit of this formula. None of the trials used traditional Chinese medicine methods of pattern diagnosis to determine the applicability of the formula. These results are an example of the challenges of taking an herb or formula out of the context of the medical model in which it has traditionally been used.

Red Clover

Like soy, red clover (*Trifolium pratense*) contains isoflavones that are thought to help menopausal symptoms because of their phytoestrogenic effects. Although some studies on red clover isoflavones have shown some positive improvements in menopausal symptoms compared to a placebo, others have found no such effects. One review, published in 2013,

Folklore

Historical Uses

Among indigenous peoples of North America, red clover is considered an excellent nutritive tonic herb, enriching and cleansing blood and tissues. It was historically used for skin conditions such as eczema and psoriasis, as well as for fever and infections. The Iroquois used red clover as a "blood medicine," and the Algonquin used it to treat whooping cough. The Iroquois and Cherokee used red clover as a gynecological aid, both for vaginal infections and during life-cycle changes such as menopause.

concluded that red clover did not decrease the incidence of hot flushes in menopausal women as compared to a placebo; an earlier review, however, found a small but significant decrease in the frequency of hot flushes. Overall, studies on red clover for hot flushes are small and of low quality, and focus exclusively on isoflavone extracts.

Sage

Sage (*Salvia officinalis*) is a very common kitchen herb, famously used to make poultry stuffing. It was immortalized in the traditional ballad "Scarborough Fair" and in the title of the Simon and Garfunkel album *Parsley, Sage, Rosemary and Thyme*. The Dutch were said to have traded sage tea at a high price, getting three times the quantity of Chinese tea in exchange.

The name *Salvia* comes from the Latin word *salvere*, which means "to be in good health." Historically, sage has been used to treat everything from sore throats to gum disease to nervousness to diarrhea to liver complaints. Sage has also been said to promote longevity in those who drink it daily as a tonic.

As an astringent, sage has been used to dry up and reduce perimenopausal hot flushes. In one clinical study, sage significantly reduced both the frequency and intensity of hot flushes in menopausal women after four weeks of treatment. Further improvements were seen after eight weeks of treatment. Menopause Rating Scale scores also decreased significantly in this study.

Another study looked at the effects of a combination of sage and alfalfa for reducing hot flushes in menopausal women. Out of thirty women in the study, twenty reported a complete disappearance of hot flushes and night sweats after three months of treatment. The other ten women reported improvements as well. There was no control group in this study.

St. John's Wort

St. John's wort (*Hypericum perforatum*) is particularly useful when perimenopause is accompanied by feelings of melancholy or depression. Because it is an herbal antidepressant, I often add St. John's wort to menopausal formulas for my patients if they are struggling to find joy as they move through this life transition.

Recent clinical trials have shown that St. John's wort, alone or in combination with other herbs, is also effective in reducing the frequency, duration and severity of hot

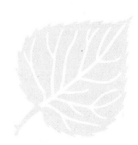

flushes. A 2014 meta-analysis concluded that St. John's wort, on its own or in combination with black cohosh and/or chaste tree, appears to be more effective than a placebo for the treatment of menopausal symptoms.

Soy

The use of soy (*Glycine max*) in the prevention and treatment of menopausal symptoms originates from observations that East Asian women whose diets consisted of large amounts of soy products experienced menopausal symptoms much less frequently than North American and European women. Early researchers hypothesized that the isoflavones in soy were responsible, as they are able to bind to estrogen receptors and mimic the natural biological estrogens that decrease postmenopausally. More recent studies have shown conflicting results, indicating that menopausal symptoms may vary across ethnicities independent of soy isoflavone intake in the diet.

CASE STUDY
Perimenopause

Parvati came to see me for help with hot flushes associated with perimenopause. At fifty-four years old, she was having ten to fifteen hot flushes a day, including several at night that woke her from sleep. Most flushes were mild enough that she became heated without intense perspiration, but sometimes the flushes were so intense that she would drench the sheets at night. She was also experiencing moderate vaginal dryness and discomfort during vaginal penetration.

Parvati's medical doctor had recommended hormone replacement therapy, but Parvati had serious concerns about taking synthetic hormones long-term. She wanted to see whether naturopathic medicine could alleviate her symptoms before she resorted to pharmaceuticals.

I encouraged Parvati to substantially increase her dietary consumption of soy products, and recommended a tea made with fenugreek, alfalfa and red clover, all of which are known to contain phytoestrogens. She alternated this phytoestrogenic tea with sage tea. (I don't usually recommend more than one tea, but she was already an avid tea drinker, so including a variety of medicinal teas worked well for her.) In addition, I recommended a tincture containing chaste tree, black cohosh, dang gui, rehmannia and shatavari, as well as the use of hyaluronic acid vaginal gel to address vaginal dryness.

Within two months, Parvati was having half as many hot flushes and her vaginal dryness had resolved. After four months, she was experiencing only one or two mild hot flushes per day.

Research does indicate that soy isoflavones can be useful in reducing the incidence of hot flushes, provided that supplements include sufficient amounts of genistein, the most predominant of soy's isoflavones. It should be noted that it appears to take a long time for soy's positive effects to be felt. While the effects of hormone replacement therapy (HRT) are seen in two to four weeks, it can take four months for a menopausal woman to feel any significant effects from the use of soy, and up to a year of use before soy's maximal effects are felt. Meta-analyses of high-quality studies on phytoestrogens have found that soy and red clover isoflavones may reduce the frequency of hot flushes when compared to a placebo but are not nearly as effective as estrogen HRT. Although soy is likely only half as effective as HRT and its effects take a long time to develop, soy is easy to implement as part of an herbal approach to hot flushes.

Two small, double-blind, randomized studies have investigated the use of a 4% soy isoflavone gel for the treatment of vaginal atrophy. Both studies found significant decreases in atrophy with the soy gel compared to a placebo. After twelve weeks of use of the soy gel, improvements in symptoms of vaginal dryness, pain during sexual activity, vaginal pH and vaginal epithelial thickness were seen. These results are promising, but more research is needed.

Valerian

Although valerian (*Valeriana officinalis*) is usually used for insomnia and anxiety, it can also be used for sleep disturbances that happen around menopause. One study that specifically looked at the impact of valerian on sleep quality in postmenopausal women found that valerian improved sleep quality significantly better than a placebo. Thirty percent of the women who took valerian, compared to 4% of the women who took a placebo, reported improvements in sleep quality.

Common Combinations

- Black cohosh, chaste tree and St. John's wort for menopausal symptoms with depression
- Black cohosh, red clover and sage for hot flushes
- Valerian, passionflower and St. John's wort for perimenopausal sleep disturbances

Conventional Medical Treatment

- Hormone replacement therapy (HRT)

Did You Know?

Natural Valium
Valerian is sometimes said to be a natural version of Valium (diazepam), a benzodiazepine drug. Although it isn't true that Valium was derived from valerian, the two may have something in common. Valium increases gamma aminobutyric acid (GABA), a neurotransmitter in the brain, which has a calming effect on anxiety. Researchers believe that valerian has a similar but weaker effect.

Further Reading

Bommer S, Klein P, Suter A. First time proof of sage's tolerability and efficacy in menopausal women with hot flushes. *Advances in Therapy*, 2011 Jun; 28 (6): 490–500.

Chen MN, Lin CC, Liu CF. Efficacy of phytoestrogens for menopausal symptoms: A meta-analysis and systematic review. *Climacteric*, 2014 Dec 1: 1–10.

Laakmann E, Grajecki D, Doege K, et al. Efficacy of *Cimicifuga racemosa*, *Hypericum perforatum* and *Agnus castus* in the treatment of climacteric complaints: A systematic review. *Gynecological Endocrinology*, 2012 Sep; 28 (9): 703–79.

Leach MJ, Moore V. Black cohosh (*Cimicifuga* spp.) for menopausal symptoms. *Cochrane Database of Systematic Reviews*, 2012 Sep 12; 9: CD007244.

Lethaby A, Marjoribanks J, Kronenberg F, et al. Phytoestrogens for menopausal vasomotor symptoms. *Cochrane Database of Systematic Reviews*, 2013 Dec 10; 12: CD001395.

Li L, Lv Y, Xu L, Zheng Q. Quantitative efficacy of soy isoflavones on menopausal hot flashes. *British Journal of Clinical Pharmacology*, 2014 Oct 15.

Lima SM, Bernardo BF, Yamada SS, et al. Effects of *Glycine max* (L.) Merr. soy isoflavone vaginal gel on epithelium morphology and estrogen receptor expression in postmenopausal women: A 12-week, randomized, double-blind, placebo-controlled trial. *Maturitas*, 2014 Jul; 78 (3): 205–11.

Liu YR, Jiang YL, Huang RQ, et al. *Hypericum perforatum* L. preparations for menopause: A meta-analysis of efficacy and safety. *Climacteric*, 2014 Aug; 17 (4): 325–35.

Mohammad-Alizadeh-Charandabi S, Shahnazi M, Nahaee J, Bayatipayan S. Efficacy of black cohosh (*Cimicifuga racemosa* L.) in treating early symptoms of menopause: A randomized clinical trial. *Chinese Medicine*, 2013 Nov 1; 8 (1): 20.

Reed SD, Lampe JW, Qu C, et al. Self-reported menopausal symptoms in a racially diverse population and soy food consumption. *Maturitas*, 2013 Jun; 75 (2): 152–58.

Taavoni S, Ekbatani N, Kashaniyan M, Haghani H. Effect of valerian on sleep quality in postmenopausal women: A randomized placebo-controlled clinical trial. *Menopause*, 2011 Sep; 18 (9): 951–55.

Wuttke W, Jarry H, Haunschild J, et al. The non-estrogenic alternative for the treatment of climacteric complaints: Black cohosh (*Cimicifuga* or *Actaea racemosa*). *Journal of Steroid Biochemistry and Molecular Biology*, 2014 Jan; 139: 302–10.

Menstrual Irregularities

Menstrual irregularities are often overlooked and go undiagnosed. Sometimes women don't even know what a physiologically normal cycle should look like. Irregular cycles may be common among girlfriends and so appear to be normal when they are, in fact, abnormal. Many women come to see me because they want help dealing with menstrual irregularities, but many more discover in their initial visit that they have been experiencing a health concern without even realizing it.

On average, a menstrual cycle is twenty-eight days long, with bleeding lasting three to five days. Most conventional medical sources state that a normal, healthy cycle ranges from twenty-one to thirty-five days long, with bleeding lasting from two to seven days. "Normal" is defined broadly to include painful and pain-free cycles, regular and somewhat irregular cycle lengths and both light and heavy bleeding.

Some researchers have suggested that menstrual irregularities are more common now than ever before. Several factors may be involved in these changes, including xenoestrogens and our connection to the earth's natural cycles.

Xenoestrogens — chemicals commonly found in plastics, personal care products and pesticides — have been shown to act as endocrine disruptors with strong estrogen-like effects on the body. Among other conditions, xenoestrogens are implicated in many estrogen-dependent conditions, such as fibroids and endometriosis.

In a world where our connection to day/night, lunar and seasonal cycles has been compromised by artificial lighting and extended or variable work/life schedules, it is often difficult for women to develop a natural menstrual cycle. The age at menarche has been steadily decreasing over the past century. Exposure to pollution, endocrine-disrupting chemicals, poor nutrition, screen time and sleep distubances have all been associated with early menarche. Taking time to reconnect with natural sunlight and sleeping in complete darkness, as well as spending time looking at the moon, may be for some women an important part of treating menstrual irregularities.

Did You Know?

The TCM Perspective

From a traditional Chinese medicine perspective, menstruation should be painless, accompanied only by minimal pre- and postmenstrual symptoms. Menstrual blood should flow freely, should be of a sufficient volume, should have a rich red color and should be free of clots. The length of the cycle should be as close to the lunar cycle of twenty-eight or twenty-nine days as possible. This is considered the goal of reestablishing a healthy menstrual cycle.

Amenorrhea and Oligomenorrhea

Amenorrhea is the absence of a period. It describes cases where a woman has not had a period by age fifteen or sixteen (often called primary amenorrhea) or when menstruation has stopped for more than three months — six months if menses was previously irregular — after it has already started (called secondary amenorrhea). A related issue, oligomenorrhea, is when a woman's menstrual cycles are consistently longer than thirty-five days.

Amenorrhea can be caused by many things, including pregnancy, breastfeeding, eating disorders, inadequate calories or fat, extreme weight loss, certain medications, premature ovarian failure, tumors, genetic conditions and birth defects, among others. In the United States, primary amenorrhea is quite rare, affecting 1% of women. Secondary amenorrhea, however, affects 5% to 7% of women each year. The most common cause of secondary amenorrhea is pregnancy.

Signs and Symptoms

Amenorrhea
- Menses has never occurred
- Menses used to be regular but has been absent for three months
- Menses was irregular and has been absent for six months

Oligomenorrhea
- Menstrual cycles longer than thirty-five days

Associated Conditions
- Anorexia nervosa
- Coronary artery disease (associated with amenorrhea related to low estrogen production)
- Diabetes
- Hyperprolactinemia
- Hypothyroidism

- Obesity
- Orthorexia
- Osteoporosis (associated with amenorrhea related to low estrogen production)
- Polycystic ovarian syndrome (PCOS)
- Primary ovarian insufficiency
- Sickle-cell anemia
- Thalassemia
- Uterine cancer
- Various mental health conditions

First-Line Herbal Care: DANG GUI

Dang gui (*Angelica sinensis*) is an important herb for treating amenorrhea and regulating menses in traditional Chinese medicine (TCM). From a TCM perspective, amenorrhea can occur as a result of insufficient blood production, and dang gui is especially useful in these cases for building blood and ensuring its optimal flow. In China and Japan, dang gui is popularly called "female ginseng."

Other Herbal Treatments

Herbal treatment, like conventional medical treatment, depends on the cause of amenorrhea or oligomenorrhea. Correct diagnosis is critical in addressing the underlying reason why a woman isn't getting her period, and each case may be treated differently. Any woman experiencing amenorrhea or oligomenorrhea should visit a licensed health-care practitioner for testing. Without a correct diagnosis, herbs may hurt rather than help.

In cases where amenorrhea is caused by genetics, birth defects and other structural abnormalities, herbal medicine has little to offer. However, when amenorrhea or oligomenorrhea is caused by hormonal imbalances in the ovaries and/or pituitary, herbal treatment can be helpful. Emmenagogues and hormone-balancing herbs are used to stimulate reproductive function, though each herb is unique and should be matched to the cause of the irregular menses and each person's individual case.

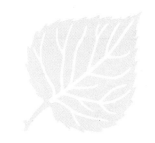

Black Cohosh

Black cohosh (*Actaea racemosa*) has long been used to regulate women's menstrual cycles. Although once believed to be phytoestrogenic, it is now understood to affect menstruation via the hypothalamus and/or pituitary. In vitro studies have shown that black cohosh stimulates ovulation via the pituitary and promotes adequate production of progesterone during the luteal phase of menstruation. It has more recently been studied for use in PCOS (see page 148).

Chaste Tree

Chaste tree (*Vitex agnus-castus*) is one of the primary herbs used in amenorrhea and oligomenorrhea. Along with dang gui and black cohosh, chaste tree is considered one of the most important menstrual regulators in traditional herbalist practice. Since it stimulates ovulation via the pituitary gland, it also indirectly raises or modulates progesterone levels. In addition, chaste tree acts as a weak dopamine agonist, reducing elevated prolactin when it is the cause of amenorrhea.

A few small, older studies suggest that chaste tree may help treat secondary amenorrhea. More research is needed in this area.

Licorice and Peony

Licorice (*Glycyrrhiza glabra* or *Glycyrrhiza uralensis*) is traditionally used alongside white peony root (*Paeonia lactiflora*) in the treatment of amenorrhea and oligomenorrhea caused by high androgens (male hormones), including testosterone. In particular, herbalists in China and Japan often use a combination of the two herbs to address high testosterone, with or without a diagnosis of PCOS.

In several small open-label studies, the combination of licorice and white peony root lowered testosterone and induced ovulation in the majority of study participants. This classic formula has also been shown in a randomized controlled trial to have comparable effects to the drug bromocriptine in addressing drug-induced high prolactin levels and resulting amenorrhea caused by risperidone, a commonly used antipsychotic medication. More research is needed to confirm these results.

Folklore

Honoring Fertility

In Ancient Greece, women adorned themselves with the boughs of chaste tree in honor of Demeter, goddess of agriculture, marriage and fertility. According to mythology, Hera, considered the protector of marriage, was said to have been born underneath a chaste tree.

Caution

Licorice is known to raise blood pressure. Anyone taking licorice should routinely monitor their blood pressure. Women with high blood pressure should avoid taking licorice.

Red Clover

Red clover (*Trifolium pratense*) is traditionally used to support women with amenorrhea when they do not produce enough estrogen on their own. The isoflavones in red clover act as phytoestrogens, weakly binding to estrogen receptors, and may be helpful for women with primary ovarian insufficiency and resultant amenorrhea.

Yarrow

Yarrow (*Achillea millefolium*) is an emmenagogue — an herb used to bring on the start of menses. In traditional use, yarrow controls the flow of blood, stopping bleeding when it is excessive, but also encouraging flow when it has stopped.

Common Combinations

- Dang gui, black cohosh and chaste tree for amenorrhea due to insufficient estrogen or irregular menses
- Licorice, peony and chaste tree for amenorrhea due to PCOS or high prolactin

Conventional Medical Treatments

- Oral contraceptives
- Hormone replacement therapy (HRT)
- Dopamine agonists
- Gonadotropins

Further Reading

Takahashi K, Kitao M. Effect of TJ-68 (shakuyaku-kanzo-to) on polycystic ovarian disease. *International Journal of Fertility and Menopausal Studies*, 1994 Mar–Apr; 39 (2): 69–76.

Takahashi K, Yoshino K, Shirai T, et al. Effect of a traditional herbal medicine (shakuyaku-kanzo-to) on testosterone secretion in patients with polycystic ovary syndrome detected by ultrasound. *Nihon Sanka Fujinka Gakkai Zasshi*, 1988 Jun; 40 (6): 789–92.

Yuan HN, Wang CY, Sze CW, et al. A randomized, crossover comparison of herbal medicine and bromocriptine against risperidone-induced hyperprolactinemia in patients with schizophrenia. *Journal of Clinical Psychopharmacology*, 2008 Jun; 28 (3): 264–370.

CASE STUDY
Amenorrhea

Astrid, a twenty-six-year old woman, came to see me three and a half months after she stopped taking oral contraceptives, when her menses had not yet returned. She had been on a variety of oral contraceptives since she was sixteen years old. Now she wanted to make sure her menstrual cycle was regular by the time she was ready to have children, so she had stopped using oral contraceptives as a method of birth control.

Although Astrid was not anemic, she had a very low appetite because of long-standing acid reflux. As a result, she was underweight. Examination and testing confirmed that her low stomach acid and low body mass index were the main reasons she was not producing adequate hormones to bring back her natural menstrual cycle.

I recommended an herbal formula with dang gui, chaste tree, centaury, black cohosh and blue cohosh. The bitterness of the herbs in the formula (especially centaury) helped return Astrid's stomach acid to normal levels and resolved her acid reflux. It also helped to improve her appetite.

I chose to include centaury in the formula because, as a flower essence, it is useful for those who have difficulty saying no, taking care of others to the detriment of their own needs. Astrid was so busy caring for her mother and younger siblings that she often put off taking care of herself — emotionally, spiritually and physically. She wasn't nourishing herself adequately with food, even though she cooked dinner for her family after coming home from work.

After two months, Astrid's menstrual cycle returned. She gained a little weight, returning to a healthy body mass index. She spent more time on self-care and started saying no to doing too much for others. Within five months, her menses normalized to a thirty-day cycle.

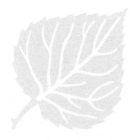

Dysmenorrhea

Too many women suffer through dysmenorrhea — pain during menstruation that interferes with daily activities — for too many years. It has become so commonplace that many women in my practice, from teenagers to women in their forties, consider it a normal and unchangeable aspect of life. The pain they experience ranges in severity from mild to severe and can interfere a little or a lot with their day-to-day routines. When severe, it can be extremely debilitating and is sometimes a sign of more severe functional or structural pathologies.

Signs and Symptoms

- Pain in the lower abdomen before and/or during menstruation (may be one-sided or may radiate to the lower back or thighs)
- Nausea and vomiting
- Diarrhea or constipation
- Fatigue, headache, dizziness
- Hypersensitivity to light, sounds or smells

Associated Conditions

- Endometriosis
- Menorrhagia
- Polycystic ovarian syndrome (PCOS)
- Uterine fibroids

First-Line Herbal Care: GINGER

Gingerroot (*Zingiber officinale*) isn't an herb most people think of for pain relief. It is more commonly known that ginger eases nausea (see Morning Sickness, page 166), but it is also an excellent herb for menstrual cramps.

Ginger contains gingerol and other anti-inflammatory constituents. Whole gingerroot has been shown in scientific studies to be on par with ibuprofen and mefenamic acid, standard pain medications for dysmenorrhea. More specifically, gingerroot powder has been shown to decrease

Did You Know?

Primary or Secondary?
Dysmenorrhea can be classified as either primary or secondary. In secondary dysmenorrhea, the pain is caused by another condition or structural abnormality (for example, endometriosis or uterine fibroids). No cause for the pain can be found in primary dysmenorrhea.

Did You Know?

A Warming Effect
In traditional Chinese medicine, ginger is used to warm the body and stop bleeding. In several studies, moxibustion (the burning of dried mugwort directly or indirectly over an acupuncture point) over a slice of ginger at specific acupuncture points was shown to reduce the symptoms associated with primary dysmenorrhea.

the intensity and duration of menstrual cramps. When cramping is accompanied by nausea or other stomach upset, ginger is definitely the herb of choice.

Other Herbal Treatments

Anti-inflammatory, antispasmodic and analgesic herbs help to address the pain in the short term. Long-term treatment should address suspected causes, such as endometriosis or an imbalance of hormones.

Cramp Bark

Cramp bark (*Viburnum opulus*) and the related species black haw (*Viburnum prunifolium*) have a long history of traditional use by indigenous peoples in North America for relieving menstrual pain. Cramp bark's common name refers to its primary use as an antispasmodic. Historical and ethnobotanical records indicate that cramp bark was also used to treat other forms of spasm in the uterus, including threatened miscarriage and prolapse. Although I frequently use cramp bark as part of acute herbal formulas for women with painful menstrual cramps and find it to be effective, scientific research is needed to confirm its traditional uses.

Fennel

In a handful of studies, fennel (*Foeniculum vulgare*) extracts have been shown to be effective in reducing menstrual pain when compared to either mefenamic acid or a placebo in cases of primary dysmenorrhea. More clinical research is needed.

Valerian

In one study, valerian (*Valeriana officinalis*) resulted in a greater reduction of pain severity than a placebo. In another study, both valerian and mefenamic acid were found to significantly reduce the pain associated with primary dysmenorrhea. More research is needed to confirm these preliminary results, but the studies support the traditional understanding of valerian as an antispasmodic herb.

Because of its sedative effects, valerian may be most useful in cases where nervous depression, anxiety or sleeping difficulties exist alongside dysmenorrhea.

CASE STUDY
Dysmenorrhea

The daughter of one of my patients came to see me about the horrible menstrual cramps she was experiencing. At seventeen years old, Yolanda had suffered through painful periods since her menses began, when she was fourteen. The pain was low in her pelvis and felt better with pressure. Rather than getting better over time, the pain was worsening. The cramping was so severe that she needed to stay home from school for one day every month. She had been prescribed naproxen, which she was taking to manage the pain.

Over the past couple of months, Yolanda had also begun to experience a worsening of premenstrual symptoms. She complained of breast tenderness, bloating and irritability for almost a week before menses. She felt that her mood swings were out of control, as were her cravings for sweets.

Together we decided that she should make some dietary changes to better manage blood sugar and hormones throughout her cycle. Yolanda avoided caffeine, simple sugars and simple carbohydrates and focused on increasing her consumption of dark green leafy vegetables to encourage better liver and bowel function. She started taking an herbal combination that included black cohosh, ginger, Jamaican dogwood and cramp bark to manage the acute pain during her period. Yolanda quickly found that she no longer needed to take naproxen.

Over the next few months, we continued to work on regulating hormones through basic lifestyle changes and counseling. In our sessions, she began to talk openly about the conflicting feelings she had about becoming an adult, as well as about cultural norms and the perceived expectations of femininity. In addition, she had unanswered questions about sex and sexuality. As her awareness and comfort with herself grew, her menses normalized and she no longer found her period to be a pain — either literally or figuratively.

Wild Yam

Wild yam (*Dioscorea villosa*) has traditionally been used as an antispasmodic in both North America and China. The Meskwaki in the United States treated both menstrual and labor pains with wild yam. Scientific research is needed to confirm these traditional uses.

Common Combinations

- Ginger, fennel and cramp bark for acute pain during the day
- Fennel, cramp bark and valerian for acute pain with anxiety or difficulty sleeping

Conventional Medical Treatments

- **Acute:** Non-steroidal anti-inflammatory drugs (NSAIDs)
- **Chronic:** Hormonal contraceptives

Further Reading

Halder A. Effect of progressive muscle relaxation versus intake of ginger powder on dysmenorrhoea amongst the nursing students in Pune. *Nursing Journal of India*, 2012 Jul–Aug; 103 (4): 152–56.

Jenabi E, Toghiri MA, Hejrati P. The comparison of the effects of antiplain of *Valeriana officinalis risom* and mefenamic acid in relief of primary dysmenorrhea. *Iranian Journal of Obstetrics, Gynecology and Infertility*, 2012 May; 15 (2): 44.

Mirabi P, Dolatian M, Mojab F, Majd HA. Effects of valerian on the severity and systemic manifestations of dysmenorrhea. *International Journal of Gynecology and Obstetrics*, 2011 Dec; 115 (3): 285–88.

Modaress Nejad V, Asadipour M. Comparison of the effectiveness of fennel and mefenamic acid on pain intensity in dysmenorrhoea. *Eastern Mediterranean Health Journal*, 2006 May–Jul; 12 (3–4): 423–27.

Omidvar S, Esmailzadeh S, Baradaran M, Basirat Z. Effect of fennel on pain intensity in dysmenorrhoea: A placebo-controlled trial. *AYU*, 2012 Apr–Jun; 33 (2): 311–13.

Ozgoli G, Goli M, Moattar F. Comparison of effects of ginger, mefenamic acid, and ibuprofen on pain in women with primary dysmenorrhea. *Journal of Alternative and Complementary Medicine*, 2009 Feb; 15 (2): 129–32.

Rahnama P, Montazeri A, Huseini HF, et al. Effect of *Zingiber officinale* R. rhizomes (ginger) on pain relief in primary dysmenorrhea: A placebo randomized trial. *BMC Complementary and Alternative Medicine*, 2012 Jul 10; 12: 92.

Sun LH, Ge JJ, Yang JJ, et al. [Randomized controlled clinical study on ginger-partitioned moxibustion for patients with cold-damp stagnation type primary dysmenorrhea]. [Article in Chinese]. *Zhen Ci Yan Jiu*, 2009 Dec; 34 (6): 398–402.

Menorrhagia

Menorrhagia refers to excessive menstrual bleeding, where the menstrual cycle is regular but blood loss is greater than the norm (over 80 milliliters per cycle) or menstrual flow lasts longer than seven days. Most women don't measure the quantity of their menstrual blood, so they and their clinicians must rely on other information for diagnosis. In practice, I ask how often women change their tampons, pads or menstrual cups and the level of absorbency they use (regular, super, super plus). If a woman is changing a super-absorbent tampon every hour or two, is emptying a full menstrual cup more than three times daily or needs more than one form of menstrual product at a time (for example, a tampon plus a pad), then she is definitely experiencing menorrhagia.

For some women, menorrhagia is manageable; for others, it disrupts their daily activities. Many women with severe menorrhagia avoid leaving home for any length of time, for fear of being too far from a washroom.

Menorrhagia may exist without any identifiable functional or structural abnormality, or it may indicate another pathology, such as fibroids, endometriosis, PCOS or even a systemic bleeding disorder. Consultation with a health-care provider is necessary to understand the cause of the excessive bleeding. Women with menorrhagia often become anemic if left untreated.

Signs and Symptoms

- Heavy menstrual bleeding (more than 80 milliliters per cycle)
- Menstrual bleeding for more than seven days

Associated Conditions

- Anemia
- Bleeding disorders
- Cervical or uterine cancer
- Endometrial polyps
- Pelvic infection
- Polycystic ovarian syndrome (PCOS)
- Uterine fibroids

First-Line Herbal Care: YARROW

Yarrow (*Achillea millefolium*) is an excellent astringent and has long been used to treat all kinds of bleeding, including menorrhagia. Although research on yarrow for menorrhagia is very limited, there is evidence to support its traditional use. Pharmacological studies show significant anti-inflammatory, astringent and antioxidant effects. Yarrow finds its way into most of my acute menorrhagia formulas in clinical practice.

Other Herbal Treatments

The herbal approach to treating menorrhagia is twofold. Over the long term, treatment is directed toward resolving any underlying conditions. For example, herbs that regulate hormones and those that support liver function are useful in the long-term treatment of fibroids and PCOS. Acutely, astringent and antihemorrhagic herbs are used to decrease blood flow during menses.

Overall, very little clinical research on herbs for menorrhagia has been performed.

Chaste Tree

Chaste tree (*Vitex agnus-castus*) is an excellent hormonal normalizer that has been used by herbalists to treat a variety of menstrual conditions, including menorrhagia. Patience is required when taking chaste tree, as its beneficial effects may take several months to become apparent.

One study on chaste tree for menorrhagia compared it to mefenamic acid, a non-steroidal anti-inflammatory drug (NSAID). Both the women taking chaste tree and the women taking mefenamic acid showed decreased quantities of menstrual blood flow and increased hemoglobin, a marker of anemia, after four months of treatment. The authors of the study concluded that chaste tree was as effective as mefenamic acid but had significantly fewer side effects.

Cinnamon

Cinnamon (*Cinnamomum verum* or *Cinnamomum cassia*) has a long history of use in menorrhagia and uterine hemorrhage around the world. Known as *guizhi* in traditional Chinese medicine, cinnamon is the main ingredient in a classic formula for treating fibroids (see page 98). It was also the subject of several letters discussing its use in menorrhagia in the medical journal *The Lancet* as early as 1853.

In both Chinese and Ayurvedic traditions, cinnamon is used to move blood where stagnation is being caused by cold. The homeopathic use of cinnamon is also applicable to cases of menorrhagia in which the woman has cold, pale extremities.

Although research on cinnamon for menorrhagia is lacking, it may be useful in cases of menorrhagia related to uterine fibroids, especially when the woman feels cold.

Dang Gui

Dang gui (*Angelica sinensis*) is one of the best-known herbal hormone regulators. From a traditional Chinese perspective, dang gui both tonifies and moves blood. It has been used to treat a wide variety of menstrual irregularities, from amenorrhea to infertility, and to regulate and normalize the menstrual cycle. In some cases, it may also be helpful in addressing anemia caused by menorrhagia (see page 49 for details).

Geranium

Geranium (*Geranium maculatum*), also known as cranesbill, is another herb that has traditionally been used to treat heavy menses. Several different varieties of geranium from Europe and Africa have been used as antihemorrhagic herbs. Like many herbs used to reduce excessive menstrual flow, geranium contains significant amounts of tannins, which act as astringents to reduce blood loss. Studies are needed to confirm geranium's traditional uses.

Shepherd's Purse

Shepherd's purse (*Capsella bursa-pastoris*) grows like a weed throughout much of North America and Europe. You have probably walked past it many times without knowing it. It is one of the most common traditional herbal remedies for excessive uterine bleeding, whether from menorrhagia or postpartum hemorrhage. Both yarrow and shepherd's purse were used in the First World War to stop bleeding when other medicines weren't available.

The German Commission E has approved shepherd's purse for use in menorrhagia and metrorrhagia (abnormal bleeding between expected menses). It has also been used in India and China to treat excessive uterine bleeding.

Caution

Although dang gui may be useful for regulating an abnormal menstrual cycle over time, it should be used cautiously during menses itself, as it may increase bleeding.

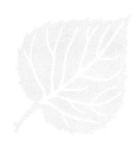

In homeopathy, shepherd's purse is used for excessive bleeding due to fibroids where there is back pain and a generalized feeling of soreness, or when every other menses is particularly heavy.

No clinical studies have been done to date on the use of shepherd's purse for the treatment of menorrhagia.

Common Combinations

- Yarrow, geranium, shepherd's purse and cinnamon for acute menorrhagia
- Dang gui and chaste tree for long-term management of menorrhagia

Conventional Medical Treatments

- Danazol
- Non-steroidal anti-inflammatory drugs (NSAIDs)
- Oral contraceptives
- Progestins
- Nonsurgical and surgical procedures: dilatation and curettage (D&C), endometrial ablation, fibroid embolization, myomectomy, hysterectomy
- Tranexamic acid

Further Reading

Bobab MZ, Farimani M, Nasr ESH. Efficacy of mefenamic acid and vitex in reduction of menstrual blood loss and HB changes in patients with a complaint of menorrhagia. *Iranian Journal of Obstetrics, Gynecology and Infertility*, 2007; 10 (1): 79–86.

El-Hemaidi I, Gharaibeh A, Shehata H. Menorrhagia and bleeding disorders. *Current Opinion in Obstetrics and Gynecology*, 2007 Dec; 19 (6): 513–20.

Shobeiri SF, Sharei S, Heidari A, Kianbakht S. *Portulaca oleracea* L. in the treatment of patients with abnormal uterine bleeding: A pilot clinical trial. *Phytotherapy Research*, 2009 Oct; 23 (10): 1411–14.

Tu X, Huang G, Tan S. Chinese herbal medicine for dysfunctional uterine bleeding: A meta-analysis. *Evidence-Based Complementary and Alternative Medicine*, 2009 Mar; 6 (1): 99–105.

CASE STUDY
Menorrhagia

Menorrhagia can happen at any time in a woman's life between menarche and menopause. I have worked with women of all ages who struggle with menorrhagia. Sometimes it is related to another condition, such as fibroids; other times, no cause is identifiable. Often menorrhagia interferes with a woman's daily activities, as it did for Francesca.

When Francesca first came to see me, she was forty-two years old and had experienced menorrhagia for most of her life. Her periods were both extremely heavy and long-lasting. Although her cycles were regular, averaging thirty to thirty-two days, her menses lasted up to eight days. On top of that, she experienced brownish spotting both before her period and after it ended. During the two to three heaviest days of her period, she wore both a tampon and a pad at the same time, changing both up to once an hour. Even so, she avoided leaving the house for fear of "accidents" — menstrual blood staining her clothes in public. She wore only dark-colored pants during menses and planned her days around proximity of a washroom. Unsurprisingly, she felt exhausted; her bloodwork showed that she had become anemic from the excessive menstrual bleeding.

Francesca had a history of fibroids, which were discovered during a routine ultrasound when she was pregnant with her first child. They decreased in size after she gave birth, but a few small fibroids remained.

Francesca's medical doctor had prescribed iron supplements and referred her to me for care. In addition to treating her anemia, our primary goal was to decrease the amount of blood lost during menses. She started taking an herbal formula made up of yarrow, shepherd's purse and geranium, taking it two days before her period was due to start, through the end of bleeding. The rest of her menstrual cycle, she took a separate formula containing yarrow, dang gui, chaste tree and dandelion root. She also did abdominal self-massage and applied castor oil packs (see pages 95–96) a few days a week.

After two months, Francesca no longer worried about leaving the house while she was on her period, as her bleeding had decreased significantly. She didn't need to change her tampons and pads quite as frequently. After another couple of months, she stopped using both tampons and pads at the same time. She felt like herself again, as her anemia had resolved. She was finally able to let go of her fear of public embarrassment, and even put on a pair of beige pants during menses.

Osteoporosis

Osteoporosis affects the quality of bones throughout the body, leading to less dense, weaker and more brittle bones. As a result, it increases the risk of fractures from even simple activities. Osteoporosis is often called a silent disease because it can go completely unnoticed until you end up in the hospital with a fracture. Depending on the location and effects of the loss of bone mass, some people may experience back pain, decreased height over time and increased curvature of the spine.

Osteoporosis is extremely common among women and increases in prevalence as women age. Globally, it affects more than 200 million women. Women are much more likely than men to be diagnosed with osteoporosis. In North America, approximately one in four women over fifty years of age has osteoporosis; comparatively, one in eight men over fifty is affected.

Several factors play a role in osteoporosis. Bone strength and density peak sometime in a woman's early thirties and are on the decline thereafter. At menopause, when estrogen levels drop, bone density decreases more rapidly. Genetics are very important as well: women whose mothers and grandmothers had osteoporosis are at greater risk for the disease themselves.

Many women in my clinical practice are concerned about current or potential osteoporosis. Although I usually recommend dietary and lifestyle changes, as well as individualized nutritional supplementation, I often include herbal support in my treatment strategy, particularly for women who are also experiencing menopausal symptoms.

Associated Conditions

- Anorexia
- Cancer
- Celiac disease
- Diabetes mellitus
- Hyperthyroidism
- Inflammatory bowel disease (IBD)
- Menopause
- Primary ovarian insufficiency
- Rheumatoid arthritis

Did You Know?

Osteopenia

"Osteopenia" refers to lower than normal bone density that is not yet low enough to be considered osteoporosis.

First-Line Herbal Care: SOY

Soy (*Glycine max*) is often touted for its role in preventing osteoporosis. The isoflavones found in soy have well-documented phytoestrogenic effects that have been used in the treatment of menopausal symptoms — and have been the source of a great deal of controversy related to breast cancer. Much of the research on soy was initially spurred by researchers who noted that osteoporosis occurs much less frequently in East Asian women, who typically eat a lot more soy foods than women in other regions.

Many studies have looked at the effects of soy supplementation on bone mineral density. One meta-analysis found that the long-term use of soy significantly increased bone mineral density — by 54% — when compared to a placebo. This increase was somewhat limited to improvements in the lumbar portion of the spine.

Soy isoflavones also consistently decrease bone resorption markers in urine. The best results appear to occur in women who are postmenopausal and those taking supplements containing over 75 milligrams of isoflavones daily. The risk and incidence of fracture with soy isoflavone supplementation have not yet been adequately investigated.

Simply eating more soy foods is an easy way to improve bone health and prevent osteoporosis. It should be noted that isoflavone content varies significantly among soy sources and even among brands. For example, according to the U.S. Department of Agriculture, boiled soybeans contain up to 65 milligrams of soy isoflavones per 100 grams; soy yogurt contains 33 milligrams per 100 grams; firm tofu contains about 25 milligrams per 100 grams; and soy nuts contain almost 150 milligrams per 100 grams. I recommend the use of nutritional tables as guides.

Other Herbal Treatments

Herbal treatment for osteoporosis focuses on prevention over treatment. Since osteoporosis tends to worsen after menopause because of decreased estrogen, the best options are either herbs that are phytoestrogenic or those that help

Did You Know?

Lifestyle Changes
Any treatment for osteoporosis or to prevent bone loss in the long term should include lifestyle measures to help promote bone mineral density, especially as women transition into their postmenopausal years. Fracture risk is decreased by weight-bearing and balance exercises and by good nutrition, including adequate intake of calcium, magnesium, potassium and vitamins D and K. Overly low body weight, smoking and excessive alcohol intake can increase fracture risk.

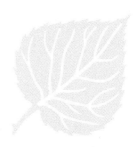

to normalize hormones. In particular, herbs may be helpful in preventing bone loss and resorption and improving certain markers of bone loss, such as bone mineral density. Traditionally, nutritive herbs such as red clover, nettles and alfalfa have also been used as an extra source of minerals.

Black Cohosh

Black cohosh (*Actaea racemosa*) is traditionally used for a variety of female reproductive health concerns, including menopause and associated conditions such as osteoporosis. Although early theories that black cohosh acts as a phytoestrogen have long since been refuted, black cohosh has shown potential in the treatment of menopause and osteoporosis.

Preliminary laboratory research suggests that black cohosh may stimulate bone growth, prevent bone density loss and protect bone strength. In two small human trials, black cohosh was shown to have effects on bone metabolism that were significantly more positive than those of a placebo and equivalent to those of estrogen replacement therapy.

Milk Thistle

Milk thistle (*Silybum marianum*) is not the first herb I think of when considering treatments to prevent osteoporosis, but recent studies have been looking at its possible use in this area. Preliminary in vitro and animal research suggests that milk thistle may increase calcium, phosphorus and parathyroid hormone levels in the blood. In a few small studies, it has also been shown to decrease alkaline phosphatase levels, a blood marker of bone loss. Some researchers have suggested that milk thistle may have mild estrogenic effects that would explain these results. Clearly, more studies are needed to gain a better understanding of how, and if, milk thistle works to prevent osteoporosis.

Red Clover

Red clover (*Trifolium pratense*) is another herb that contains a significant amount of isoflavones and has a long history of use in menopause and related conditions. Experimental animal research may support the use of red clover isoflavones in the prevention of fractures and osteoporosis in postmenopausal women. In several studies, ovariectomized rats given red clover isoflavones showed improvements in osteoporosis markers, likely through inhibition of bone resorption and thus reduction of bone turnover.

Researchers note that other constituents in red clover may contribute to its medicinal effects, and that these contributions cannot be captured by studies that focus on extracts of isoflavones alone. Red clover has significant nutritive qualities and is a plant source of calcium, magnesium, phosphorus, potassium and other vitamins and minerals that are important for bone health. If these minerals or red clover's other plant chemicals have a potential medicinal impact, more research on whole herb extracts is needed.

Common Combination

- Black cohosh and red clover for osteoporosis in postmenopausal women

Conventional Medical Treatments

- Bisphosphonates
- Calcitonin
- Estrogen
- Parathyroid hormone
- Selective estrogen receptor modifiers (SERMs)

Further Reading

Cui G, Leng H, Wang K, et al. Effects of Remifemin treatment on bone integrity and remodeling in rats with ovariectomy-induced osteoporosis. *PLoS One*, 2013 Dec 9; 8 (12): e82815.

El-Shitany NA, Hegazy S, El-Desoky K. Evidences for antiosteoporotic and selective estrogen receptor modulator activity of silymarin compared with ethinylestradiol in ovariectomized rats. *Phytomedicine*, 2010 Feb; 17 (2): 116–25.

Taku K, Melby MK, Nishi N, et al. Soy isoflavones for osteoporosis: An evidence-based approach. *Maturitas*, 2011 Dec; 70 (4): 333–38.

Wei P, Liu M, Chen Y, Chen DC. Systematic review of soy isoflavone supplements on osteoporosis in women. *Asian Pacific Journal of Tropical Medicine*, 2012 Mar; 5 (3): 243–48.

Wuttke W, Gorkow C, Seidlová-Wuttke D. Effects of black cohosh (*Cimicifuga racemosa*) on bone turnover, vaginal mucosa, and various blood parameters in postmenopausal women: A double-blind, placebo-controlled, and conjugated estrogens–controlled study. *Menopause*, 2006 Mar–Apr; 13 (2): 185–96.

Did You Know?

Red Clover Flower Essence

Red clover is frequently used by bees for honey production. This relationship with bees is mirrored in the flower essence of red clover, which can be used to separate someone from a panicked or hysterical "hive mentality" during a family crisis, public emergency or other crowded situation. Red clover helps users maintain individuality and avoid the influence of a strong group energy, protecting them from being carried away by the emotions of the crowd.

Polycystic Ovarian Syndrome

Polycystic ovarian syndrome (PCOS) is a variable condition that may present in different ways in different women. Originally known as Stein-Leventhal syndrome, PCOS was initially described as a hormonal imbalance that resulted in amenorrhea, hirsutism (abnormal hair growth), obesity and ovaries with multiple cysts. Over the years, doctors' understanding of the condition grew to encompass the metabolic, cardiovascular and reproductive effects associated with PCOS.

Between 4% and 12% of women have PCOS. (Some sources put the prevalence rate at 20%, depending on the diagnostic criteria used.) Many women don't even know they have it. Some women are diagnosed when they seek out

Signs and Symptoms

PCOS may include some or all of the following signs and symptoms. Having two of the three key signs and symptoms is considered diagnostic for PCOS.

Key Signs and Symptoms
- Amenorrhea or oligomenorrhea
- Androgen excess, including symptoms of abnormal facial or body hair growth, adult acne or male pattern baldness
- Polycystic ovaries (discovered through ultrasound)

Other Signs and Symptoms
- Weight gain or difficulty gaining weight
- Difficulty conceiving
- Depression
- Higher than normal blood sugar or insulin levels
- Insulin resistance
- Darkening of the skin in the armpits or other skin folds
- High blood pressure
- Sleep apnea

fertility testing to help explain why they are having difficulty conceiving. Others may become aware that something is wrong thanks to signs of androgen excess (an overabundance of male hormones). Still others may be thankful for physical changes more consistent with their gender identity.

Associated Conditions

- Anxiety
- Depression
- Diabetes
- Disordered eating
- Dyslipidemia (abnormal cholesterol levels)
- Endometrial cancer
- Heart disease
- Infertility
- Metabolic syndrome
- Obesity

First-Line Herbal Care: CINNAMON

Cinnamon (*Cinnamomum verum* or *Cinnamomum cassia*) is an effective and generally safe herbal treatment for treating type 2 diabetes (see page 83). Since blood sugar dysregulation is a common factor in PCOS, cinnamon may also play an important role in an herbal approach to treating PCOS.

Only a small number of studies have looked at the role of cinnamon in women with PCOS. One study showed significantly more frequent and more regular menstrual cycles in women taking 1.5 grams of cinnamon supplements daily compared to a placebo. Another pilot study showed positive effects on blood sugar and insulin resistance compared to a placebo with 1 gram daily. Larger studies performed specifically on women diagnosed with PCOS are needed.

Other Herbal Treatments

Herbal treatment for PCOS largely depends on how the condition manifests in a particular woman and what her goals are at that stage of life. Regulating blood sugar and improving insulin response are often important. For some women, the priority is decreasing androgen excess. Others may want to regulate their menstrual cycles because they are trying to conceive.

In general, hormone-normalizing herbs, such as chaste tree and black cohosh, are used to regulate menstrual cycles and resolve amenorrhea. Spearmint, green tea, peony and nettle can be useful in decreasing excess male hormones. Cinnamon and barberry work to improve blood sugar levels and insulin responses.

Did You Know?

Lifestyle Changes
Any herbal treatment for PCOS must be balanced with lifestyle changes. Blood sugar regulation through a low-glycemic-index and/or low-carbohydrate diet is an important starting point, along with exercise. The Mediterranean diet has been shown to reduce cardiovascular risk and may be recommended for some women.

Berberine

Berberine is an alkaloid found in some plants, including barberry, Oregon grape root, goldenseal and coptis. Traditionally, berberine-containing herbs have been used to stimulate digestive functions through the release of pancreatic enzymes and bile from the gallbladder, and to address everything from fat malabsorption to diabetes to urinary tract infections to skin conditions. As cholagogues that stimulate gallbladder function, berberine-containing herbs help to bind excess hormones for excretion through stool. As bitters, they encourage the release of and sensitization to pancreatic enzymes, such as insulin.

Because several berberine-containing herbs have been known to have hypoglycemic effects, researchers have looked at the use of berberine for PCOS. A small number of studies have shown that berberine decreases waist circumference, waist-to-hip ratio, triglycerides and low-density lipoprotein (LDL), or "bad," cholesterol. In addition, berberine increases sex hormone–binding globulin and high-density lipoprotein (HDL), or "good," cholesterol and improves blood sugar regulation in women with PCOS. In fact, all of these markers were significantly improved compared to either no treatment or treatment with a placebo. In one randomized trial, the changes were shown to be comparable to the effects of metformin.

The dosage of berberine in clinical trials is usually 500 milligrams, either twice or three times a day.

Chaste Tree

Chaste tree (*Vitex agnus-castus*) has been used to regulate hormones in both women and men ever since herbalists noticed that it reduces male libido and wondered how it might affect testosterone and other hormones. It was traditionally used for a variety of female conditions where hormonal imbalances were thought to be in play, including premenstrual breast pain, or cyclic mastalgia (see page 91).

As for the use of chaste tree in PCOS, research is very limited. Since chaste tree is believed to act through the pituitary to decrease prolactin release, it may indirectly increase follicle-stimulating hormone and estrogen production, which could benefit women with PCOS. It may also have antiandrogen effects, but these haven't been well studied.

Chaste tree is best used in cases of PCOS where prolactin is high and there is a history of anovulation, premenstrual syndrome, premenstrual breast pain and/or progesterone deficiency.

Folklore

Monk's Pepper

Once known as monk's pepper, chaste tree was used by monks in their cooking because it was associated with decreased libido in men. It was called chaste tree for the same reason — it helped monks to stay chaste.

Green Tea

Green tea's catechins have been studied for their use in many conditions. For women with PCOS, green tea (*Camellia sinensis*) may act as an antiandrogen by inhibiting the enzyme 5-alpha reductase, which reduces the impact of testosterone on the body. Green tea has also been investigated for its role in weight loss and its cardiovascular effects. In one meta-analysis, which included a study specifically on women with PCOS, green tea was shown to induce a small but non-significant weight loss. Although research is only preliminary, green tea may be a helpful addition to an herbal approach to PCOS.

Licorice

Licorice (*Glycyrrhiza glabra* or *Glycyrrhiza uralensis*) and white peony root (*Paeonia lactiflora*) are components of a traditional Chinese medicine formula that was shown, in a couple of small Chinese studies, to decrease testosterone levels in women with PCOS. Following these early trials, in vitro studies showed that licorice may have been the ingredient responsible. In high doses, licorice appears to inhibit the conversion of androstenedione (a precursor hormone) to testosterone. More recently, a preclinical study showed that a daily dose of 3.5 grams of licorice lowered testosterone levels in healthy women.

For women with PCOS who are taking spironolactone, an antiandrogen drug, licorice may help to reduce unwanted side effects. In one small study, licorice reduced the negative side effects associated with spironolactone's diuretic effect, kept blood pressure stable and decreased breakthrough bleeding during the women's menstrual cycles.

> **Caution**
>
> Licorice is known to raise blood pressure. Anyone taking licorice should routinely monitor their blood pressure. Women with high blood pressure should avoid taking licorice.

Spearmint

The potential of spearmint (*Mentha spicata*) for PCOS was discovered almost accidentally. Clinicians in Turkey noted that male patients who drank a lot of spearmint tea complained about a reduction in libido. Animal studies found that spearmint had antiandrogen-like effects that might explain the diminished libido. It occurred to these clinicians that, although antiandrogen effects aren't often desirable in men, women with symptoms of androgen excess might benefit from taking spearmint.

A very small open-label study found that two cups of spearmint tea per day decreased free testosterone and increased luteinizing hormone, follicle-stimulating hormone and estradiol in twenty-one women with hirsutism. A more recent, randomized trial confirmed these results, concluding

that two cups of spearmint tea per day for thirty days significantly reduced free and total testosterone, increased luteinizing hormone and follicle-stimulating hormone, and improved women's subjective assessment of hirsutism, compared to a placebo of chamomile tea. More research is needed, particularly trials that last longer than thirty days, as hirsutism is likely to take much longer than that to resolve. In the meantime, spearmint tea is an easy and delicious way to treat hirsutism in PCOS.

Common Combinations

- Spearmint, green tea and licorice for androgen excess in PCOS
- Cinnamon, barberry and fenugreek for insulin resistance in PCOS
- Chaste tree, licorice and white peony for menstrual regulation in PCOS with high prolactin

Conventional Medical Treatments

- Antiandrogens
- Clomiphene
- Metformin
- Oral contraceptives

Further Reading

Grant P. Spearmint herbal tea has significant anti-androgen effects in polycystic ovarian syndrome: A randomized controlled trial. *Phytotherapy Research*, 2010 Feb; 24 (2): 186–88.

Grant P, Ramasamy S. An update on plant derived anti-androgens. *International Journal of Endocrinology and Metabolism*, 2012 Spring; 10 (2): 497–502.

Jurgens TM, Whelan AM, Killian L, et al. Green tea for weight loss and weight maintenance in overweight or obese adults. *Cochrane Database of Systematic Reviews*, 2012 Dec 12; 12: CD008650.

Kort DH, Lobo RA. Preliminary evidence that cinnamon improves menstrual cyclicity in women with polycystic ovary syndrome: A randomized controlled trial. *American Journal of Obstetrics & Gynecology*, 2014 Nov; 211 (5): 487.e1-6.

Wang JG, Anderson RA, Graham GM 3rd, et al. The effect of cinnamon extract on insulin resistance parameters in polycystic ovary syndrome: A pilot study. *Fertility and Sterility*, 2007 Jul; 88 (1): 240–43.

Wei W, Zhao H, Wang A, et al. A clinical study on the short-term effect of berberine in comparison to metformin on the metabolic characteristics of women with polycystic ovary syndrome. *European Journal of Endocrinology*, 2012 Jan; 166 (1): 99–105.

CASE STUDY
PCOS

Like many of the women I see in my practice, Charlotte came to see me for fertility support. She had been trying unsuccessfully for the past five months to conceive through intravaginal insemination with a friend's sperm. Although she had a history of infrequent and sometimes absent menses, she hadn't been diagnosed with PCOS.

During her twenties and early thirties, Charlotte hadn't really kept track of her periods, since she had sexual contact only with women and therefore wasn't concerned about getting pregnant. If anything, she considered it a blessing not to have regular menstrual cycles. It never occurred to her that her irregular cycles might later have an impact on her ability to get pregnant.

When she was thirty-seven years old, Charlotte and her partner, Ayesha, decided they were ready to have children. A friend was willing to donate sperm, and they proceeded to use an at-home method of intravaginal insemination. When several attempts were unsuccessful, Charlotte came to see me for testing and naturopathic fertility care. After taking a through history and giving her a physical examination, I suspected that PCOS was a factor in her difficulty conceiving. Bloodwork showed preliminary signs of insulin resistance and abnormally high levels of prolactin in her blood, and a pelvic ultrasound showed multiple cysts on her ovaries.

We started with eliminating dairy and limiting carbohydrates in Charlotte's diet, to normalize her blood sugar levels. I recommended a concentrated chaste tree extract to help reduce her prolactin, along with a high-quality prenatal multivitamin and myo-inositol. After three months, her prolactin was reduced to normal levels and her blood sugar had normalized. Five months after our first appointment, she was pregnant, and she gave birth to a healthy baby nine months later.

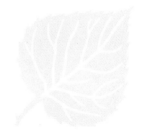

Pregnancy and Breastfeeding

Women often come see me when they are pregnant or breastfeeding, for general wellness checks and for more specific health concerns that typically arise during these times. Symptoms during pregnancy may come and go. Some may be more prevalent at a certain stage of pregnancy, while others may last the entire time. Often women are looking for guidance about what kinds of herbs and supplements are safe to take during pregnancy or lactation for non-baby-related issues such as a common cold or flu.

Safety

Recommending herbs for conditions related to pregnancy and breastfeeding presents many challenges with regards to safety. In fact, the subject of herbal medicine for pregnancy and breastfeeding deserves an entire book on its own. For some herbs, the risks of use during pregnancy are well documented and absolute; for others, dangers are theorized based on the herbs' known actions. Some herbs are known to cause birth defects; others may cause uterine contractions or miscarriage; others have been related to premature birth.

You should always consult a licensed health-care provider before taking any herb, but this caution is even more important when you are pregnant or breastfeeding. Although some herbs have a long history of safe use by herbalists and midwives, very few have been studied in clinical trials to evaluate safety during pregnancy. Nonetheless, some herbs have been identified by various health agencies as "likely safe" or "possibly safe." Other herbs may be deemed "possibly unsafe" or "likely unsafe." Caution and consultation are advised, especially during the first trimester.

Constipation

Constipation is a very common concern during pregnancy. Anywhere from 10% to 40% of pregnant women experience it. Normal changes during pregnancy to women's anatomy and physiology make them predisposed to constipation. For example, the hormone progesterone increases transit time, the time stool spends in the bowel. Water absorption from the intestines increases, which then dries stool, making it more difficult to pass. Later in pregnancy, pressure from an expanded uterus may also contribute.

Constipation can also be related to taking prenatal vitamins, which contain supplemental iron, known to cause constipation. Certain forms of iron are more likely to cause constipation than others.

Signs and Symptoms

- Infrequent bowel movements
- Straining or discomfort with the passage of stool

Associated Conditions

- Heartburn
- Hemorrhoids
- Nausea and vomiting

First-Line Herbal Care: DANDELION

Dandelion root (*Taraxacum officinale*) has been used for years by herbalists, naturopaths and midwives to treat constipation in the second and third trimesters of pregnancy. However, right now there is insufficient scientific evidence available to clearly state that dandelion is safe in pregnancy. In small doses, dandelion may be considered in resistant cases of constipation. It may be helpful to eat dandelion leaf in culinary amounts, as a source of fiber with gentle laxative properties.

Conventional Medical Treatments

- Bulk-forming agents
- Lubricant laxatives
- Osmotic laxatives
- Stimulant laxatives
- Stool softeners

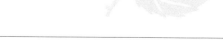

Heartburn

Heartburn is another extremely common symptom in pregnancy. Pregnancy hormones can relax the lower esophageal sphincter, allowing acid to come up from the stomach and cause irritation in the esophagus. As the uterus expands and takes up more space, it can apply upward pressure on the stomach and esophagus. Heartburn most often occurs in the second and third trimesters, but it may happen at any time. More than 50% of pregnant women report heartburn at some point in their pregnancies.

Signs and Symptoms

- Discomfort, heaviness or burning pain under the breastbone
- Acid taste in the mouth
- Regurgitation of food
- Burping, gas or bloating

Associated Conditions

- Constipation
- Nausea and vomiting

First-Line Herbal Care: SLIPPERY ELM

The inner bark of slippery elm (*Ulmus fulva*) contains a lot of mucilage (a thick, gelatinous substance made by plants). When slippery elm powder is added to water, it makes a tea that coats the throat, protecting it from acid reflux.

There is limited scientific evidence on whether slippery elm is safe in pregnancy, but it has a long history of use by midwives. There are some concerns that slippery elm can increase uterine contractions. It is likely that the caution is due to the potential for contamination by the outer bark of slippery elm.

Other Herbal Treatments

The primary herbs used to relieve the symptoms of heartburn are demulcent herbs that coat and soothe irritated mucous membranes.

Licorice

Licorice (*Glycyrrhiza glabra* or *Glycyrrhiza uralensis*) is generally not recommended in pregnancy. In fact, there is some evidence that licorice consumption during pregnancy is associated with preterm births. So why am I mentioning it in the section on pregnancy? The problems associated with licorice consumption, including increased blood pressure and preterm births, are attributed to glycyrrhizin, one of the constituents in the plant. This suggests that deglycyrrhizinated licorice (DGL), in which the glycyrrhizin component has been removed, may be safe in pregnancy. In vitro and human studies on DGL in non-pregnant people have shown that it improves symptoms of reflux, heartburn, nausea and bloating, particularly if these symptoms are associated with a *Helicobacter pylori* infection. Human clinical trials on DGL for peptic ulcer disease and canker sores have also shown positive results. Research is needed to confirm the safety of DGL in pregnancy.

> ### Did You Know?
> **TCM**
> In traditional Chinese medicine, licorice is added to almost all formulas for its ability to harmonize the herbs in the formula and lead them into the appropriate channels (also known as meridians).

Conventional Medical Treatments

- Alginates
- Antacids
- Omeprazole
- Ranitidine

Further Reading

Stapleton H. The use of herbal medicine in pregnancy and labour. Part I: An overview of current practice. *Complementary Therapies in Nursing and Midwifery*, 1995 Oct; 1 (5): 148–53.

Strandberg TE, Andersson S, Järvenpää AL, McKeigue P. Preterm birth and licorice consumption during pregnancy. *American Journal of Epidemiology*, 2002; 156 (9): 803–5.

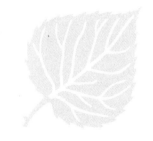

Hemorrhoids

Prolonged constipation and straining can lead to hemorrhoids, as the increased pressure on the rectum creates stress and may weaken the blood vessels in the area. Sitting or standing for long periods of time can worsen symptoms. About 25% to 35% of women experience hemorrhoids during pregnancy. The incidence is highest in the third trimester, when the expanded uterus increases pressure inside the abdomen and pelvis. Although hemorrhoids sometimes resolve on their own after delivery, it isn't uncommon for them to linger, or even worsen, postpartum. Hemorrhoids can also develop during the second stage of labor, especially if prolonged pushing is required during delivery.

Hemorrhoids are basically varicose veins in the rectum, and as with varicose veins (see page 169), the likelihood of developing hemorrhoids is greater with each additional pregnancy. They are sometimes painful and can be a cause of distress, especially if they bleed. In some cases, women may mistake the blood released from hemorrhoids as a sign of fetal distress or miscarriage.

Thankfully, hemorrhoids are easy to diagnose with a simple physical exam. In most women, hemorrhoids resolve on their own after the baby is born.

Signs and Symptoms

- Discomfort or pain in the anus or rectum
- Swollen, inflamed veins in the anus or rectum

Associated Conditions

- Constipation
- Varicose veins

First-Line Herbal Care: HORSE CHESTNUT

Horse chestnut seed extract (*Aesculus hippocastanum*) is a well-accepted treatment for venous insufficiency (see the section on varicose veins, page 169), and in a sense, hemorrhoids are a localized manifestation of venous insufficiency in which the veins in the rectum become enlarged and engorged.

Few studies have been conducted on horse chestnut for hemorrhoids. One double-blind, placebo-controlled trial showed significant improvements in pain, itching, burning, swelling and bleeding after one week of treatment with horse chestnut. The dosage in this trial was standardized to 40 milligrams of aescin, taken three times daily. Although this trial was not done specifically on pregnant women, other research suggests that there is minimal risk during pregnancy.

Other Herbal Treatments

The first step in treating hemorrhoids is to resolve any constipation or straining with bowel movements by increasing water and fiber intake and partaking in moderate exercise. Sitz baths in warm water alone may help to reduce the pain associated with hemorrhoids. If not, astringent and other blood vessel–tonifying herbs can be added to the bath.

Alternatively, astringent and other blood vessel–tonifying herbs can be applied topically through compresses or gels to help relieve symptoms. Local topical applications are generally safer in pregnancy, as there is minimal absorption into the bloodstream in most cases. Although this approach will not address underlying causes, such as constipation or chronic venous insufficiency, it will help to resolve local symptoms while a systemic approach is addressed through diet and lifestyle measures.

Astringent herbs help to tonify the blood vessel walls and prevent blood vessel fragility by constricting and tightening (like the puckered mouthfeel you get from eating a not-quite-ripe banana or persimmon). Other blood vessel–tonifying herbs work by decreasing the fragility of the capillaries (the smallest blood vessels) and increasing microcirculation. Some examples of herbs used to treat hemorrhoids include horse chestnut, pine bark, grape seed, gotu kola and butcher's broom.

Ginkgo

The main plant constituents in ginkgo are flavonoids, which promote the integrity and strength of blood vessel walls and are known to decrease inflammation. Ginkgo has traditionally been included in formulas for hemorrhoids to support blood vessel integrity.

One small open-label study investigating a combination herbal product containing ginkgo for the treatment of hemorrhoids found improvements in bleeding, pain and discharge after one week of use. More research is needed.

Caution

Ginkgo should be used cautiously in the later stages of pregnancy, as its blood-thinning effects may increase bleeding during delivery. Since hemorrhoids are more common in the third trimester, topical preparations and other herbs such as horse chestnut are safer choices.

Dowsing

Witch hazel may have gotten its name from the historical use of Y-shaped witch hazel twigs in dowsing, an ancient method of divining for water underground. The "witch" part of the name does not imply that the herb was often used by witches, but rather it comes from the Old English word *wych*, referring to the pliability of the branches. The "hazel" part likely arose because the common hazel (*Corylus* species) was also used for dowsing in Europe.

Witch hazel's ability to find fluids underground is akin to its ability to find the unhealthy seepage of blood and fluids within the body. Therapeutically, witch hazel astringes unnecessary or excess fluids, such as those found in hemorrhoids, varicose veins, bruises, diarrhea, weeping wounds and leucorrhea. Eclectic herbalists used witch hazel specifically for passive hemorrhages — cases where blood or another fluid leaks slowly, much like the elusive underground springs sought by dowsers.

Witch Hazel

Witch hazel (*Hamamelis virginiana*) is a gentle, effective astringent that also has antiseptic properties. The astringency of witch hazel extracts applied topically to external hemorrhoids helps to tone the blood vessel walls, and the antiseptic action helps to prevent local infections.

Although witch hazel has a long history of use for treating hemorrhoids and varicose veins, and witch hazel distillates can easily be found for sale on pharmacy shelves, few studies have been conducted to confirm its therapeutic use. Researchers believe that witch hazel works because it contains proanthocyanidins that tone and improve the integrity of blood vessels. (Grapeseed extract, pine bark extract and gotu kola, other herbs used to treat hemorrhoids and varicose veins, also contain proanthocyanidins.)

Commercially distilled witch hazel is used in many personal products, including toners, cleansers, makeup removers, acne products, vaginal washes and, of course, hemorrhoid treatment products. Witch hazel is listed as the active ingredient in several Preparation H products, including Medicated Wipes for Women, which are advertised specifically for use postpartum.

Yarrow

Yarrow (*Achillea millefolium*) is used topically and internally for bleeding of all kinds. As both an astringent and a regulator of blood flow, yarrow can treat conditions where there is excessive bleeding and conditions where blood is stagnant and does not flow as it should. Yarrow is particularly useful in conditions such as uterine fibroids and hemorrhoids, where both actions are needed. In hemorrhoids, blood stagnates in the pooling and swelling of the veins in the anus/rectum, and the fragile blood vessels can sometimes break open and bleed.

Common Combination

- Yarrow, witch hazel and horse chestnut applied topically

Conventional Medical Treatments

- Antihemorrhoidal analgesics
- Stool softeners

Further Reading

[No authors listed]. *Aesculus hippocastanum* (Horse chestnut). Monograph. *Alternative Medicine Review*, 2009 Sep; 14 (3): 278–83.

Sumboonnanonda K, Lertsithichai P. Clinical study of the *Ginkgo biloba* — Troxerutin-heptaminol Hce in the treatment of acute hemorrhoidal attacks. *Journal of the Medical Association of Thailand*, 2004 Feb; 87 (2): 137–42.

CASE STUDY
Hemorrhoids

Maya, a thirty-two-year-old woman whom I had seen throughout her pregnancy, made an appointment to see me about her hemorrhoids. Although she had first noticed them toward the tail end of her third trimester, she hadn't mentioned them because they weren't all that bothersome. But now, at five weeks postpartum, she was seeing blood in the toilet after bowel movements. Her bowel movements were regular, but she did occasionally need to strain to pass stool.

I recommended that Maya increase her soluble fiber intake by eating chia pudding and oatmeal, to help with the passage of stool. In addition, I reminded her that she needed to drink adequate amounts of water in order to keep up with the production of breast milk. She used a concentrated witch hazel extract topically to stop the bleeding and tonify her rectal blood vessels. A couple of days later, she was already feeling better and the bleeding had stopped.

Low Milk Supply

Low milk supply — and perceived low milk supply — can be a major source of stress for breastfeeding mothers. Unfortunately, many people have not had the opportunity to witness how a normal breastfed infant behaves and have not had this knowledge passed down from older generations. Lack of breastfeeding support, incomplete education and sociocultural factors may all contribute to misunderstandings of what to expect in terms of infant feeding and sleeping schedules. As a result, some mothers question their body's ability to produce adequate breast milk. They may lack confidence or wonder whether their baby is getting enough.

Parents sometimes mistake an infant's desire for frequent nursing, fussiness in the evening, a poor breastfeeding latch or a decreased sensation of fullness in breast tissue for insufficient supply. Postpartum depression or anxiety can exacerbate both the perception of low supply and the actual milk supply. A good rule of thumb is this: if your baby is gaining weight and producing enough wet and dirty diapers, your milk supply is just fine.

In cases where there really isn't enough breast milk being produced and the baby is not gaining weight appropriately, supplementation with donor breast milk or infant formula may be recommended, at least until milk supply increases. Lactation support is essential to promote frequent, efficient nursing and facilitate the normal supply-and-demand cycle of milk production.

Signs and Symptoms
- Insufficient wet and dirty diapers
- Baby not gaining weight as expected

Associated Conditions
- Anemia
- Hypothyroidism
- Insulin resistance
- Polycystic ovarian syndrome (PCOS)
- Postpartum hemorrhage
- Previous breast injury or surgery
- Retained placenta

First-Line Herbal Care: FENUGREEK

The Ancient Greeks and Romans grew fenugreek (*Trigonella foenum-graecum* L.) as cattle fodder, and the *foenum-graecum* portion of the Latin binomial means "Greek hay." Fenugreek is still fed to dairy cows today to increase their milk production. Although breastfeeding mothers might not love the idea of being given the same treatment as cows, fenugreek has also been used traditionally to support human breast milk production. In some regions of India, a porridge made of fenugreek seeds and rice is given to new mothers to promote lactation.

Although research is lacking, fenugreek continues to be widely used to stimulate milk supply, and few adverse effects (such as digestive upset or diarrhea) have been reported. One study evaluated the effectiveness of a combination herbal product containing fenugreek for breast milk production. Breast milk production increased in the treatment group, but not significantly more than in the control group.

A randomized clinical trial compared the effects of an herbal galactagogue tea containing fenugreek to the same tea containing apple, with a control group drinking no tea at all. The study was conducted on women with healthy, full-term infants who were exclusively breastfed. Three days postpartum, the fenugreek tea group showed a significantly greater volume of pumped milk than the other two groups. In addition, the infants who were breastfed by women drinking fenugreek tea had significantly lower weight loss and faster recovery of their birth weight than either the apple tea group or the control group.

The dose of fenugreek from traditional sources and clinical studies ranges from 3 to 6 grams daily in divided doses. As a tincture (at a 1:5 concentration ratio), it is usually given as 1 to 2 milliliters, three times daily. Occasionally fenugreek can cause loose stools at higher doses and can lead to urine and/or sweat that smells like maple syrup.

Caution

Fenugreek may cause hypoglycemia. Women with diabetes mellitus who are taking hypoglycemic medications should be cautious about also taking this herb. Fenugreek should not be used by people with allergies to peanuts or chickpeas, as it comes from the same family of plants.

Other Herbal Treatments

Traditionally, herbal treatment for low breast milk supply consists primarily of galactagogues — herbs that increase breast milk production. Nutritive herbs and adaptogens may also be used to support the mother's increased nutritional needs while breastfeeding and to better handle physical stresses after childbirth. If anxiety or depression

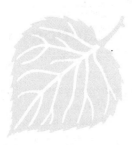

is having an impact on breast milk supply, gentle nervine tonics may be appropriate.

Chaste Tree

Although chaste tree (*Vitex agnus-castus*) has been shown in numerous studies to reduce prolactin in cases of hyperprolactinemia, some animal studies have also shown it to *increase* prolactin. Some herbalists have suggested that chaste tree has a normalizing effect on prolactin, increasing and decreasing its levels as needed. One study on a proprietary extract of chaste tree improved breast milk production in women compared to controls. More research is definitely needed to resolve questions of whether chaste tree would be harmful or might be helpful in cases of insufficient breast milk.

Milk Thistle and Blessed Thistle

Milk thistle (*Silybum marianum*) is best known for its ability to support liver detoxification and heal liver damage, but it has also been used as a galactagogue. One small placebo-controlled trial compared a milk thistle extract to a placebo. The milk thistle treatment group had significant increases in breast milk production compared to the placebo group. No evidence of the milk thistle passing into the breast milk was found.

Blessed thistle (*Cnicus benedictus*), a relation of milk thistle, has also been used to help increase breast milk production. Although there have been no clinical trials on the use of blessed thistle as a galactagogue, literature reviews and participant surveys on herbal galactagogues frequently note its traditional use for this purpose and indicate that more research is needed.

Nettle

From the perspective of traditional Chinese medicine, both blood and yin energy are lost through the process of childbirth. In many cultures, certain foods and herbs are used after birth to help replenish lost fluids, blood and vitality. Nettle (*Urtica dioica*) is one of those nutritive herbs.

Because nettle contains iron and other minerals, it may be helpful in supporting healthy breast milk supply, particularly when a woman has lost a lot of blood or has a history of anemia. Care should be taken to source nettle from land known to have high-quality soil and good growing conditions, as nettles can pull heavy metals out of the soil they grow in.

Shatavari

Shatavari (*Asparagus racemosus*) is an herb from the Ayurvedic tradition. Considered a female tonic herb, shatavari is given to women to increase fertility, libido and breast milk supply.

Studies on shatavari have shown mixed results. One randomized clinical trial on breastfeeding mothers who reported low milk production found no significant differences between a placebo and a combination product containing shatavari. A second randomized trial found that shatavari on its own in a higher dosage (20 milligrams per kilogram of the mother's body weight, taken three times daily) significantly increased prolactin levels and infant weight gain compared to a placebo of rice powder. More research is needed.

Did You Know?

Word Origin

In Sanskrit, *shatavari* means "able to have one hundred husbands," a reference to the use of the herb to support vitality, fertility and sex drive.

Common Combination
- Fenugreek and blessed thistle

Conventional Medical Treatment
- Domperidone, a dopamine antagonist

Further Reading

Abascal K, Yarnell E. Botanical galactagogues. *Alternative and Complementary Therapies*, 2008 December; 14 (6): 288–94.

Forinash AB, Yancey AM, Barnes KN, Myles TD. The use of galactogogues in the breastfeeding mother. *Annals of Pharmacotherapy*, 2012 Oct; 46 (10): 1392–404.

Mortel M, Mehta SD. Systematic review of the efficacy of herbal galactogogues. *Journal of Human Lactation*, 2013 May; 29 (2): 154–62.

Zapantis A, Steinberg JG, Schilit L. Use of herbals as galactagogues. *Journal of Pharmacy Practice*, 2012 Apr; 25 (2): 222–31.

Morning Sickness

Morning sickness — nausea and vomiting of pregnancy — is inaccurately named since it can happen at any time of the day. It is extremely common, especially in the first trimester. Between 50% and 90% of women have some degree of nausea, either with or without vomiting. Nausea and vomiting may even be a sign of a strong pregnancy: research shows that women with mild nausea and vomiting experience fewer miscarriages and stillbirths.

Although nausea and vomiting of pregnancy (NVP) is normal and doesn't harm the fetus, it is unpleasant and can interfere with daily activities. In some cases, it can make eating and drinking difficult, which can be a problem if dehydration or malnutrition result. Weight loss, dark-colored urine, vomiting multiple times daily, cramping pain or other signs of dehydration indicate a severity that may require hospitalization. When NVP is extreme and persistent, it is called hyperemesis gravidarum.

Signs and Symptoms

- Nausea
- Vomiting

Caution

In some cases, ginger consumption can lead to acid reflux. Heartburn may be caused by the ginger, as opposed to occurring independently.

First-Line Herbal Care: GINGER

Ginger (*Zingiber officinale*) is effective for nausea caused by everything from chemotherapy to motion sickness to pregnancy. It is well studied and in clinical trials consistently results in a significant reduction in NVP. Some trials have shown it to be as effective as vitamin B_6 or dimenhydrinate (Gravol).

Two recent systematic reviews of the literature concluded that ginger is a safe and effective treatment for nausea and vomiting during pregnancy. The dosage used in the trials reviewed ranged from 1 to 2 grams per day of encapsulated ginger powder, in divided doses of 250 milligrams. This dosage does not appear to pose any risk of heartburn, drowsiness or miscarriage, in spite of ginger's potential anticoagulant effects.

Other Herbal Treatments

Herbal treatment for NVP focuses on antinausea herbs such as ginger and peppermint, which are often very effective.

Peppermint

Peppermint tea (*Mentha piperita*) has long been used as a gentle digestive aid and antinausea herb. It is best for mild nausea with bloating or gas and has been shown to be effective for nausea after surgery and nausea induced by chemotherapy in human clinical trials. Peppermint is considered relatively safe in pregnancy, especially in culinary amounts.

No specific research has been conducted on peppermint tea for NVP, but one small study on mint oil aromatherapy had positive results. In the double-blind, randomized trial, women with NVP placed either four drops of mint essential oil or four drops of saline in a bowl of water beside their bed before falling asleep. The severity and intensity of nausea decreased in the mint group after four days of treatment, but the trend was not statistically significant.

Common Combination

- Ginger and peppermint tea

Conventional Medical Treatments

- Diphenhydramine
- Doxylamine plus vitamin B_6 and/or dicyclomine (Diclectin, Bendectin, Debendox)

> **Did You Know?**
>
> **Tea as Aromatherapy**
> The positive effects of aromatherapy can be felt when you make and drink peppermint tea. After the tea steeps, the volatile oils that give peppermint its pleasing scent evaporate and are released into the air. As you drink the tea, you benefit from the smell as much as from the taste and internal antinauseant effects.

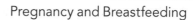

CASE STUDY
Morning Sickness

Lin came in to see me to share some exciting news — and some not so great news. She was five weeks pregnant and had already started feeling nauseated. The previous morning, she had vomited for the first time. Her nausea was worse in the morning and when she smelled food cooking or freshly cooked food. The smell of cigarette smoke also bothered her. In general, most food was unappealing, and her appetite had plummeted as a result.

I recommended that Lin eat small, frequent meals and snacks and eat immediately upon waking, before even getting out of bed. Lin also drank small cups of ginger tea throughout the day. Her nausea was barely noticeable as long as she ate regularly and continued drinking the ginger tea. She didn't vomit again, and the nausea had passed by the end of the first trimester.

Further Reading

Ding M, Leach M, Bradley H. The effectiveness and safety of ginger for pregnancy-induced nausea and vomiting: A systematic review. *Women and Birth*, 2013 Mar; 26 (1): e26–30.

Matthews A, Haas DM, O'Mathúna DP, et al. Interventions for nausea and vomiting in early pregnancy. *Cochrane Database of Systematic Reviews*, 2014 Mar 21; 3: CD007575.

Pasha H, Behmanesh F, Mohsenzadeh F, et al. Study of the effect of mint oil on nausea and vomiting during pregnancy. *Iranian Red Crescent Medical Journal*, 2012 Nov; 14 (11): 727–30.

Thomson M, Corbin R, Leung L. Effects of ginger for nausea and vomiting in early pregnancy: A meta-analysis. *Journal of the American Board of Family Medicine*, 2014 Jan–Feb; 27 (1): 115–22.

Viljoen E, Visser J, Koen N, Musekiwa A. A systematic review and meta-analysis of the effect and safety of ginger in the treatment of pregnancy-associated nausea and vomiting. *Nutrition Journal*, 2014 Mar 19; 13: 20.

Varicose Veins

Varicose veins — visibly enlarged, twisted veins — are a common complaint during and after pregnancy, thanks to weight increase, pressure increase, and hormonal changes. The incidence of varicose veins increases with each subsequent pregnancy; in other words, you're more likely to get varicose veins when you are pregnant with a second or third child than with your first.

Pregnant or not, women are twice as likely as men to have varicose veins. Varicose veins develop when the walls of the veins become weakened or the valves in the veins no longer work as well to help pump blood back to the heart (also called venous insufficiency). Blood then begins to pool in the lower limbs, especially when one is standing for long periods of time.

Signs and Symptoms

- Dull aching, heaviness, cramping, itching or tingling pain in the legs
- Enlarged, sometimes twisted veins near the surface of the skin
- Swelling in the legs and feet
- Redness or other skin color changes around the ankles
- Thickening or hardening of the skin

Associated Condition

- Hemorrhoids

First-Line Herbal Care: HORSE CHESTNUT

Horse chestnut seed extract (*Aesculus hippocastanum*) has been well studied for its use in the treatment of chronic venous insufficiency in non-pregnant people. Research has shown it to be safe and effective at resolving swelling and pain. A recent meta-analysis concluded that horse chestnut seed extract significantly reduces leg volume, leg circumference, pain, edema and itching in people with chronic venous insufficiency.

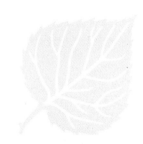

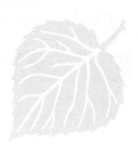

Horse chestnut seed extract has also been used internally for pregnancy-induced venous insufficiency and appears to have minimal risks associated with it. One randomized trial on pregnant women found no serious adverse effects after two weeks of horse chestnut seed extract use.

Other Herbal Treatments

Herbal treatment for varicose veins is very similar to the herbal approach for hemorrhoids (see page 158). In both cases, priority is given to herbs that tonify the venous system by strengthening blood vessel walls. Astringent herbs that contain tannins, proanthocyanidins and other bioflavonoids are most effective for decreasing capillary fragility and preventing the development or worsening of varicose veins.

Calendula

Traditional herbalists have long used calendula (*Calendula officinalis*) to treat varicose veins, but no human clinical research has been performed specifically on its use for this condition. However, calendula contains flavonoids and volatile oils that have demonstrated anti-inflammatory and wound-healing effects in vitro and in animal studies. Calendula ointment applied topically to venous leg ulcers has been shown to significantly speed up skin healing compared to a saline dressing in a small, non-blinded human study. While these results are promising, more research is needed.

Ginkgo

Like horse chestnut and witch hazel, ginkgo contains flavonoids, which help improve blood vessel integrity and decrease inflammation. Ginkgo has historically been used in combination herbal formulas for varicose veins.

A few open-label trials have been conducted in Russia on a combination product containing ginkgo for the treatment of varicose veins and chronic venous insufficiency. Although these studies reported decreased symptoms when ginkgo was taken orally, the study quality was poor. More research is needed.

Caution

Ginkgo should be used cautiously in the later stages of pregnancy, as its blood-thinning effects may increase bleeding during delivery. Since varicose veins are more common in the third trimester, topical preparations and other herbs such as horse chestnut are safer choices.

Witch Hazel

As witch hazel (*Hamamelis virginiana*) is high in tannins and also contains flavonoids and volatile oils, it has a history of internal and topical use for the treatment of hemorrhoids and varicose veins. Although it isn't safe for internal use during pregnancy, witch hazel extracts and tinctures can be used topically to help ease the throbbing pain of varicose veins and prevent worsening of the condition.

No human clinical research has been conducted on witch hazel for varicose veins, but pharmacological studies show that it promotes the integrity of blood vessel walls and acts as a local anti-inflammatory.

Common Combination

- Horse chestnut, witch hazel and calendula applied topically to varicose veins as a compress

Conventional Medical Treatments

Compression stockings are usually recommended by obstetricians. Saline injections, laser surgery, sclerotherapy (use of a liquid chemical to close off the affected vein) and ablation (use of heat or radio waves to close off a vein) are other potential treatments.

Did You Know?

Native Uses

The Cherokee, Osage, Iroquois and Chippewa used witch hazel to treat sores, scratches and skin ulcers. The Iroquois also used it to prevent hemorrhage after childbirth and to prevent bleeding and miscarriage in pregnant women who had fallen or been hurt. Other Native American uses include treatment for sore throat, colds, sore muscles, diarrhea, tuberculosis and painful menses.

Further Reading

Duran V, Matic M, Jovanović M, et al. Results of the clinical examination of an ointment with marigold (*Calendula officinalis*) extract in the treatment of venous leg ulcers. *International Journal of Tissue Reactions*, 2005; 27 (3): 101–6.

Mills E, Duguoa JJ, Koren G. *Herbal Medicines in Pregnancy and Lactation: An Evidence-Based Approach*. London: Taylor & Francis, 2006.

Pittler MH, Ernst E. Horse chestnut seed extract for chronic venous insufficiency. *Cochrane Database of Systematic Reviews*, 2012 Nov 14; 11: CD003230.

Zhukov BN, Kukol'nikova EL. [Clinical response to Ginkor-Fort in the treatment of chronic venous insufficiency in varicosity]. [Article in Russian]. *Terapevticheskiĭ arkhiv*, 2004; 76 (12): 48–50.

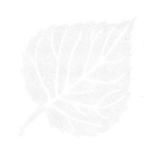

Weaning

Weaning is the process of discontinuing breast milk production, whether lactation is naturally tapering off through baby-led weaning, breastfeeding is no longer possible or no longer desired, or a baby has died (late in the third trimester or sometime after delivery). Regardless of the reasons for weaning, the process is frequently emotional and may involve physical symptoms.

Signs and Symptoms

- Feeling of fullness or engorgement in breast tissue
- Plugged ducts or mastitis
- Grief, loss, depression, emotional lability
- Nausea
- Headaches

Associated Conditions

- Depression
- Mastitis

First-Line Herbal Care: SAGE

Regular or excessive use of sage (*Salvia officinalis*) is to be avoided during breastfeeding because it can dry up milk supply. However, sage can be useful when weaning a child, for the same reason.

The traditional dosage is 1 tablespoon (15 mL) of dried sage per 1 cup (250 mL) of boiled water, steeped for five to ten minutes. Drinking 2 to 6 cups (500 mL to 1.5 L) daily is recommended to decrease milk supply. Research is needed to back up the use of sage in weaning.

Other Herbal Treatments

Weaning does not require any treatment as long as it is slow and steady. However, it can lead to significant pain, both emotional and physical, especially if it is abrupt. Nervines, such as chamomile or lavender, can help ease anxiety related to weaning, while adaptogens with positive effects on mood, such as rhodiola, can provide additional emotional support. For the physical pain, astringent herbs can help decrease breast milk production without negative side effects. Green cabbage leaves, chilled and rolled to break their hard spine, can be put inside a bra or directly against a breast to relieve the discomfort of engorgement or mastitis and support the weaning process. Hand-expressing a little milk is also useful, to relieve pressure.

Peppermint

Peppermint oil (*Mentha piperita*) has traditionally been given to women to help decrease milk supply during weaning, administered as a tea, in capsules or through inhalation. Some women have even used peppermint candies to help lower milk supply. There is no research to support the effectiveness of these approaches.

Common Combination

- Sage, rhodiola and peppermint for weaning with fatigue and/or depression

Conventional Medical Treatments

Pharmaceutical treatment is generally not recommended for weaning, but it may include oral contraceptives and pseudoephedrine.

Further Reading

Mangesi L, Dowswell T. Treatments for breast engorgement during lactation. *Cochrane Database of Systematic Reviews*, 2010 Sep 8; (9): CD006946.

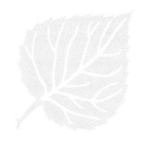

Premenstrual Syndrome

Did You Know?

Self-Care

When it comes to PMS, self-care can go a long way. Exercise, adequate sleep and increased protein intake all help to alleviate premenstrual symptoms, as does avoiding refined and added sugar. Vitamin B_6 and magnesium supplements may also help.

Did You Know?

Premenstrual Dysphoric Disorder

When PMS is so severe that it includes suicidal thoughts and even psychosis, it is called premenstrual dysphoric disorder (PMDD).

Premenstrual syndrome (PMS) is a collection of a wide range of symptoms that occur during the luteal phase of the menstrual cycle, up to two weeks before the start of menses. These symptoms stop one or two days after menses begins. Possible causes of PMS include changes in blood glucose, high prolactin or abnormal levels of estrogen or progesterone.

PMS is one of the most common health concerns cited by women who visit my office, and up to 75% of women experience PMS at some point in their lives. Many women consider PMS a normal part of menses and believe it is just something they must tolerate or medicate. But a number of researchers in the medical humanities field have criticized the concept of PMS, and the pharmaceutical treatments developed around it, as pathologizing normal body functions and variations in mood, hormones, weight and metabolism. In one study on women who believed they were more emotionally volatile premenstrually, daily mood records failed to show a pattern of moods related to their menstrual cycles. A recent review of studies on PMS likewise concluded that there is no scientific support for the existence of a premenstrual mood syndrome.

Other studies have investigated the role of sociocultural factors on a woman's experience of PMS. Women from certain cultural backgrounds, women with a history of sexual abuse and women who are overburdened at work and at home are more likely to report symptoms of PMS. As a result, many medical professionals and anthropologists argue that PMS is, by and large, a socially constructed disease.

Regardless of the ongoing scientific and philosophical debates surrounding whether PMS really exists, women continue to express distress about PMS symptoms, especially when those symptoms interfere with the activities of daily living.

Premenstrual symptoms may worsen with age, as women approach menopause. Since PMS can be a result of hormone changes, it may signal more serious hormonal imbalances that should be investigated and addressed.

Signs and Symptoms

- Breast pain (cyclic mastalgia), tenderness or swelling
- Bloating, gas, water retention
- Constipation or diarrhea
- Emotional lability: moodiness, irritability, sadness, hopelessness, tension
- Clumsiness, forgetfulness, confusion, poor concentration
- Headaches
- Food cravings
- Feelings of guilt, lowered self-esteem, fear
- Difficulty sleeping

Associated Conditions

- Depression
- Dysmenorrhea
- Endometriosis
- Fibroids
- Menstrual irregularities
- Polycystic ovarian syndrome (PCOS)

First-Line Herbal Care: EVENING PRIMROSE

Evening primrose oil (*Oenothera biennis*) contains the omega-6 fatty acid gamma-linolenic acid (GLA), which is involved in promoting an anti-inflammatory pathway. GLA derived from evening primrose has been used to relieve premenstrual breast pain (cyclic mastalgia), tenderness and swelling.

Research studies generally support the use of evening primrose oil for alleviating cyclic mastalgia. In randomized trials, it has been shown to reduce pain better than a placebo and as well as non-steroidal anti-inflammatory drugs (NSAIDs). Formulas that combine evening primrose oil with vitamin E and vitamin B_6 also appear to improve premenstrual breast pain, mood and behavior.

Some studies, however, have found no difference in effect between evening primrose oil and a placebo. Although these studies may appear contradictory, it is important to note that the oils used as placebos may themselves have had

Folklore

Moon Plant

Evening primrose is best known nowadays for the use of its seed oil. Historically, however, evening primrose roots and flowers were used medicinally for physical and spiritual treatments. Long considered a moon plant, evening primrose blooms at night and appears to glow in the dark. Associated with the yin/feminine aspects, evening primrose is said to stimulate the solar plexus and heart, allowing the user to experience love without fear of rejection or betrayal.

The energetics of evening primrose may help provide the space and security for the expression of potentially challenging emotions, such as frustration, irritability and vulnerability, without fear of rejection or betrayal. It may allow space for emotionality to be a sign of health rather than disease.

Did You Know?

Underlying Causes

If a known reproductive health condition, such as fibroids (page 94), endometriosis (page 87) or PCOS (page 148), is causing or contributing to PMS symptoms, herbs that address the specific underlying causes should be used.

Did You Know?

TCM Perspective

From a traditional Chinese medicine perspective, PMS that is characterized by cyclic mastalgia, anger, depression and distending pain is associated with a stagnation of liver qi. *Xiao yao wan*, a traditional formula used to address PMS when it is caused by liver qi stagnation, includes bupleurum, dang gui, poria, atractylodes, white peony, ginger, mint and licorice.

anti-inflammatory action. In other cases, the studies may not have been long enough. It may take up to four to six months of evening primrose oil use before significant improvements in cyclic breast pain can be seen.

Evening primrose oil is best used when the primary symptom of PMS is breast pain or swelling, or when a woman doesn't get enough essential fatty acids in her diet. If, on the other hand, a woman tends to consume a large amount of pro-inflammatory fats, evening primrose oil may help to shift the balance toward less inflammation overall.

Other Herbal Treatments

Herbal treatment for PMS is often focused on regulating hormones throughout the menstrual cycle. Hormone-regulating herbs such as dang gui, black cohosh and chaste tree all have a long history of use in PMS. Since hormones are metabolized through the liver, herbs for liver detoxification are also often included in formulas for PMS. Dandelion and milk thistle are two examples of liver herbs used to treat premenstrual symptoms, especially estrogen dominance, constipation or irritability.

If PMS symptoms are primarily weight gain and water retention, diuretic herbs (such as dandelion leaf) or herbs that stimulate digestion (such as ginger or centaury) can help. If depression and feelings of hopelessness and low self-esteem predominate, St. John's wort is a good choice. Sometimes, PMS symptoms are associated with anemia and fatigue, in which case dang gui, nettles, rehmannia, yellow dock and dandelion may be used.

Chaste Tree

Chaste tree (*Vitex agnus-castus*) is a well-known hormonal regulator with a long history of use in the treatment of PMS symptoms. It is particularly effective in cases of PMS associated with latent hyperprolactinemia (abnormally high prolactin levels) and cyclic mastalgia.

Chaste tree is one of the most thoroughly studied herbs for PMS. It has been shown to consistently reduce psychological and physical PMS symptoms compared to a placebo, especially where breast tenderness and swelling are among the major complaints. Several systematic reviews have all concluded that chaste tree is a safe and effective treatment for PMS.

Other studies have found that chaste tree results in a greater reduction in premenstrual symptoms than vitamin B6 (pyridoxine) and magnesium oxide. Mixed results have been found in studies comparing the use of chaste tree to the use of fluoxetine in premenstrual dysphoric disorder.

The dose of chaste tree used in most clinical trials is 20 to 40 milligrams, once or twice daily.

Dandelion

Both dandelion root and dandelion leaf (*Taraxacum officinale*) are useful in addressing premenstrual symptoms. Dandelion root is a liver herb and gentle laxative that can help in cases of PMS where there is an excess of hormones circulating in the body. In some cases, this excess may be the result of constipation, as hormones that are not excreted through stool get reabsorbed in the intestines and travel back to the liver through a process called enterohepatic circulation. When PMS symptoms include constipation, dandelion root can help.

Dandelion leaf, alone or in combination with dandelion root, is used when premenstrual symptoms include water retention. The leaf supports the movement and elimination of excess fluids, relieving bloating in the abdomen due to water retention. Unlike pharmaceutical diuretics, dandelion leaf and root help the body excrete extra fluid without upsetting the balance of minerals such as potassium. Since dandelion is a source of minerals itself, it does not carry the potential side effects of conventional diuretic drugs.

Although there is very little clinical research on dandelion, it is a generally safe herb with a long history of use.

Ginkgo

Although ginkgo (*Ginkgo biloba*) is not traditionally used for PMS, one small clinical trial looked at its use in treating PMS symptoms and found that taking 40 milligrams of ginkgo, three times a day, during the luteal phase for two cycles significantly reduced overall and psychological symptoms. More research is needed.

St. John's Wort

Since the conventional medical approach to PMS often includes antidepressant drugs, it only makes sense to consider the use of St. John's wort (*Hypericum perforatum*), often seen as an herbal antidepressant.

Two separate randomized, controlled clinical trials found that St. John's wort was significantly more effective than a placebo at reducing behavioral and physical premenstrual symptoms. Case reports and preliminary studies also

support the use of St. John's wort for premenstrual dysphoric disorder, particularly in cases where standard pharmaceutical antidepressants lead to undesirable side effects.

Although St. John's wort appears to be a promising treatment for some of the most common symptoms of PMS, it is not appropriate for everyone because of its well-documented herb–drug interactions.

Common Combinations

- Chaste tree, St. John's wort and evening primrose oil for PMS with cyclic mastalgia and psychoemotional symptoms
- Dandelion leaf and root, white peony and chaste tree for PMS with PCOS and constipation
- Dandelion root, milk thistle, bupleurum and ginger for PMS with digestive symptoms, irritability and estrogen dominance

Conventional Medical Treatments

- Antidepressants for psychoemotional symptoms
- Aspirin, ibuprofen and other non-steroidal anti-inflammatory drugs (NSAIDs) for aches and pains
- Bromocriptine and danazol for breast pain
- Diuretics for weight gain and edema
- Oral contraceptives

Further Reading

Canning S, Waterman M, Orsi N, et al. The efficacy of *Hypericum perforatum* (St. John's wort) for the treatment of premenstrual syndrome: A randomized, double-blind, placebo-controlled trial. *CNS Drugs*, 2010 Mar; 24 (3): 207–25.

Jang SH, Kim DI, Choi MS. Effects and treatment methods of acupuncture and herbal medicine for premenstrual syndrome/premenstrual dysphoric disorder: Systematic review. *BMC Complementary and Alternative Medicine*, 2014 Jan 10; 14: 11.

Kashani L, Saedi N, Akhondzadeh S. Femicomfort in the treatment of premenstrual syndromes: A double-blind, randomized and placebo controlled trial. *Iranian Journal of Psychiatry*, 2010 Spring; 5 (2): 47–50.

Ozgoli G, Selselei EA, Mojab F, Majd HA. A randomized, placebo-controlled trial of *Ginkgo biloba* L. in treatment of premenstrual syndrome. *Journal of Alternative and Complementary Medicine*, 2009 Aug; 15 (8): 845–51.

Romans S, Clarkson R, Einstein G, et al. Mood and the menstrual cycle: A review of prospective data studies. *Gender Medicine*, 2012 Oct; 9 (5): 361–84.

CASE STUDY
PMS

PMS is a very common concern in my practice. Even when it is not the primary health concern, most of my female patients report PMS symptoms when asked. In some cases, these symptoms can feel quite debilitating and interfere with normal daily activities.

Emma came to see me specifically to address symptoms of PMS. While some people experience PMS on some cycles and not others, Emma struggled with symptoms for a full two weeks every month, without fail. Her bloating was so intense that she gained ten pounds each month, only to lose it again once her period started. She had bought what she called a "PMS wardrobe" because she needed to wear clothing one size larger for half the month.

Emma's other major concern was her mood. She found that she was extremely impatient and irritable, lashing out at her partner over the smallest things. This created a cycle of rage and depression in which she felt guilty about her anger and unattractive because of the excess bloating. She often found herself either screaming or crying.

Emma also experienced constipation, fatigue, carbohydrate and sugar cravings, decreased interest in sex and breast pain. She was now thirty-nine and, like many women as they approach menopause, felt that her symptoms had worsened over the past year or so.

We started with changes to diet and lifestyle. I recommended that Emma avoid dairy, coffee, alcohol, sugar and chocolate. She started exercising four times a week, and I helped her develop tools to better manage everyday stressors through breathing, visualization and basic cognitive behavioral techniques. In addition to vitamin B_6, magnesium and evening primrose oil, I recommended an herbal formula that included St. John's wort, chaste tree, dandelion, bupleurum and yarrow.

After one month, Emma noticed substantial differences in her symptoms, especially in terms of her emotional lability. Her partner noticed too, which made a big difference in their relationship. Within three months, she no longer needed her "PMS wardrobe" and happily donated it to charity.

Schellenberg R, Zimmermann C, Drewe J, et al. Dose-dependent efficacy of the *Vitex agnus castus* extract Ze 440 in patients suffering from premenstrual syndrome. *Phytomedicine*, 2012 Nov 15; 19 (14): 1325–31.

van Die MD, Burger HG, Teede HJ, Bone KM. *Vitex agnus-castus* extracts for female reproductive disorders: A systematic review of clinical trials. *Planta Medica*, 2013 May; 79 (7): 562–75.

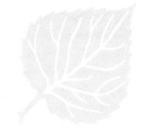

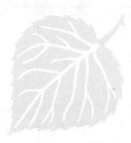

Sexual Dysfunction

Did You Know?

Treatment Strategies

The emotional, psychological and relationship aspects of sexual function cannot be overlooked or underestimated. Sociocultural expectations regarding women, gender, sexuality and aging are also very important in many cases. Depending on the factors contributing to sexual dysfunction, increasing exercise, encouraging intimacy and communication between partners, individual and/ or couples counseling and stress management techniques can be helpful. If medication or other physical conditions are possible causes, treatment strategies should address those factors too.

"Sexual dysfunction" is an umbrella term that describes a variety of difficulties related to sexual activity. The word "dysfunction" often makes people feel like something is horribly wrong or that it is their fault, but it really just refers to sexual health that is less than optimal in some way. In other words, sexual function is completely individual. There's nothing wrong unless the person feels there is. There is no "right" amount of desire or arousal. In practice, I prefer to use positive words even when discussing challenges to health. I first ask patients if they are satisfied with their sex life, and only later follow up with more specific questions about potential challenges or sexual dysfunction.

Sexual dysfunction encompasses everything from low libido to decreased vaginal lubrication to pain during sexual activities to difficulties with orgasm. Sexual function or dysfunction involves many different factors. Physiology, hormonal changes, emotions, sociocultural beliefs, sexuality, gender identity and past history are all factors that contribute to sexual health. Pregnancy and breastfeeding, relationships that are beginning or ending, and stress at work or in other parts of life may all play a role. Certain medications, such as some antidepressants, are known to decrease sexual arousal and response in some people.

Since sexual function naturally fluctuates over each month and over years, determination of sexual function is largely based on the individual's experience and personal perspective. The alignment or misalignment of sexual interest and arousal between partners is also an important factor. Where there is misalignment, it may create strain in relationships. If dissatisfaction persists and causes personal distress, potential causes and treatments should be discussed with a health-care practitioner. Sometimes sexual dysfunction may be diagnosed as hypoactive sexual desire disorder (an older term) or female sexual interest/arousal disorder.

Statistics on the prevalence of sexual dysfunction or dissatisfaction are difficult to find, as many patients find it difficult to talk about the subject with their health-care practitioner and few large-scale surveys have been conducted. Likewise, many health-care practitioners shy away from asking about sexual health satisfaction in a general health screening. Many patients may be missed because of social stigma. A recent survey in the United States concluded that more than 30% of women had lacked sexual interest for several months in the past year. It is estimated that anywhere from 25% to 60% of women experience sexual dysfunction at some point in their lives.

Signs and Symptoms

Dissatisfaction or distress caused by any of the following:

- Decreased sexual arousal, desire or response
- Decreased vaginal lubrication
- Pain during sexual activity
- Difficulty achieving orgasm

Associated Conditions

- Arthritis
- Depression
- Diabetes
- High blood pressure and heart disease
- Hormonal imbalances
- Hypothyroidism
- Menopause
- Pregnancy and breastfeeding

First-Line Herbal Care: GINSENG

Korean ginseng (*Panax ginseng*) has been traditionally used to improve libido and sexual function in both women and men. In traditional Chinese medicine, ginseng is an adaptogen and a stimulating tonic, used to increase energy and stimulate sexual function.

Three studies have looked at the use of ginseng in menopausal women. Two of them showed significant improvements in overall menopausal symptoms compared to a placebo. The other trial looked at the use of ginseng specifically to improve sexual function in postmenopausal women. In this study, women who took 3 grams of ginseng daily reported improvements in sexual arousal compared to a placebo. Animal studies support these findings.

Did You Know?

Energetics

Ginseng's Chinese name, *ren shen*, translates as "person roots." This name refers to the shape of the plant's roots, which are forked in a way that looks like a human body, complete with head, arms and legs. Ginseng looks like a whole person and is used as a tonic, or panacea, to treat the whole person. In fact, the plant's Latin name, *Panax*, comes from the same Greek root as "panacea," which means "all-healing."

In vitro and animal studies show that ginseng may work in a similar way to sildenafil — better known as Viagra — as both increase nitric oxide, which dilates blood vessels and allows for better blood flow through the sexual organs. Other studies suggest that ginseng contains constituents that act indirectly like phytoestrogens.

Other Herbal Treatments

Herbal treatment to improve sexual function can take many forms. While male sexual dysfunction has been reasonably well studied, researchers are just beginning to focus on treatment for female sexual dysfunction. If decreased estrogen and/or testosterone in perimenopause is a factor, phytoestrogenic and/or androgenic herbs are typically recommended, as are herbs that regulate hormones more generally, such as dang gui, black cohosh and chaste tree. See the section on menopause (page 122) for more details.

Adaptogens such as ginseng, shatavari, ashwagandha, maca, schisandra and rhodiola may be helpful when chronic stress has had a negative impact on arousal, desire or endurance. Herbs such as ginkgo improve circulation to help get blood where it is needed — in this case, to sexual organs. When vaginal dryness is the primary concern, I recommend herbal phytoestrogens and natural lubricants containing aloe vera and calendula.

Dang Gui

Dang gui (*Angelica sinensis*) has been called the "female ginseng." As an herb that helps to build and move blood, it works to improve both reproductive and sexual function. Since dang gui is also used for menstrual irregularities, anemia and menopausal symptoms, it is best used when sexual dysfunction occurs alongside one of these other conditions.

No studies have looked specifically at dang gui for sexual function, but traditional Chinese formulas that include dang gui appear to have positive effects on other menopausal symptoms. More research is needed.

Evening Primrose

Evening primrose oil (*Oenothera biennis*), and other oils like borage and coconut oil, contain healthy fats that provide lubrication and soothe inflamed tissues. They can be used on their own or in combination. Sometimes they are infused with other herbs that act as phytoestrogens, like dang gui, or increase circulation, like cinnamon and ginseng.

Two clinical studies on a topical combination product made up of evening primrose oil, borage oil, dang gui root and coleus showed significant improvements in arousal, satisfaction, sensation and ability to orgasm compared to a placebo. Women with healthy sexual function also noted improvements, though less substantial ones than those reported by women who had been diagnosed with sexual dysfunction.

Evening primrose oil and all other oils are compatible with sexual activity, including the use of sex toys. However, oils are not appropriate for use with latex condoms, as the oil will degrade the latex, making the condom ineffective.

Ginkgo

Ginkgo (*Ginkgo biloba*) has been around for millions of years. Ginkgo trees existed during the time of the dinosaurs. Fossils of ginkgo have been found from as early as the Paleolithic era. Ginkgo's longevity on earth is reflected in its traditional medicinal uses to improve memory, circulation throughout the body and overall longevity.

Early clinical studies show that ginkgo may also be useful in improving the longevity of sexual health. In one study, a combination product of ginkgo and muira puama improved sexual desire and satisfaction as well as the ability to reach orgasm and the intensity of orgasm. Other preliminary studies support this use. More research is needed.

Shatavari

Shatavari (*Asparagus racemosus*) is a tonic herb from both the Ayurvedic and Chinese traditions. In Mandarin it is known as *tian men dong*. *Shatavari* is the plant's name in Sanskrit, and many translate it as "having 100 husbands." As a traditional yin tonic, shatavari has been used in both India and China to increase fertility and act as a female sexual tonic. More studies are needed to better understand the specific medicinal uses of shatavari.

Tribulus

The use of tribulus (*Tribulus terrestris*) to increase sexual interest dates back to Avicenna's *Canon of Medicine*, written in 1025. In the Unani medical tradition, tribulus is used to increase libido in both men and women. Ayurvedic practitioners use tribulus to tonify and strengthen the whole body, especially the reproductive tissues.

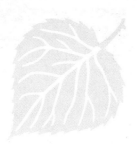

In laboratory studies, tribulus has been shown to increase testosterone in animals. It has also displayed aphrodisiac effects in some animal studies. In a recent study in premenopausal women diagnosed with hypoactive sexual desire disorder, the use of tribulus for four weeks significantly improved desire, arousal, lubrication, satisfaction and pain compared to a placebo.

Common Combinations

- Evening primrose, black cohosh and chaste tree for sexual dysfunction with menopausal symptoms
- Shatavari and dang gui for vaginal dryness and decreased libido with anemia or yin deficiency
- Ginseng and ginkgo for sexual dysfunction related to circulation

Conventional Medical Treatments

Currently there are no pharmaceutical treatments available in the United States or Canada for female hypoactive sexual desire disorder (HSDD) or female sexual interest/arousal disorder (FSIAD). Treatment usually consists of therapy and lubricants or gels to heighten sensation during sex. Hormone replacement therapy may be used orally or vaginally to improve lubrication and decrease discomfort, but it has not been shown to improve desire. In Europe, transdermal testosterone is available for women who experience HSDD after surgical removal of both ovaries. Other pharmaceutical treatments are currently being investigated.

Further Reading

Akhtari E, Raisi F, Keshavarz M, et al. *Tribulus terrestris* for treatment of sexual dysfunction in women: Randomized double-blind placebo-controlled study. *DARU Journal of Pharmaceutical Sciences*, 2014 Apr 28; 22: 40.

Ferguson DM, Steidle CP, Singh GS, et al. Randomized, placebo-controlled, double blind, crossover design trial of the efficacy and safety of Zestra for Women in women with and without female sexual arousal disorder. *Journal of Sex & Marital Therapy*, 2003; 29 Suppl 1: 33–44.

Kim MS, Lim HJ, Yang HJ, et al. Ginseng for managing menopause symptoms: A systematic review of randomized clinical trials. *Journal of Ginseng Research*, 2013 Mar; 37 (1): 30–36.

Kotta S, Ansari SH, Ali J. Exploring scientifically proven herbal aphrodisiacs. *Pharmacognosy Reviews*, 2013 Jan; 7 (13): 1–10.

CASE STUDY
Sexual Dysfunction

Decreased libido is a common concern among parents during the postpartum period. Between the physical exhaustion from giving birth (or supporting someone through labor and delivery), the frequent nighttime waking that is par for the course with newborns, and the emotional focus on caring for the newest member of the family, women (and men!) often say they are too tired to even think about sex. Sometimes the fatigue and decreased desire lasts well into the postpartum period.

Caitlyn, a thirty-five-year-old woman, came to see me with concerns about her sex drive. Her baby was just over a year old and was sleeping through the night, but she still had little interest in or desire for sex. Adding to the problem, when she and her partner did engage in sexual activity, she felt that she produced less vaginal lubrication than before the birth of her child. Overall, she felt exhausted. Sex, she said, just felt like more work.

I encouraged Caitlyn to use a natural lubricant during masturbation and sex play to move away from the idea that she wasn't producing enough lubrication on her own. Normalizing the use of lubricants was transformative in her case (as it is for many people). It is often necessary to dispel self-deprecating and often grossly inaccurate ideas about what a normal amount of vaginal lubrication is, as well as other myths about women and sex. We spent a lot of time talking about her relationship, communication and sexual desire, and how to reignite the desire that she felt had gone by the wayside while caring for an infant.

In addition to sexual health promotion and counseling, I recommended a botanical formula that included schisandra, shatavari, rehmannia and maca. Within a couple of months, Caitlyn felt that she had more energy overall, and she was once again having more regular and more enjoyable sex.

Mazaro-Costa R, Andersen ML, Hachul H, Tufik S. Medicinal plants as alternative treatments for female sexual dysfunction: Utopian vision or possible treatment in climacteric women? *Journal of Sexual Medicine*, 2010 Nov; 7 (11): 3695–714.

Oh KJ, Chae MJ, Lee HS, et al. Effects of Korean red ginseng on sexual arousal in menopausal women: Placebo-controlled, double-blind crossover clinical study. *Journal of Sexual Medicine*, 2010 Apr; 7 (4 Pt 1): 1469–77.

Waynberg J, Brewer S. Effects of Herbal vX on libido and sexual activity in premenopausal and postmenopausal women. *Advances in Therapy*, 2000 Sep–Oct; 17 (5): 255–62.

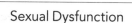

Stress

Stress is hard to describe and sometimes difficult to even identify. Most of us would agree that events like the death of a loved one or a car accident are stressful. It is easy to pick out the extreme examples. Sometimes, however, even joyous events like weddings can be stressful, and many people experience low-grade chronic stress in their daily lives due to concerns about money, health, work or family.

In response to stress in our lives and environments, our bodies activate the sympathetic nervous system through what many know as the "fight or flight" response. Blood vessels in muscles dilate and skin pores open to encourage sweating. The heart beats faster, raising both pulse rate and blood pressure. This brings blood to where it is needed for action and away from areas working on internal regulatory functions such as digestion or reproduction. Pupils and lung airways dilate too, and the breath rate quickens. Stress hormones, such as cortisol and epinephrine, are released and then act to move blood sugar and fats into the bloodstream for immediate use. Blood also flows to the brain, increasing alertness, so that you become more aware of the sounds, smells and sights around you.

This physiological response is designed for acute, short-lived situations like being attacked by a bear. When we experience prolonged or chronic stress, however, this response can lead to high blood pressure, diabetes, hormone dysregulation and obesity. Long-term stress can damage brain cells, impair memory and make us more susceptible to anxiety, depression and addictive behaviors. It leads to premature brain aging. Everyone responds to stress differently, and small amounts of stress can motivate in positive ways. Unfortunately, even low-grade chronic stress can be detrimental to health.

According to surveys conducted by the American Psychological Association, over 20% of Americans feel that they are experiencing extreme stress. People of color, people who identify as LGBT and people of lower socioeconomic status experience more stress. Women are more likely than men to report stress, especially higher levels of stress, as well as physical symptoms of stress. Overall, women say their degree of stress is on the rise, and married women report more stress than single women. All women appear to connect with family and friends more than men do, using these social supports as a strategy for managing stress.

Signs and Symptoms

In general, symptoms are often vague and vary from one person to the next. The symptoms of chronic stress are often condensed into the saying "wired and tired" but may include some or all of the following:

- Fatigue, lack of motivation or interest
- Emotional or muscular tension
- Headaches
- Anxiety or depression

- Poor memory or concentration
- Change in appetite
- Upset stomach or indigestion
- Difficulty sleeping, insomnia

Associated Conditions

- Addiction
- Anxiety
- Depression
- Diabetes
- High blood pressure
- Hypothyroidism

- Maldigestion
- Obesity
- Polycystic ovarian syndrome (PCOS)
- Sexual dysfunction

First-Line Herbal Care: RHODIOLA

Rhodiola (*Rhodiola rosea*) is an herb that grows in difficult climates and helps people adapt to environmental, physical and emotional stress. It is native to cold, mountainous regions and sea cliffs at high altitudes in Scandinavia, Russia and Tibet. Rhodiola has traditionally been used to mitigate the negative effects of living at high altitudes in cold climates, helping people to better use the limited oxygen available. The Vikings used it to increase physical endurance; in Siberia, it was used by newlyweds to increase fertility.

Some studies on rhodiola have confirmed its effectiveness in improving physical performance. One placebo-controlled trial showed that rhodiola plus starch delayed time to exhaustion and increased oxygen intake during strenuous physical exercise compared to starch alone. Another trial showed that rhodiola hastened muscle recovery after exercise. Other studies have failed to show significant effects compared to a placebo.

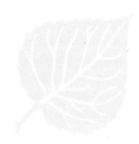

Caution

The combination of rhodiola with ginseng may cause headaches and overstimulation in some people. From a traditional Chinese medicine perspective, both herbs are more yang in nature. They are best paired with yin adaptogens for balance, especially when taken long-term.

In terms of mental performance, research on rhodiola has found that it conveys significant improvements in measures of attention and fatigue, or "burnout." One study on students during examination periods found that rhodiola improved their hand–eye coordination and delayed mental fatigue. A study on night-shift workers found that rhodiola enhanced their visual perception, short-term memory and perception of order compared to a placebo.

As for its role in reducing stress, animal models show that rhodiola suppresses a number of stress-activated molecules, including cortisol. Various studies have looked at different physical manifestations of stress, but there is wide variability among the studies in terms of the dosage used, who was taking the rhodiola and what was measured. This lack of consistency makes it difficult to state conclusively whether rhodiola is effective for stress.

In one open-label trial, a combination of rhodiola, eleuthero and schisandra improved cardiovascular responses to stress. In other studies, the combination also reduced fatigue, helped cosmonauts adjust to new environments and helped maintain high performance standards in extreme work situations.

The dosage of rhodiola in clinical studies has ranged from 150 milligrams per day to over 1,500 milligrams per day, which suggests a wide margin of safe use. There are few side effects reported from taking rhodiola. Minor side effects include headaches and insomnia.

Did You Know?

Take a Break

It is often important to take a break from herbal adaptogens every four to eight weeks, or to switch the herbs used, to avoid side effects.

Other Herbal Treatments

Herbal treatment to address chronic stress relies heavily on adaptogens and nervines. Adaptogens help people better adapt to their environment, decrease exaggerated stress responses and increase vitality and resistance to stress. They prevent and delay exhaustion. Many adaptogens help to decrease blood sugar and cortisol and increase physical endurance. Nervines support the work of adaptogens by relieving anxiety and tension. See the sections on anxiety (page 51) and depression (page 77) for details.

Ashwagandha

Ashwagandha (*Withania somnifera*) is often called "Indian ginseng" because it has been used as a tonic and adaptogen in India the way ginseng has been used in China. In Ayurvedic medicine, ashwagandha is considered a *rasayana* herb: a rejuvenating and tonifying herb used to conserve and revive youthfulness and increase longevity. It has historically been used for stress, fatigue, infertility and insomnia and to generally promote health and longevity.

Preclinical and animal studies support the use of ashwagandha as an adaptogen. In these trials, ashwagandha appears to produce significant anti-stress activity, improve memory and learning, and protect the body from oxidative damage.

Clinical trials are lacking in number, but the few conducted appear to be positive. In one, participants were given either 300 milligrams of ashwagandha or a matched placebo, twice daily. After sixty days of treatment, the ashwagandha group had significantly lower scores on the perceived stress scale, representing a 44% reduction in their stress. Their scores on the General Health Questionnaire were also significantly decreased. In addition, the ashwagandha group had significantly lower cortisol scores compared to baseline. More trials are needed to confirm these results.

Eleuthero

Eleuthero (*Eleutherococcus senticosus*), also known as Siberian ginseng, is another plant native to northern, cold climates in China and Siberia. Like rhodiola, it has been used as a tonic for fatigue and to build resistance to stress.

Animal studies support the traditional use of eleuthero to increase physical endurance, improve cognition and prevent the long-term effects of stress. In clinical studies, eleuthero has been shown to significantly improve memory, fatigue, stamina, mood and other cognitive functions. In patients with chronic fatigue, eleuthero substantially reduced physical and mental fatigue compared to a placebo. These effects were more pronounced in a sub-group of people with mild to moderate fatigue. After two months the effects diminished, showing that eleuthero's effects may fade over time.

Schisandra

Schisandra (*Schisandra chinensis*) is known in traditional Chinese medicine as *wu wei zi*, or "five-flavored seed," referring to the fact that the berries contain all five flavors: sweet, salty, sour, bitter and pungent. Chinese medical practitioners use schisandra to calm the spirit and prevent the loss of fluids. It has long been considered an aphrodisiac, increasing sexual desire by improving overall health. Schisandra has also been used to decrease the side effects of drugs such as amitriptyline, to improve social

markers in schizophrenics, to help addicts safely withdraw from opiate use and to treat chronic hepatitis C.

Pharmacological and animal studies demonstrate that schisandra helps to modulate the stress response and acts as a detoxifier for the liver. Schisandra has also been shown to reduce oxidative stress in schizophrenics. Older Russian studies and clinical experience suggest that schisandra may improve stress symptoms such as fatigue, weakness and decreased physical performance and endurance. More research is need to confirm these results.

Common Combinations

- Rhodiola, ginkgo and eleuthero to improve memory and overall mental capacity
- Rhodiola, eleuthero and schisandra to increase physical endurance
- Schisandra and ashwagandha for stress with insomnia and/or depression

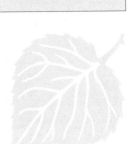

Conventional Medical Treatments

There are no pharmaceutical treatments available for treating stress, but medical doctors may prescribe antianxiety and/or antidepressant medications. Exercise and behavioral and lifestyle changes are generally recommended. Stress reduction techniques, such as mindfulness, may be suggested by some medical doctors.

Further Reading

Chandrasekhar K, Kapoor J, Anishetty S. A prospective, randomized double-blind, placebo-controlled study of safety and efficacy of a high-concentration full-spectrum extract of ashwagandha root in reducing stress and anxiety in adults. *Indian Journal of Psychological Medicine*, 2012 Jul; 34 (3): 255–62.

Hung SK, Perry R, Ernst E. The effectiveness and efficacy of *Rhodiola rosea* L.: A systematic review of randomized clinical trials. *Phytomedicine*, 2011 Feb 15; 18 (4): 235–44.

Ishaque S, Shamseer L, Bukutu C, Vohra S. *Rhodiola rosea* for physical and mental fatigue: A systematic review. *BMC Complementary and Alternative Medicine*, 2012 May 29; 12: 70.

Panossian AG. Adaptogens in mental and behavioral disorders. *Psychiatric Clinics of North America*, 2013 Mar; 36 (1): 49–64.

Ross SM. *Rhodiola rosea* (SHR-5), Part I: A proprietary root extract of *Rhodiola rosea* is found to be effective in the treatment of stress-related fatigue. *Holistic Nursing Practice*, 2014 Mar–Apr; 28 (2): 149–54.

Urinary Tract Infections

Urinary tract infections (UTIs) are an uncomfortable reality for many women. More than 50% of women will experience at least one UTI by their mid-thirties. Most of the time, UTIs are acute, short-lived illnesses. Sometimes, however, they can recur time and time again, leading to a cycle of chronic recurring infection and pelvic pain. Since 30% to 40% of UTIs return within six months of the initial infection, even after treatment with antibiotics, women often come to see me to break the cycle of infection and antibiotic use.

Urinary tract infections are much more common in women than in men — up to fifty times more common. Anatomy and physiology are primarily to blame. The urethral opening is physically closer to the anus in women than men. Bacteria from the anus can travel to the urethra, disrupting its normal bacterial flora and causing an infection. The urethra itself is also shorter, which means that bacteria need travel only a short distance before infecting the bladder. *Escherichia coli* (*E. coli*) is the most common cause of UTIs, accounting for 75% to 95% of cases.

Signs and Symptoms

- Burning or pain before, during or after urination
- Increased urinary frequency or urgency to urinate
- Pressure, cramping or pain in the lower abdomen and pelvis
- Cloudy, strong-smelling or discolored urine
- Pain during sexual activity
- Back pain, fever, chills and/or nausea (which can indicate that the infection has moved to the kidneys)

Associated Conditions

- Diabetes
- Menopause
- Pregnancy
- Sexually transmitted infections

First-Line Herbal Care: CRANBERRY

Researchers tend to agree that cranberry (*Vaccinium macrocarpon*) is the most effective option for treating women with recurrent UTIs. Cranberry products may need to be taken long-term, for up to a year, before maximum benefits are seen. Because sugar has been shown to increase infection by encouraging bacteria to replicate (and generally suppresses immune function), sugar-free juices or extracts are best.

A 2012 systematic review on cranberry juice, tablets and capsules found that, overall, there was no significant decrease in the occurrence of UTIs when cranberry products were taken preventatively. However, the studies did not account for large differences in the concentration of proanthocyanidins, widely recognized as the key chemical constituent responsible for protecting against adherence of bacteria in the urinary tract. Many juices, tablets and capsules fall very short of the recommended daily dose of proanthocyanidins (72 milligrams per day) found in studies to be most effective.

A 2011 meta-analysis concluded that cranberry products were very effective in reducing the occurrence of UTIs, especially for women with recurrent UTIs. The results were greatest in people who took higher doses of cranberry.

The recommended dose is 1 cup (250 mL) of cranberry juice three times daily, 50 milliliters of unsweetened cranberry concentrate three times daily, 50 grams of dried cranberries three times daily or 400 milligrams of cranberry extract three times daily.

Hygiene and Other Lifestyle Changes

As for many conditions, an ounce of prevention is worth a pound of cure. Wiping toward the back (urethra to anus) after urination will prevent the potential transfer of fecal matter to the urethra. Washing hands, sex toys or genitals and changing condoms or gloves when moving from anal play to vaginal play is another important way to prevent bacterial transfer.

Since many women experience UTIs after sexual activity, using lubrication to avoid irritating the urethral opening and urinating immediately after sex can help flush bacteria out of the urethra. Increasing intake of water and other fluids helps to dilute and flush out bacteria. Other recommendations include avoiding caffeine, wearing cotton underwear, sleeping naked and eliminating the use of irritating soaps, body washes or spermicides. Certain nutritional supplements are also helpful, including d-mannose, a sugar that prevents *E. coli* from adhering to cell walls (this may sound counterintuitive, but it's true).

Other Herbal Treatments

Diuretic herbs, such as yarrow, nettles and dandelion leaf, help to encourage the flushing of bacteria. I usually recommend taking these as teas, to increase overall fluid intake at the same time. Antimicrobial herbs and those that prevent bacteria from sticking to the walls of the urethra, such as uva ursi, are particularly useful in treating UTIs.

Corn Silk

While most people compost the silky hairs that surround a corn of cob when they remove the husk before cooking or eating, herbalists save that silk to treat UTIs and other irritations to the urethra or ureters.

Traditionally, corn silk (*Zea mays*) is believed to soothe the urinary tract during a UTI. It is also seen as a urinary sedative or painkiller. It has long been added to formulas to help ease the passage of urine during a UTI as the infection is being resolved.

In vitro studies have shown that corn silk decreases adhesion of *E. coli* bacteria on bladder cell surfaces. In one small open-label trial, a corn silk infusion significantly decreased urinary symptoms, such as frequency, urgency and pain, as well as laboratory signs of UTIs.

Dandelion

Dandelion leaf (*Taraxacum officinale*) is an excellent herbal diuretic used in many different conditions, from high blood pressure to constipation to acne to urinary tract infections. I often wonder if its wide range of uses is reflected in how readily available it is: dandelion can be found on almost every continent, often growing in cracks in the sidewalk or along roadsides.

Dandelion's diuretic action is reflected in its French name, *pissenlit*, literally meaning "urine in bed." In vitro studies and one small human study support dandelion's diuretic use. The resulting increase in urinary frequency helps to flush the urinary system during an infection, encouraging faster resolution. It has also been shown to decrease the ability of bacteria to stick to bladder cells in vitro.

Goldenseal

Goldenseal (*Hydrastis canadensis*), one of several herbs that contains berberine, has an affinity for mucous membranes in general, and the mucous membranes of the genitourinary tract in particular. It restores tone and helps to recreate a healthy barrier on sensitive tissues like the urethra and bladder walls.

Goldenseal and other berberine-containing herbs, such as Oregon grape root, barberry and coptis, are frequently used at the first sign of a UTI. In vitro research has shown that berberine interferes with the ability of bacteria to adhere. When it comes in contact with *E. coli*, berberine appears to stop the bacteria from forming little hair-like appendages, called fimbriae, that help it to stick to bladder cell walls. Berberine has also been found to have antimicrobial effects against a number of bacteria, including *E. coli*, *Staphylococcus aureus* and *Pseudomonas aeruginosa*. It even appears to work against resistant strains.

In part, berberine's action may be connected to its ability to treat *E. coli*–related diarrhea. Human studies have shown that berberine resolves diarrhea caused by *E. coli* faster than a placebo, making a transfer of bacteria from the anus to the urethra less likely.

Caution

Because nettles pull minerals — and heavy metals — out of the soil, care should be taken when sourcing them. Whether you are buying nettles or wildcrafting them (harvesting them from the wild), be cautious about their soil quality and growing conditions. Don't pick nettles from land that is known to be toxic or that was previously used for industrial purposes.

Nettle

Nettle (*Urtica dioica*), like dandelion, has a long history of use for conditions of the urinary tract. Both herbs are diuretics that increase the output of urine while replenishing minerals, such as potassium, that are usually depleted by pharmaceutical diuretics.

In vitro studies show that nettle in the presence of *E. coli* reduces the ability of the bacteria to move and helps break down biofilms that protect the bacteria from being destroyed. More studies are needed to better understand how nettles work in the treatment of UTIs.

Uva Ursi

Uva ursi (*Arctostaphylos uva-ursi*), also known as bearberry, is a low-growing plant native to North America and a cousin of cranberry, another plant used in urinary tract infections. Related species are also found in Europe and Asia. Uva ursi's colloquial name derives from the fact that bears are partial to eating it. It is one of my favorite herbs for the treatment of UTIs, though it is the leaf, not the berry, that is used medicinally.

The main antimicrobial constituent in uva ursi appears to be arbutoside, which converts to hydroquinone in the body. As long as urine is sufficiently alkaline, hydroquinone is able to act directly as an antimicrobial in the urinary tract. If the urine isn't alkaline enough to allow uva ursi to work, decreasing acidic foods and adding alkalizing foods and supplements can help. Uva ursi also contains tannins that reduce inflammation and tissue irritation.

Nettle Flower Essence

Nettle flower essence is used when someone feels angry and powerless to change a situation, particularly one that is stressful and relates to close relationships. This is a good reminder of the mental–emotional connection in urinary tract infections. UTIs can be a manifestation of unresolved or unexpressed anger or irritation, especially anger related to sexual relationships. This irritation parallels the physical pain and inflammation during urination. On the flip side, experiencing a UTI may lead to feelings of anger or resentment.

In the Cree tradition, nettles are related to a feeling of being taken for granted and a subsequent reaction of anger. In my clinical experience, nettle is best used when someone with a UTI also expresses anger, powerlessness or resentment.

Although uva ursi is traditionally used acutely to treat UTIs, one double-blind study investigated the long-term use of uva ursi and dandelion leaf to prevent recurrent cystitis. After one year of use, none of the participants who took uva ursi and dandelion leaf had experienced a UTI. Among those taking a placebo, over 20% had experienced at least one bladder infection during the twelve-month period.

Common Combinations

- Uva ursi, corn silk and goldenseal for acute or chronic UTIs
- Nettle, dandelion leaf and cranberry to gently prevent recurrence

Conventional Medical Treatments

- Antibiotics

Further Reading

Head KA. Natural approaches to prevention and treatment of infections of the lower urinary tract. *Alternative Medicine Review*, 2008 Sep; 13 (3): 227–44.

Howell AB, Botto H, Combescure C, et al. Dosage effect on uropathogenic *Escherichia coli* anti-adhesion activity in urine following consumption of cranberry powder standardized for proanthocyanidin content: A multicentric randomized double blind study. *BMC Infectious Diseases*, 2010 Apr 14; 10: 94.

Jepson RG, Williams G, Craig JC. Cranberries for preventing urinary tract infections. *Cochrane Database of Systematic Reviews*. 2012 Oct 17; 10: CD001321.

Folklore

New World and Old World Alike

Uva ursi has been used for thousands of years — and independently by healers separated by oceans and thousands of miles — to treat urinary tract conditions. Native Americans used it for urinary tract and kidney infections. Legend says that Marco Polo learned about using uva ursi for kidney and urinary tract infections from Chinese physicians.

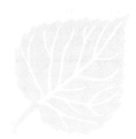

Rossi R, Porta S, Canovi B. Overview on cranberry and urinary tract infections in females. *Journal of Clinical Gastroenterology*, 2010 Sep; 44 Suppl 1: S61–62.

Wang CH, Fang CC, Chen NC, et al. Cranberry-containing products for prevention of urinary tract infections in susceptible populations: A systematic review and meta-analysis of randomized controlled trials. *Archives of Internal Medicine*, 2012 Jul 9; 172 (13): 988–96.

Wojnicz D, Kucharska AZ, Sokół-Łętowska A, et al. Medicinal plants extracts affect virulence factors expression and biofilm formation by the uropathogenic *Escherichia coli*. *Urological Research*, 2012 Dec; 40 (6): 683–97.

CASE STUDY
Urinary Tract Infections

A single urinary tract infection is bad enough, but they are even worse when they have a tendency to recur. Sexual activity can often trigger an acute infection, as in Isabella's case. Before she came to see me, the twenty-two-year-old had experienced three UTIs in the preceding six months, all treated with antibiotics. Having already identified sex as a potential trigger, she was careful to urinate after intercourse but was still getting UTIs.

Two days before our first appointment, Isabella had had sex with an ex-partner and was already feeling the symptoms of infection. The sex had been unexpected, and she felt ashamed and angry about giving in to his desires even though it wasn't truly what she wanted. She had felt pressured to have sex, and now she felt angry as a result. This pressure and anger were mirrored in her physical symptoms: she felt pressure around her urinary meatus (the external opening of the urethra) and was experiencing pain at the end of urination. She also felt like she couldn't completely empty her bladder. A quick urine test in my office showed signs of an acute infection.

I recommended an herbal tea with uva ursi, corn silk, goldenrod and yarrow, as well as a homeopathic remedy made from delphinium flowers (staphysagria). Isabella also took d-mannose and cranberry supplements. Her symptoms subsided quickly, and repeat urine testing was negative. She continued with the herbal tea for another two weeks while she worked on setting healthy boundaries with her ex-partner. She kept taking the cranberry supplements for another three months, to prevent a future infection. As of a year later, she hadn't gotten another UTI.

Vaginitis

Vaginitis is a common inflammatory condition of the vagina that many women struggle with over and over again. Vaginitis encompasses different infections caused by a variety of bacteria, fungi and parasites. Decreased estrogen after menopause can also lead to vaginitis (this is called atrophic vaginitis).

The microenvironment and bacterial flora of the vagina vary over time, at different life stages and from one person to another. The vaginal flora is incredibly resilient, keeping infections at bay and keeping the pH, or acidity level, stable and normal. Premenopausal women normally have a vaginal pH of somewhere between 3.8 and 4.5. Nonetheless, certain things can upset the ecosystem balance, leading to vaginitis. Antibiotics and spermicides can trigger vaginal infections by changing the pH of the vagina. Semen can also affect the pH level of the vagina and may be a contributing factor in some cases. Personal care products, such as perfumed soaps, douches and scented detergents, and menstrual care products (feminine hygiene products) can also cause irritation and infection. Oral contraceptives, intrauterine devices (IUDs), pregnancy, sexually transmitted infections and stress can all create imbalances in the vaginal environment.

When they experience vulvar itchiness and redness, most women blame a yeast infection (vaginal candidiasis, caused by the fungus *Candida albicans*). In fact, approximately 75% of women will experience at least one bout of vaginal candidiasis in their lifetime. About half of those women will have at least one recurrence. Candida infections can lead to infection in other parts of the body, including the mouth, folds of the skin and nails. When candida is present in the mouth, it is called thrush. Because of widespread use of antifungal medications for both treatment and prevention, resistance to commonly used drugs is becoming more and more common.

Bacterial vaginosis is caused by an overgrowth of some of the bacteria normally found in the vagina in smaller quantities. When certain bacteria overtake others, the imbalance leads to vaginitis. Bacterial vaginosis is the most common cause of vaginitis, associated with 40% to 50% of all cases, but many people don't even know they have it, as it is frequently asymptomatic.

Trichomoniasis, a sexually transmitted infection caused by the parasite *Trichomonas vaginalis*, also causes vaginitis.

Did You Know?

Hygiene and Other Lifestyle Changes

Avoiding the use of tampons and perfumed personal care products reduces irritation in bacterial, fungal and parasitic cases. Bacteria and fungi thrive in dark, moist environments, so it is very important to keep the vagina dry with thorough toweling after showering, bathing or swimming, and by wearing breathable cotton underwear. Vaginal probiotics can replenish healthy vaginal bacteria or shift the balance back to normal in cases of bacterial vaginosis. The use of vaginal lubricants and probiotics can also help prevent infection and can acidify the vagina in postmenopausal atrophic vaginitis.

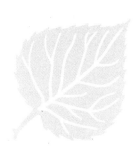

Signs and Symptoms

- Itchiness, irritation, burning or discomfort on the inside or outside of the vagina
- A change in the color, consistency or smell of vaginal discharge: white, thick, curdled, cottage cheese–like discharge is associated with candida infections; grayish, thick, foul-smelling discharge is associated with bacterial vaginosis (many people describe the smell as "fishy"); greenish yellow frothy discharge is associated with *Trichomonas*
- Painful urination
- Pain during sexual activity
- Spotting or light bleeding

Associated Conditions

- Diabetes
- Menopause
- Oral contraceptive use
- Pregnancy
- Sexually transmitted infections

First-Line Herbal Care: GARLIC

Since its antimicrobial properties have been well documented for millennia, garlic (*Allium sativum*) has historically been used both topically and orally to treat vaginal infections, regardless of the cause.

A recent randomized trial of 120 women compared garlic and metronidazole in the treatment of bacterial vaginosis and found that garlic was significantly more effective in terms of clinical improvement of symptoms. In terms of laboratory improvement and overall improvement, garlic and metronidazole worked equally well. Although garlic was associated with nausea and heartburn, the side effects of metronidazole were significantly greater. The dose of garlic in the trial was 1 gram of garlic powder in tablet form, twice daily for seven days.

In another recent study on women without symptoms but with candida found in laboratory testing, oral garlic was not found to be effective at preventing a symptomatic infection when taken for fourteen days premenstrually.

The authors noted that future studies should consider topical applications or longer time spans.

A small, older study compared garlic and thyme in a vaginal cream to clotrimazole cream in premenopausal women with vaginal yeast infections. The garlic-thyme cream inserted for seven nights was found to be just as effective as the clotrimazole cream applied for the same duration. In addition, the women using the clotrimazole cream complained of vaginal redness and irritation, whereas the women using the garlic-thyme cream did not.

In vitro, garlic at a moderate to high dosage has been shown to be as effective as metronidazole in eradicating *Trichomonas*. The researchers suggested that garlic taken orally may be used in the treatment of *Trichomonas vaginalis* instead of metronidazole, which is known to have unpleasant side effects.

A Natural Antibiotic

Garlic is well known to repel bacteria and fungi (and even vampires). It has been given nicknames like "Russian penicillin" in honor of its broad-spectrum use in fighting infections and its widespread use in Russia during the Second World War, even once penicillin was available. Garlic was mentioned in the Vedas of ancient India and was widely used in ancient China and Egypt. Hippocrates (one of the major figures in the history of medicine, after whom the Hippocratic Oath is named) wrote about the use of garlic in treating intestinal parasites. Much later, Louis Pasteur extolled garlic's abilities to kill bacteria, even bacteria that appeared resistant to other forms of treatment.

Other Herbal Treatments

Herbal treatment of vaginitis is focused on resolving the infection and decreasing the amount of abnormal vaginal discharge through the use of antibacterial and antifungal herbs such as goldenseal and tea tree oil. Astringent herbs help to decrease discharge and restore normal tone to vaginal tissues. If vaginitis is due to tissue atrophy, as is common after menopause, topical lubrication with calendula or evening primrose may be helpful. See the sections on menopause (page 122) and sexual dysfunction (page 180) for more details.

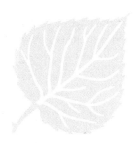

Goldenseal

Goldenseal (*Hydrastis canadensis*) has antiseptic, antimicrobial and astringent properties and is specifically indicated for chronic recurrent vaginitis. It has been used in the treatment of vaginitis of all kinds, including sexually transmitted infections such as gonorrhea. Goldenseal is a good choice when there is profuse vaginal discharge, as it contains tannins that help to reduce secretions. It can be applied externally, as a topical powder, added to a sitz bath or included as an ingredient in an herbal suppository.

No clinical studies have been conducted on goldenseal for vaginitis. Numerous in vitro studies, however, support the use of goldenseal in vaginal *Candida albicans* and *Trichomonas vaginalis* infections. In both cases, berberine, one of the main active constituents of goldenseal, has been found to be comparable to standard pharmaceutical treatment. Berberine also appears to act synergistically with miconazole and fluconazole in the treatment of drug-resistant candida infections.

CASE STUDY
Vaginitis

Fatima came to see me for help with long-standing vaginitis. Now forty-five, she had experienced symptoms off and on for a couple of years. She had taken many courses of antifungal vaginal suppositories, but they seemed to work only temporarily; within a couple of weeks, she would notice the return of a thick, grayish, smelly vaginal discharge. She felt very self-conscious about the smell. She exclusively wore pants and kept her legs close together at all times, as she was worried that people would notice. Unsurprisingly, her sex life had been affected: she didn't want to start dating when she knew she would eventually have to disclose her ongoing infection.

A vaginal culture swab confirmed my working diagnosis of bacterial vaginosis. I recommended that Fatima alternate between diluted tea tree oil and vaginal probiotic suppositories to rebalance her vaginal flora. In addition, she removed all added sugar from her diet and increased her intake of raw garlic.

When I saw Fatima two months later, she exclaimed that her life had changed dramatically. She was wearing skirts again and wasn't worried about vaginal odor. She had even gone on a date the week before. Another vaginal culture swab confirmed what she already knew: she no longer had bacterial vaginosis.

Tea Tree Oil

Tea tree oil (*Melaleuca alternifolia*) has demonstrated antibacterial, antiparasitic and antifungal properties in vitro. It has also been shown to be particularly effective against drug-resistant strains and the specific bacteria associated with bacterial vaginosis. These findings support the traditional use of external and internal vaginal applications of plants high in volatile oils, such as tea tree, to treat vaginitis and other infections.

Common Combinations

- Garlic, calendula, goldenseal and tea tree oil for bacterial, fungal or parasitic vaginitis
- Calendula and aloe vera for atrophic vaginitis

Conventional Medical Treatments

- Clotrimazole
- Fluconazole
- Metronidazole
- Miconazole
- Vaginal estrogen creams (for atrophic vaginitis)

Further Reading

Bahadoran P, Rokni FK, Fahami F. Investigating the therapeutic effect of vaginal cream containing garlic and thyme compared to clotrimazole cream for the treatment of mycotic vaginitis. *Iranian Journal of Nursing and Midwifery Research*, 2010 Dec; 15 (Suppl 1): 343–49.

Dhamgaye S, Devaux F, Vandeputte P, et al. Molecular mechanisms of action of herbal antifungal alkaloid berberine, in *Candida albicans*. PLoS One, 2014 Aug 8; 9 (8): e104554.

Ibrahim AN. Comparison of in vitro activity of metronidazole and garlic-based product (Tomex®) on *Trichomonas vaginalis*. *Parasitology Research*, 2013 May; 112 (5): 2063–67.

Mohammadzadeh F, Dolatian M, Jorjani M, et al. Comparing the therapeutic effects of garlic tablet and oral metronidazole on bacterial vaginosis: A randomized controlled clinical trial. *Iranian Red Crescent Medical Journal*, 2014 Jul; 16 (7): e19118.

Watson CJ, Grando D, Fairley CK, et al. The effects of oral garlic on vaginal candida colony counts: A randomised placebo controlled double-blind trial. *BJOG: An International Journal of Obstetrics and Gynaecology*, 2014 Mar; 121 (4): 498–506.

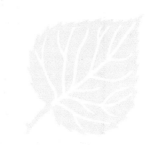

Part 3

Women's Medicinal Herbs

🍃 Ashwagandha

Current Medicinal Uses

In Ayurvedic medicine, ashwagandha is viewed as a general tonic, or *rasayana*, used to support learning and improve memory, aid with recovery from illness, ward against premature aging and promote fertility. In other herbal traditions, ashwagandha is considered an adaptogen, an herb that helps one adapt to the physical consequences of chronic stress and aging. It has also been used to promote healthy immune system responses, treat asthma and other chronic respiratory conditions, relieve arthritis pain and support normal thyroid function. Recently, research has shown that ashwagandha can play an important role in adjunctive cancer care.

History and Energetics

The name "ashwagandha" comes from Sanskrit and can be roughly translated as "the smell and strength of a horse." It's certainly true that most people would find its aroma quite unpleasant. Historical sources agree that the reference to a horse's strength is related to ashwagandha's ability to improve sexual function in both men and women.

Ashwagandha has often been compared to tonic herbs from other cultures and is sometimes called "Indian ginseng." Like ginseng and other *rasayana* herbs, it supports healthy aging, imbuing users with the muscle strength, vitality, mental faculties and sexual stamina of their younger self.

Ashwagandha's Latin species name, *somnifera*, means "sleep-inducing," an indication of its use in promoting healthy sleep patterns and relieving insomnia.

In Ayurvedic medicine, ashwagandha's bitter, pungent taste works to reduce vata and kapha as needed. Ashwagandha has an affinity for the bone marrow, nervous, reproductive and respiratory systems, and increases strength, vitality, intellect and sexual potency.

Research Evidence

Interest in ashwagandha outside of India is relatively recent. As a result, research into its medicinal uses is sparse but beginning to build. Human studies have seen positive results for the use of ashwagandha in increasing cognitive function in patients with bipolar disorder and improving cholesterol and blood glucose levels in people with diabetes and schizophrenia.

Latin name
- *Withania somnifera*

Part Used
- Root

Common Combinations
- **For anxiety and/or insomnia:** Passionflower, lavender and valerian
- **For sexual dysfunction:** Shatavari and ginseng
- **For iodine-deficiency hypothyroidism:** Seaweed
- **For stress management:** Eleuthero and schisandra

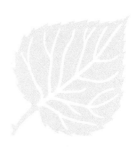

Anxiety and Stress

A recent review of five human clinical trials found that ashwagandha significantly reduced both anxiety and stress levels compared to controls. In one of these studies, both perceived levels of stress and cortisol levels in the blood were substantially lowered. Similarly, in the other trials, the participants experienced decreased levels of stress and anxiety. These results are promising. Further high-quality studies will help bolster the evidence supporting the use of ashwagandha in anxiety and stress.

Cancer

Ashwagandha has been shown to reduce fatigue in women undergoing chemotherapy for breast cancer. Animal and in vitro studies have demonstrated additional anticancer effects. In mice, ashwagandha increased white blood cell markers negatively affected by chemotherapeutic drugs. In vitro, the use of ashwagandha led to apoptosis (the death of cancer cells) in various tissues, without affecting normal cells.

Hypothyroidism

In animal studies, ashwagandha appears to increase the production of thyroid hormones. One case study reported a case of thyrotoxicosis (an overload of thyroid hormones, also known as hyperthyroidism) in a woman taking an ashwagandha supplement.

In a study investigating the potential cognitive-enhancing abilities of ashwagandha for people with bipolar disorder, the researchers noted that ashwagandha may increase levels of thyroxine (T4), the major form of thyroid hormone secreted into the blood. Since this study tested thyroid hormone levels only for safety reasons, conclusions cannot be made about ashwagandha's potential thyroid effects. More human clinical studies should be conducted to confirm the potential role of ashwagandha in treating hypothyroidism.

Sexual Dysfunction

Traditionally, ashwagandha has been considered an aphrodisiac. In this regard, it has been used mostly to improve sexual function and sperm parameters in men. Some preliminary research supports the use of ashwagandha in treating low sperm counts and erectile dysfunction in men.

Did You Know?

***Rasayana* Herbs**

In Sanskrit, *rasayana* means "path of essence." The term refers to the science of restoring youthfulness and promoting longevity through the use of medicines. *Rasayana* herbs, such as ashwagandha, shatavari and amla, are used to return someone to a state of health, and then maintain that health. These herbs are often combined with ghee and honey in a traditional preparation called *chyawanprash*.

To date, no research has been undertaken to look at how ashwagandha might impact sexual arousal or desire in women. However, adaptogens such as ashwagandha have traditionally been used to improve sexual function in women, especially where stress and/or fatigue are contributing factors.

Health Condition	Level of Scientific Evidence
Anxiety and stress	Fair
Cancer	Fair
Hypothyroidism	Poor
Sexual dysfunction	Fair for men; poor for women

Safety

Overall, ashwagandha is a safe herb. Caution is advised in pregnancy, as ashwagandha's safety has not yet been determined and it can act as an emmenagogue in larger doses. Women with hyperthyroidism should avoid this herb, as it has been linked to hyperthyroidism in a handful of cases.

Further Reading

Agnihotri AP, Sontakke SD, Thawani VR, et al. Effects of *Withania somnifera* in patients of schizophrenia: A randomized, double blind, placebo controlled pilot trial study. *Indian Journal of Pharmacology*, 2013 Jul–Aug; 45 (4): 417–18.

Biswal BM, Sulaiman SA, Ismail HC, et al. Effect of *Withania somnifera* (ashwagandha) on the development of chemotherapy-induced fatigue and quality of life in breast cancer patients. *Integrative Cancer Therapies*, 2013 Jul; 12 (4): 312–22.

Gannon JM, Forrest PE, Roy Chengappa KN. Subtle changes in thyroid indices during a placebo-controlled study of an extract of *Withania somnifera* in persons with bipolar disorder. *Journal of Ayurveda and Integrative Medicine*, 2014 Oct–Dec; 5 (4): 241–45.

Jatwa R, Kar A. Amelioration of metformin-induced hypothyroidism by *Withania somnifera* and *Bauhinia purpurea* extracts in type 2 diabetic mice. *Phytotherapy Research*, 2009 Aug; 23 (8): 1140–45.

Pratte MA, Nanavati KB, Young V, Morley CP. An alternative treatment for anxiety: A systematic review of human trial results reported for the Ayurvedic herb ashwagandha (*Withania somnifera*). *Journal of Alternative and Complementary Medicine*, 2014 Dec; 20 (12): 901–8.

Did You Know?

Nightshades

Ashwagandha is also known as winter cherry and is a member of the nightshade family of plants, which includes tomatoes, potatoes, belladonna (*Atropa belladonna*) and bittersweet nightshade (*Solanum dulcamara*), a poisonous invasive plant found growing throughout North America.

Did You Know?

Pitta Caution

Although ashwagandha is considered a calming adaptogen, it has the opposite effect on some people. In my experience, these are typically people with internal heat — or a pitta constitution, from an energetic perspective — as ashwagandha is a warming herb.

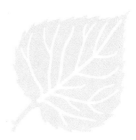

🍂 Barberry

Latin Name
- *Berberis vulgaris*

Parts Used
- Root
- Bark
- Fruit

Common Combinations
- **For acne:** Dandelion and green tea
- **For breast cancer or menopause with high cholesterol:** Soy
- **For high cholesterol:** Milk thistle

Current Medicinal Uses

Barberry is well known as an herbal remedy for skin conditions such as acne, psoriasis and eczema and has also been used to treat liver disease, gallstones and viral hepatitis. Because it tastes bitter and stimulates liver function, it is sometimes included in formulas for depression, to enliven the spirit and overall metabolic function of the body, and thus brighten the mood.

History and Energetics

Historically, Native North Americans used barberry to treat colds, fevers, sore throats, sluggish digestion, jaundice and other liver diseases. The Ancient Egyptians and Ayurvedic physicians both used barberry to treat dysentery.

When classified according to taste and energetics, barberry is a bitter plant. Like all bitters, barberry has a cooling effect on the digestive system, draining internal heat that manifests externally as inflammation, redness and yellowish secretions. If you picture the kind of acne that looks like red pustules filled with yellowish sebum, you have an idea of the type of conditions barberry is most suitable for.

People who would benefit from barberry often have a thick, yellowish coating on the tongue. This yellowish color is mirrored in the color of the bark and roots, imparted by the plant's main constituent, berberine. From a Doctrine of Signatures perspective, this coloring is an indicator of barberry's uses: for jaundice, where the skin and eyes turn yellow, and for conditions such as acne, eczema and psoriasis where there is yellowish tinge to skin lesions.

Barberry's homeopathic remedy is used for stitching and cutting pains in the kidneys and liver with nausea and indigestion, and for itchy skin conditions, such as eczema. A sensation of bubbling water coming up through the skin is associated with barberry homeopathically.

Research Evidence

Barberry wasn't very well researched until recently, but reports of its blood-sugar-reducing and lipid-lowering effects have led to multiple clinical trials on one of its chemical constituents, berberine. Preclinical trials have found that barberry has anti-inflammatory, antioxidant and antimicrobial properties that may be useful in a number of conditions.

Acne

A couple of small trials have investigated the use of barberry for acne. One randomized, controlled trial of teenagers with acne found that 200 milligrams of barberry extract, taken three times daily for four weeks, significantly reduced both the number and severity of acne lesions. The group of teens taking a placebo did not experience any significant changes. In another small trial, on teens and young adults with mild to moderate acne, barberry fruit juice also significantly reduced the total number of acne lesions and the number of inflamed acne lesions.

Breast Cancer

Preliminary research suggests that barberry, and its constituent berberine, may have potent anticancer effects. In vitro studies have shown that berberine enhances the effects of some common chemotherapy drugs and estrogen-receptor antagonist drugs in estrogen-receptor-positive breast cancer cells. More research is needed in this area.

Diabetes

Through its work in the liver, barberry has beneficial impacts on blood sugar by reducing the production of glucose and improving insulin sensitivity. In preclinical trials, berberine has been shown to have activity similar to sulfonylureas or metformin. A recent but small double-blind, randomized clinical trial found that barberry significantly decreased blood sugar, insulin, insulin resistance and cholesterol compared to a placebo in people with type 2 diabetes.

High Cholesterol

A recent randomized trial that looked at the use of barberry in people with metabolic syndrome found that barberry significantly improved both cholesterol profiles and C-reactive protein, a marker of inflammation found in the blood, compared to a placebo. Other trials have had similar results. One study on menopausal women found that barberry combined with isoflavones significantly reduced total cholesterol, low-density lipoprotein (LDL), or "bad," cholesterol, triglycerides and menopausal symptoms compared to treatment with calcium and vitamin D. Similar results have been found in studies on people with diabetes.

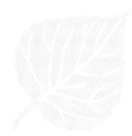

Health Condition	Level of Scientific Evidence
Acne	Fair
Breast cancer	Poor
Diabetes	Fair
High cholesterol	Fair

Safety

Although barberry has traditionally been used to treat liver and gallbladder diseases, it may not be suitable for this purpose in all cases. Because of its stimulating effects, it can actually make these conditions worse and, in some cases, may lead to bile duct obstruction, an emergency condition. Barberry is not safe for use in pregnancy or while breastfeeding.

Further Reading

Cianci A, Cicero AF, Colacurci N, et al. Activity of isoflavones and berberine on vasomotor symptoms and lipid profile in menopausal women. *Gynecological Endocrinology*, 2012 Sep; 28 (9): 699–702.

Fouladi RF. Aqueous extract of dried fruit of *Berberis vulgaris* L. in acne vulgaris: A clinical trial. *Journal of Dietary Supplements*, 2012 Dec; 9 (4): 253–61.

Johnson M, Rafikhah N. *Berberis vulgaris* juice and acne vulgaris: A placebo-controlled study. *Asian Journal of Clinical Nutrition*, 2014; 6(2): 47–52.

Shidfar F, Ebrahimi SS, Hosseini S, et al. The effects of *Berberis vulgaris* fruit extract on serum lipoproteins, apoB, apoA-1, homocysteine, glycemic control and total antioxidant capacity in type 2 diabetic patients. *Iranian Journal of Pharmaceutical Research*, 2012 Spring; 11 (2): 643–52.

Zilaee M, Kermany T, Tavalaee S, et al. Barberry treatment reduces serum anti-heat shock protein 27 and 60 antibody titres and high-sensitivity C-reactive protein in patients with metabolic syndrome: A double-blind, randomized placebo-controlled trial. *Phytotherapy Research*, 2014 Aug; 28 (8): 1211–15.

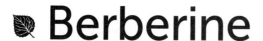# Berberine

Current Medicinal Uses

Extracts of berberine are used to treat diarrhea and other gastrointestinal infections, diabetes, cancer, polycystic ovarian syndrome (PCOS) and some cases of infertility.

History and Energetics

Plants containing berberine have traditionally been used for a variety of different illnesses, including infectious diarrhea, urinary tract and vaginal infections, liver and gallbladder conditions and skin conditions such as eczema and psoriasis. In China, berberine has been extracted and used to treat infectious diarrhea in cases of cholera and dysentery. Its use in the treatment of giardia and candida, among other microbial infections, has also been investigated. Many products have been formulated for these uses and continue to be available for purchase today.

From a traditional Chinese medicine perspective, berberine-containing plants are all classified as herbs that clear heat and dry dampness. They are used in conditions such as burning diarrhea, acid reflux, gum disease, liver pain, headaches, ulcers on the tongue, urinary tract infections with scanty yellow urine, boils and other inflammatory skin lesions.

Research Evidence

Although berberine was not traditionally used specifically to reduce blood sugar and blood lipids, these results were well known as side effects of herbs containing berberine. This has led researchers to study berberine for conditions such as diabetes, cancer and PCOS.

Diabetes and High Cholesterol

Reviews on berberine have concluded that it is an effective form of treatment for type 2 diabetes, high cholesterol and even high blood pressure. One recent review found that berberine lowers fasting blood sugar levels and hemoglobin A1c to a degree that is significantly greater than a placebo or lifestyle interventions alone, and is comparable to the effect of standard oral pharmaceutical drugs used to treat type 2 diabetes.

Latin Name
- Not applicable; berberine is a constituent found in a variety of plants, including barberry (*Berberis vulgaris*), Oregon grape root (*Mahonia aquifolium*), goldthread (*Coptis chinensis*), goldenseal (*Hydrastis canadensis*) and phellodendron (*Phellodendron amurense*)

Parts Used
- Not applicable

Common Combinations
- **For diabetes, with or without high cholesterol:** Cinnamon and fenugreek
- **For PCOS:** Green tea and chaste tree

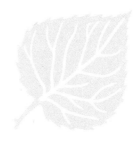

In terms of its effects on blood lipids, berberine lowers low-density lipoprotein (LDL), or "bad," cholesterol and total cholesterol and increases high-density lipoprotein (HDL), or "good," cholesterol when combined with lifestyle changes or cholesterol-lowering drugs. Berberine also appears to decrease triglycerides and increase HDL cholesterol more effectively than standard pharmaceutical drugs.

Berberine also appears to decrease blood pressure in clinical trials.

Polycystic Ovarian Syndrome

In studies on PCOS, berberine appears to decrease waist circumference, waist-to-hip ratio, triglycerides and LDL cholesterol. As in studies for high cholesterol, berberine was also demonstrated to increase HDL cholesterol.

In terms of its direct effects on hormones, berberine has been shown to increase sex hormone–binding globulin and decrease testosterone. It also improves blood sugar regulation comparably to metformin, a pharmaceutical drug used in the treatment of PCOS, especially in cases of PCOS-related infertility. In women with PCOS who were undergoing IVF, treatment with berberine was shown to increase pregnancy rates and reduce ovarian hyperstimulation. These results are very promising, but more research is needed to confirm them.

Health Condition	Level of Scientific Evidence
Diabetes	Good
High cholesterol	Good
Polycystic ovarian syndrome	Fair

Safety

Information about the safety of berberine comes from traditional knowledge about the plants that contain it, as well as from clinical studies. Overall, berberine extracts appear safe for most adults in the short term. In the long term, berberine-containing herbs are too cooling to be used on their own and are best combined with warming digestive herbs, such as fennel, ginger or turmeric. Berberine should be avoided in pregnancy, as it is known to cause uterine contractions. It should also be avoided by women who are breastfeeding, as animal studies have implicated it in cases of jaundice in newborns.

Further Reading

An Y, Sun Z, Zhang Y, et al. The use of berberine for women with polycystic ovary syndrome undergoing IVF treatment. *Clinical Endocrinology* (Oxford), 2014 Mar; 80 (3): 425–31.

Dong H, Zhao Y, Zhao L, Lu F. The effects of berberine on blood lipids: A systemic review and meta-analysis of randomized controlled trials. *Planta Medica*, 2013 Apr; 79 (6): 437–46.

Lan J, Zhao Y, Dong F, et al. Meta-analysis of the effect and safety of berberine in the treatment of type 2 diabetes mellitus, hyperlipemia and hypertension. *Journal of Ethnopharmacology*, 2015 Feb 23; 161C: 69–81.

Li Z, Geng YN, Jiang JD, Kong WJ. Antioxidant and anti-inflammatory activities of berberine in the treatment of diabetes mellitus. *Evidence-Based Complementary and Alternative Medicine*, 2014; 2014: 289264.

Wei W, Zhao H, Wang A, et al. A clinical study on the short-term effect of berberine in comparison to metformin on the metabolic characteristics of women with polycystic ovary syndrome. *European Journal of Endocrinology*, 2012 Jan; 166 (1): 99–105.

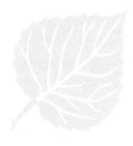

🍂 Black Cohosh

Latin Name
- *Actaea racemosa* (synonym *Cimicifuga racemosa*)

Part Used
- Root

Common Combinations
- **For infertility:** Chaste berry
- **For irregular menses:** Chaste berry and dang gui
- **For menopausal symptoms, especially with depression and/or anxiety:** St. John's wort and valerian

Current Medicinal Uses

Black cohosh is most frequently used for menopausal symptoms and irregular menstrual cycles, especially when these are accompanied by depression and/or rheumatic diseases (painful inflammatory conditions involving the joints and/or muscles). It may also be used to support and encourage fertility.

History and Energetics

Black cohosh is one of the many herbs that Europeans learned about from the indigenous peoples of eastern North America. It is possibly the most important herb for women's health from this area, as is reflected in one of its older common names, squaw root. "Squaw" is an English variant of an Algonquin word meaning "woman"; however, the term has been used in a derogatory manner and is now generally considered offensive. Another name for black cohosh is snake root or rattle root. The seeds rattle inside their pods when the stalk is shaken, making a sound like that of a rattlesnake. Black cohosh was thus used by Native Americans for snakebites and as snake medicine.

Native women used black cohosh for menstrual pain and to help speed childbirth and ease labor pains, as well as for rheumatism, measles and respiratory diseases such as tuberculosis and whooping cough. Many of these uses have been confirmed in modern clinical trials.

The black root represents the dark, depressed or brooding mental state associated with black cohosh in energetic and homeopathic descriptions. From this perspective, black cohosh is especially useful for women whose menstrual or menopausal symptoms are accompanied by moping, gloominess or despondency.

Black cohosh's thin, rigid flower stalk reaches high above the leaves. In the wind, the stalk appears to whip back and forth. Both the rigidity of the stalk and the whipping motion serve as a reminder of black cohosh's traditional use for the treatment of spasms and rheumatic pains of all kinds.

Black cohosh was one of the ingredients in Lydia E. Pinkham's Vegetable Compound, a very popular patented remedy sold in the nineteenth century for women's

menstrual pains and complaints. The original formula was made up of black cohosh, unicorn root, pleurisy root, life root and fenugreek in an alcohol extract. Although many of the original ingredients have been replaced by safer, more effective herbs, black cohosh remains in most modern versions of the formula.

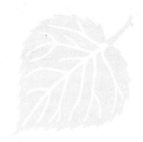

Research Evidence
Amenorrhea/Oligomenorrhea

Black cohosh (*Actaea racemosa*) has long been used to regulate women's menstrual cycles. Although once believed to be phytoestrogenic, it is now understood to affect menstruation via the hypothalamus and/or pituitary. In vitro studies have shown that black cohosh stimulates ovulation via the pituitary and promotes adequate production of progesterone during the luteal phase of menstruation. As such, it may be effective in resolving amenorrhea or oligomenorrhea in some cases. More research is needed.

Fibroids

In a randomized, controlled trial comparing black cohosh to the drug tibolone for menopausal symptoms, it was noted that women with fibroids who took black cohosh experienced a reduction in fibroid volume, while the women taking tibolone experienced fibroid growth. Although these are the results of only one study, black cohosh may be helpful in reducing fibroid size, particularly in perimenopausal women.

Infertility

Two similar studies of women with unexplained infertility showed significant improvement in clomiphene citrate induction cycles when black cohosh was supplemented during the follicular phase. Further research is needed to confirm these results and explore the role of black cohosh in fertility treatment.

Menopause

Although many studies on black cohosh show promising results for perimenopausal and postmenopausal women, a recent systematic review concluded that insufficient scientific evidence exists to support the clinical use of black cohosh for menopausal symptoms. The authors cited poor trial quality, studies that were difficult to compare and inadequate reporting as some of the problems.

Another review, however, concluded that black cohosh was effective in treating hot flushes of mild to moderate severity. Since that review was published, several new positive studies have been conducted. The majority of these clinical trials demonstrated significant reductions in hot flushes, mood variability and other physical and sexual symptoms associated with menopause. Observational studies have produced similarly positive results.

European studies using the commercial preparation Remifemin have consistently shown black cohosh to be effective in treating menopausal symptoms. Several studies that used a combination of black cohosh with St. John's wort also found significant decreases in menopausal symptoms.

Osteoporosis

Animal studies show that extracts of black cohosh slow or inhibit the development of osteoporosis. These results have not been replicated in human trials. Further research in this area is needed.

Health Condition	Level of Scientific Evidence
Amenorrhea/ oligomenorrhea	Poor
Fibroids	Fair
Infertility	Fair
Menopause	Fair/mixed
Osteoporosis	Poor

Safety

Early concerns that black cohosh produced estrogenic-like effects, and therefore should not be used in women with estrogen-positive breast cancers, have been refuted. Reviews of the scientific literature show few side effects. Caution is advised during pregnancy and breastfeeding, as safety has not been demonstrated.

Further Reading

Bai W, Henneicke-von Zepelin HH, Wang S, et al. Efficacy and tolerability of a medicinal product containing an isopropanolic black cohosh extract in Chinese women with menopausal symptoms: A randomized, double blind, parallel-controlled study versus tibolone. *Maturitas*, 2007 Sep 20; 58 (1): 31–41. Epub 2007 Jun 22.

Drewe J, Zimmermann C, Zahner C. The effect of a *Cimicifuga racemosa* extracts Ze 450 in the treatment of climacteric complaints: An observational study. *Phytomedicine*, 2013 Jun 15; 20 (8–9): 659–66.

Jacobson JS, Troxel AB, Evans J, et al. Randomized trial of black cohosh for the treatment of hot flashes among women with a history of breast cancer. *Journal of Clinical Oncology*, 2001 May 15; 19 (10): 2739–45.

Laakmann E, Grajecki D, Doege K, et al. Efficacy of *Cimicifuga racemosa*, *Hypericum perforatum* and *Agnus castus* in the treatment of climacteric complaints: A systematic review. *Gynecological Endocrinology*, 2012 Sep; 28 (9): 703–9.

Leach MJ, Moore V. Black cohosh (*Cimicifuga* spp.) for menopausal symptoms. *Cochrane Database of Systematic Reviews*, 2012 Sep 12; 9: CD007244.

Mohammad-Alizadeh-Charandabi S, Shahnazi M, Nahaee J, Bayatipayan S. Efficacy of black cohosh (*Cimicifuga racemosa* L.) in treating early symptoms of menopause: A randomized clinical trial. *Chinese Medicine*, 2013 Nov 1; 8 (1): 20.

Ross SM. Menopause: A standardized isopropanolic black cohosh extract (Remifemin) is found to be safe and effective for menopausal symptoms. *Holistic Nursing Practice*, 2012 Jan–Feb; 26 (1): 58–61.

Shahin AY, Ismail AM, Zahran KM, Makhlouf AM. Adding phytoestrogens to clomiphene induction in unexplained infertility patients — A randomized trial. *Reproductive BioMedicine Online*, 2008 Apr; 16 (4): 580–88.

Wuttke W, Jarry H, Haunschild J, et al. The non-estrogenic alternative for the treatment of climacteric complaints: Black cohosh (*Cimicifuga* or *Actaea racemosa*). *Journal of Steroid Biochemistry and Molecular Biology*, 2014 Jan; 139: 302–10.

Xi S, Liske E, Wang S, et al. Effect of isopropanolic *Cimicifuga racemosa* extract on uterine fibroids in comparison with tibolone among patients of a recent randomized, double blind, parallel-controlled study in Chinese women with menopausal symptoms. *Evidence-Based Complementary and Alternative Medicine*, 2014; 2014: 717686.

Blessed Thistle

Latin Name
- *Cnicus benedictus* (formerly *Carduus benedictus*)

Parts Used
- Aerial parts (everything above the ground)

Common Combination
- To increase breast milk supply: Fenugreek and fennel

Current Medicinal Uses

Blessed thistle is used to support lactation and bolster milk supply levels in breastfeeding women. It also supports healthy digestion and liver metabolism, much like a related plant, milk thistle (see page 299).

History and Energetics

According to legend, a plague infected the medieval king Charlemagne's troops. While he was asleep, an angel appeared to Charlemagne and told him to shoot an arrow into the air and use the plant pierced by the arrow to heal his troops. The arrow fell into a patch of *Cnicus benedictus*, which Charlemagne gave to his soldiers. The herb did, indeed, save the lives of his soldiers, and it became known as blessed thistle, or holy thistle, as a result.

The Ancient Greeks and Romans used blessed thistle to lift curses and protect people from evil spirits (as is the case with many thorny plants). During the Middle Ages, blessed thistle was seen as a cure-all. In particular, it was used to treat the bubonic plague, which is likely the illness referred to in the story about Charlemagne's troops. Monks also grew blessed thistle as a cure for smallpox.

In Shakespeare's *Much Ado about Nothing*, Margaret says, "Get you some of this distilled *Carduus benedictus*, and lay it to your heart: it is the only thing for a qualm." Scholars believe that Shakespeare intended "qualm" to refer to both a misgiving and the historical use of blessed thistle in treating plague.

Research Evidence

Low Milk Supply

To date, there have been no clinical trials conducted on the use of blessed thistle to increase breast milk supply. Several literature reviews and participant surveys on herbal galactagogues note blessed thistle's traditional use for this purpose and indicate that more research is needed to confirm its efficacy and safety.

Health Condition	Level of Scientific Evidence
Low milk supply	Poor

Safety

Caution is advised for those who are allergic to other Asteraceae plants, such as daisies and ragweed.

Further Reading

Low Dog T. Smart talk on supplements and botanicals. *Alternative and Complementary Therapies*, 2008 Dec; 14 (6): 272–74.

Westfall RE. Galactagogue herbs: A qualitative study and review. *Canadian Journal of Midwifery Research and Practice*, 2003; 2 (2): 22–27.

🍃 Boswellia

Latin Name
- *Boswellia serrata*

Part Used
- Gum resin

Common Combination
- **For osteoarthritis:** Turmeric, devil's claw and ginger

Current Medicinal Uses

Boswellia is used in Ayurvedic medicine as an anti-inflammatory herb for arthritis, inflammatory bowel disease (IBD) and asthma. Recently it has been investigated for its use in cancer, and specifically for reducing inflammation and edema in the brain.

History and Energetics

Boswellia — more commonly known as frankincense or Indian frankincense, depending on the exact species — has been used since the beginning of written history in religious and cultural ceremonies. It was used as incense by the Egyptians, Jews, Greeks and Romans and is referred to in the Hebrew Bible.

Frankincense was exported from the Arabian peninsula to Europe and even China, where it is known medicinally as *ru xiang* and used for blood stasis resulting in pain, arthritis, dysmenorrhea, gastrointestinal issues and traumatic injuries with swelling.

As a favorite food of elephants, boswellia's Sanskrit name is *gajabhakshya*, meaning "the elephants eat its leaves with great interest." An elephant's ability to walk long distances despite its heavy weight is mirrored in boswellia's traditional use for treating arthritis, thereby helping humans to walk more freely and with less pain.

Research Evidence
Osteoarthritis and Rheumatoid Arthritis

Evidence from high-quality studies on boswellia indicates that it significantly decreases pain in people with osteoarthritis. Daily physical functioning also improved significantly, including the ability to walk up and down stairs, stand up from a lying down or seated position, put on or take off socks, and other regular activities that are often restricted by arthritis. Boswellia was also shown to reduce degradation of cartilage in the joint, a degenerative process common in osteoarthritis. Lower-quality trials have found similar results.

In addition, some clinical studies have noted that boswellia decreases swelling around arthritic joints and reduces the amount of ibuprofen needed to manage pain. Studies on boswellia in combination with other Ayurvedic herbs for osteoarthritis have found similar results. In some cases, boswellia extracts have been found to be as effective as celecoxib, a COX-2 inhibitor that is commonly used in the treatment of arthritis.

Several case studies on the use of boswellia extracts to treat rheumatoid arthritis suggest that boswellia may improve pain, swelling and stiffness and decrease the use of pain-relieving medications. High-quality human clinical studies are needed to confirm these findings.

Health Condition	Level of Scientific Evidence
Osteoarthritis	Good
Rheumatoid arthritis	Poor

Did You Know?

Enriched Extracts
Enriched standardized extracts may be more effective in the treatment of osteoarthritis than non-enriched forms of boswellia. It may take up to three months for boswellia's positive effects on pain to be noted.

Safety

Boswellia may cause stomach irritation and upset in some people. No research has evaluated the effects of boswellia during pregnancy or breastfeeding; therefore, it is best avoided, since there is no clear evidence of its safety.

Further Reading

Cameron M, Chrubasik S. Oral herbal therapies for treating osteoarthritis. *Cochrane Database of Systematic Reviews*, 2014 May 22; 5: CD002947.

Etzel R. Special extract of *Boswellia serrata* (H 15) in the treatment of rheumatoid arthritis. *Phytomedicine*, 1996 May; 3 (1): 91–94.

Sengupta K, Alluri KV, Satish AR, et al. A double blind, randomized, placebo controlled study of the efficacy and safety of 5-Loxin for treatment of osteoarthritis of the knee. *Arthritis Research & Therapy*, 2008; 10 (4): R85.

Sengupta K, Krishnaraju AV, Vishal AA, et al. Comparative efficacy and tolerability of 5-Loxin and Aflapin against osteoarthritis of the knee: A double blind, randomized, placebo controlled clinical study. *International Journal of Medical Sciences*, 2010 Nov 1; 7 (6): 366–77.

Vishal AA, Mishra A, Raychaudhuri SP. A double blind, randomized, placebo controlled clinical study evaluates the early efficacy of Aflapin in subjects with osteoarthritis of knee. *International Journal of Medical Sciences*, 2011; 8 (7): 615–22.

🍃 Calendula

Latin Name
- *Calendula officinalis*

Part Used
- Flower

Common Combinations
- **For acne:** Tea tree oil or green tea (topically)
- **For atrophic vaginitis:** Aloe vera
- **For gum disease and mouth ulcers:** Boswellia
- **For microbial vaginitis and leukorrhea:** Goldenseal
- **For varicose veins:** Horse chestnut and witch hazel

Folklore

Weather Prediction

Calendula flowers are said to predict the weather for the days ahead: the flowers stay closed if a storm is coming. When its flowers open, calendula invites us to share in the brightness and energy of the sun.

Current Medicinal Uses

Calendula, or marigold, is best known for its topical uses in a range of skin conditions, from acne and eczema to varicose veins, cuts, scrapes and burns. It is also used as a gargle for gum infections and canker sores and as a compress for pink eye (conjunctivitis) and vaginitis. Internally, calendula is used for stomach ulcers and indigestion.

History and Energetics

The name "calendula" derives from the Latin word for "calendar" or "monthly ledger." Some believe this is because pot marigolds flower at the beginning of the month. Others say it is related to the fact that the flower can bloom every month of the year in certain climates. Still others suggest that, because calendula's flowers open and turn toward the sun, the Latin name refers to the plant's ability to tell time, like a sundial.

The Ancient Egyptians, Romans and Greeks used calendula to help rejuvenate skin. In India, it was strung in wreaths for weddings and other religious ceremonies.

Research Evidence

Acne

Calendula contains several plant chemicals that are known to be anti-inflammatory, most notably flavonoids. Since acne is primarily an inflammatory condition of the sebaceous glands and follicles in the skin, calendula has been incorporated in many topical treatments for acne. Little research in the form of clinical trials has been conducted, but in vitro research shows antimicrobial and anti-inflammatory actions. Several poor-quality case reports support the use of calendula as a topical treatment for acne. Other studies show that calendula helps to decrease irritation and damage due to chemicals or ultraviolet light.

Vaginitis

Research on calendula for vaginitis is lacking. Studies tend to be of poor quality and rely on in vitro studies. One small study found that calendula decreased leukorrhea (vaginal discharge) and itchiness in women with recurrent vaginal candida infections. Another challenge is that calendula oil is sometimes used as a filler, or non-medicinal ingredient, in preparations for vaginal atrophy and infections. With multiple ingredients, it is difficult to evaluate which ones are working to create positive health effects.

Varicose Veins

Traditional herbalists have long used calendula to treat varicose veins, but no human clinical research has been performed specifically on its use for this condition. However, calendula contains flavonoids and volatile oils that have demonstrated anti-inflammatory and wound-healing effects in vitro and in animal studies. Calendula ointment applied topically to venous leg ulcers has been shown to significantly speed up skin healing compared to a saline dressing, in a small non-blinded human study. While these results are promising, more research is needed.

Did You Know?

Culinary Uses
Calendula flowers make a good food dye and have been used historically to color butter and cheese yellow. Calendula has also been used as a less expensive substitute for saffron.

Health Condition	Level of Scientific Evidence
Acne	Poor
Vaginitis	Poor
Varicose veins	Poor

Safety

Overall, calendula is an extremely safe herb, especially when used topically. People with sensitivities to plants in the Asteraceae family should be cautious when using calendula. Calendula should not be used during early pregnancy, as it may act as an emmenagogue or abortifacient.

Further Reading

Nand P, Drabu S, Gupta RK, et al. In vitro and in vivo assessment of polyherbal topical gel formulation for the treatment of acne vulgaris. *International Journal of Drug Delivery*, 2012; 4 (4): 434–42.

Priyanka M, Patidar A, Gupta D, Agrawal S. Treatment of acne with herbal remedie — *Calendula officinalis*: An overview. *International Journal of Pharmaceutical & Biological Archives*, 2011; 2 (4): 1020–23.

Milián Vázquez PM, Seife Rodríguez JM, Morales Ojeda R, et al. [*Calendula officinalis* L. for the topical treatment of recurrent vaginal candidiasis]. [Article in Spanish]. *Boletín latinoamericano y del Caribe de plantas medicinales y aromáticas*, 2011; 9 (5): 344–52.

Castor Oil

Latin Name
- *Ricinus communis*

Part Used
- Seed oil

Common Combination
- **For acne:** Tea tree oil (topically, as a spot treatment)

Folklore

What's in a Name?

The name "castor oil" is believed to originate from its use as a replacement for castoreum, a perfume base extracted from the pineal glands of beavers (known as *castor* in Latin). Castor oil is also called *palma Christi*, or palm of Christ, in honor of its reputed healing powers.

Current Medicinal Uses

Castor oil is used topically as an anti-inflammatory. Internally, it works as a stimulant laxative. In certain cases it is also used internally by midwives to induce labor in pregnancies past their due date.

History and Energetics

Castor oil was first documented in the Ebers Papyrus from Ancient Egypt, where it was used for lamp oil and as an ointment base. Dioscorides noted its external medicinal uses for skin conditions, and the Aztecs also used it topically for skin irritations.

Castor oil is used in many places around the world to help ensure regular bowel movements and prevent intestinal parasites, so it may have a bad reputation among some who were given it orally as children.

Castor oil's topical use for a variety of purposes regained popularity through the work of Edgar Cayce, an early-nineteenth-century medical intuitive, and later through the efforts of Dr. William A. McGarey.

Research Evidence

Although castor oil has been used topically for thousands of years, very little evidence exists to support its use. A review of its topical applications suggests that castor oil may increase certain white blood cells and have a positive effect on liver function and cholesterol levels. Studies have shown that castor oil packs applied for three consecutive days improved some symptoms of constipation in the elderly. Topical castor oil may also reduce pain associated with inflammation and may be useful as a form of artificial tears.

Fibroids

Castor oil's effects on the immune system, pain and inflammation may provide clues as to why castor oil packs have long been used for conditions such as fibroids. More research is needed to confirm these preliminary results.

Labor Induction

In studies on the use of castor oil to induce labor, women took castor oil orally, took a placebo or received no treatment.

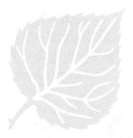

There were no differences among the different groups in terms of rates of Caesarean section, use of forceps during delivery, Apgar score or mortality of either the mothers or their babies. All of the women who took castor oil reported feeling nauseated afterward. Research on other outcomes, such as length of labor, may be useful.

Health Condition	Level of Scientific Evidence
Fibroids	Poor
Labor induction	Poor

Safety

The castor plant contains ricin, a highly toxic poison that was studied by various governments in the twentieth century for its potential use as a chemical or biological warfare agent. However, cold-pressed castor oil is non-toxic to humans in normal doses, whether taken internally or used externally.

As a laxative, castor oil may induce severe cramps, nausea and even vomiting while stimulating a bowel movement. Diarrhea is common. It should not be used by children or for extended periods of time, as it can cause electrolyte losses.

Castor oil should not be used during pregnancy, except at the very end — and only under the advice and care of a licensed medical professional.

Did You Know?

Non-medicinal Uses

Castor oil has also been used in manufacturing, in paints, varnishes and soaps, and as mechanical lubrication.

Further Reading

Arslan GG, Eşer I. An examination of the effect of castor oil packs on constipation in the elderly. *Complementary Therapies in Clinical Practice*, 2011 Feb; 17 (1): 58–62.

Boel ME, Lee SJ, Rijken MJ, et al. Castor oil for induction of labour: Not harmful, not helpful. *Australian and New Zealand Journal of Obstetrics and Gynaecology*, 2009 Oct; 49 (5): 499–503.

Grady H. Immunomodulation through castor oil packs. *Journal of Naturopathic Medicine*, 1998; 7 (1): 84–89.

Kelly AJ, Kavanagh J, Thomas J. Castor oil, bath and/or enema for cervical priming and induction of labour. *Cochrane Database of Systematic Reviews*, 2013 Jul 24; 7: CD003099.

Kennedy DA, Keaton D. Evidence for the topical application of castor oil. *International Journal of Naturopathic Medicine*, Apr 2012; 5 (1).

Cayenne Pepper

Latin Name
- *Capsicum frutescens*

Part Used
- Fruit, dried and ground

Common Combination
- **For arthritis:** Ginger and devil's claw

Current Medicinal Uses

Cayenne pepper is used to increase heat and stimulate blood circulation, whether taken internally or applied topically. It is also used topically as a counterirritant or rubefacient to reduce pain in cases of arthritis and other musculoskeletal conditions. Other uses include the treatment of diabetic neuropathy and post-shingles neuropathy, as well as migraines. Because it stimulates metabolism, cayenne may also promote weight loss.

History and Energetics

A member of the nightshade family, cayenne peppers are related to potatoes, tomatoes, eggplant and ashwagandha. Native to South America, the pepper was named for a city in French Guiana. Cayenne peppers were imported to Europe as a cheaper alternative to black pepper. Because it is a good source of vitamin C, cayenne pepper juice was used as a treatment for scurvy by some military units.

Research Evidence
Osteoarthritis

Research supports the topical use of cayenne pepper to treat arthritis. Pharmacological studies show that cayenne decreases substance P, a compound involved in the transmission and thus experience of pain. Clinical studies have found that cayenne applied topically to painful joints in osteoarthritis is significantly more effective than a placebo at reducing the intensity of pain.

Study participants commonly experience redness and burning, making it difficult to eliminate the placebo effect, as participants may guess whether they are receiving cayenne cream or a placebo, based on the side effects or lack thereof.

The creams used in studies range in concentration from 0.0125% to 0.075% weight per volume. Effectiveness may depend on dosage and how often the cream is applied.

Health Condition	Level of Scientific Evidence
Osteoarthritis	Fair

Safety

Applied topically, cayenne powder can irritate or possibly even burn the skin if it is too concentrated or left on for too long. Fairer-skinned individuals may be more susceptible. Caution is warranted: as with other counterirritants and rubefacients, a little cayenne goes a long way. Avoid inhaling the powder or applying cayenne near the eyes or other mucous membranes. Do not use cayenne on broken skin.

Internally, cayenne may irritate mucous membranes and aggravate a dry cough. In large quantities (much larger than anyone would dare add to food), cayenne may cause nausea, vomiting, pain and ulceration. Cayenne should not be used internally during pregnancy, as it may aggravate nausea or heartburn or cause uterine contractions because of its stimulating effects.

Did You Know?

Toasty Toes

As a heat-inducer, cayenne powder has been used to improve circulation — even being sprinkled inside socks to help keep toes warm during the winter.

Further Reading

Cameron M, Chrubasik S. Topical herbal therapies for treating osteoarthritis. *Cochrane Database of Systematic Reviews*, 2013 May 31; 5: CD010538.

De Silva V, El-Metwally A, Ernst E, et al; Arthritis Research UK Working Group on Complementary and Alternative Medicines. Evidence for the efficacy of complementary and alternative medicines in the management of osteoarthritis: A systematic review. *Rheumatology* (Oxford). 2011 May; 50 (5): 911–20.

❧ Chamomile

Latin Name
- *Matricaria recutita*

Part Used
- Flower

Common Combinations
- For anxiety: Lavender, lemon balm and passionflower
- For indigestion: Peppermint

Current Medicinal Uses

Chamomile is used primarily to calm digestion, easing symptoms such as bloating, gas and colic in infants. It may also be used to calm the nerves in cases of mild anxiety and insomnia. The essential oil of chamomile, taken internally in tea form or concentrated and applied topically, is used as an anti-inflammatory for the digestive tract and skin, respectively.

History and Energetics

The Ancient Egyptians used chamomile for fevers and associated the plant with the sun god Ra. Over time, chamomile has been used for a wide variety of conditions, including digestive concerns, menstrual pain, irritable bowel syndrome, hay fever and eye infections.

From a homeopathic and eclectic perspective, chamomile is appropriate for irritable, nervous people who are oversensitive to pain and may be inconsolable. They may want something and be angry if they don't get it, but they may also vehemently reject it when it is offered. Notably, one cheek may be red and hot while the other is normal. The homeopathic remedy is often used for teething infants but is equally applicable for adults, especially those with digestive complaints accompanied by pain, diarrhea and gas that smells of rotten eggs. Similarly, the flower essence of chamomile is used in people with nervous irritability and impatience that manifests as emotional tension in the solar plexus.

As an herbal medicine, chamomile is most suitable in cases of anxiety with digestive symptoms — in other words, a "nervous stomach." In addition to settling digestion, its side benefits include emotional balance, integration of self and a more peaceful, sunny disposition.

Research Evidence

Anxiety

A small randomized trial investigated the use of a chamomile extract in people diagnosed with generalized anxiety disorder (GAD). After eight weeks, the group taking chamomile experienced a significant decrease in symptoms of anxiety compared to the group taking a placebo.

A second clinical trial compared chamomile extract to a placebo in people with either anxiety alone or anxiety accompanied by depression. In this trial, chamomile significantly reduced symptoms of depression and improved mood in the group taking it.

More research is needed, but chamomile may be an effective treatment for mild to moderate anxiety, with or without accompanying depression.

Did You Know?

A Popular Drink
Researchers estimate that, worldwide, over 1 million cups of chamomile tea are drunk every day.

Health Condition	Level of Scientific Evidence
Anxiety	Fair

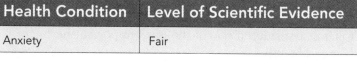

Safety

Overall, chamomile is a relatively safe herb. Caution is advised for people who are allergic to members of the Asteraceae family. Chamomile tea is likely safe in pregnancy in normal amounts.

Further Reading

Amsterdam JD, Li Y, Soeller I, et al. A randomized, double-blind, placebo-controlled trial of oral *Matricaria recutita* (chamomile) extract therapy for generalized anxiety disorder. *Journal of Clinical Psychopharmacology*, 2009 Aug; 29 (4): 378–82.

Amsterdam JD, Shults J, Soeller I, et al. Chamomile (*Matricaria recutita*) may provide antidepressant activity in anxious, depressed humans: An exploratory study. *Alternative Therapies in Health and Medicine*, 2012 Sep–Oct; 18 (5): 44–49.

Chaste Tree

Latin Name
- *Vitex agnus-castus*

Part Used
- Berries

Common Combinations
- **For androgenic acne, male-pattern hair loss and hirsutism:** Licorice and white peony
- **For menorrhagia:** Yarrow, cramp bark and raspberry
- **For irregular menses, especially amenorrhea:** Black cohosh, blue cohosh and dang gui
- **For menopause:** Motherwort, lemon balm, red clover and St. John's wort

Current Medicinal Uses

Chaste tree may be used to regulate hormones in a multitude of women's health conditions, including premenstrual syndrome, mastalgia, irregular menses, menorrhagia, infertility, hyperprolactinemia, insufficient lactation, menopause and acne.

History and Energetics

Chaste tree's botanical name derives from the Greek word *agnos*, meaning purity and innocence. It may refer either to lambs, a symbol of purity, or to another Greek word that means chastity. Either etymology is likely connected to the historical use of chaste tree by monks to help them stay abstinent. Although the herb may also be of use to men, it is now considered one of the most important herbs for women's health.

In Ancient Greece, women adorned themselves with the boughs of chaste tree in honor of Demeter, goddess of agriculture, marriage and fertility. According to mythology, Hera, considered the protector of marriage, was said to have been born underneath a chaste tree.

Research Evidence
Amenorrhea

A few small, older studies suggest that chaste tree may help treat secondary amenorrhea (when menstruation has stopped for more than three months — six months if menses was previously irregular — after it has already started). Since hyperprolactinemia is one potential cause of amenorrhea, chaste tree's known and presumed hormonal effects (see hyperprolactinemia and PCOS, below) provide a therapeutic rationale for why it may work to help menses resume a normal schedule. More research is needed in this area.

Hyperprolactinemia and Infertility

In trials looking at the use of chaste tree for latent hyperprolactinemia (high prolactin levels), one study found it comparable to bromocriptine, while another resulted in reduced prolactin secretion, longer luteal phases and higher

levels of mid-luteal progesterone and estrogen. The use of chaste tree to improve female fertility is likely related to these effects.

Low Milk Supply

Although chaste tree has been shown in numerous studies to reduce prolactin in cases of hyperprolactinemia, some animal studies have shown it to *increase* prolactin. Some herbalists have suggested that chaste tree has a normalizing effect on prolactin, increasing and decreasing its levels as needed. One study on a proprietary extract of chaste tree found that it improved breast milk production in women compared to controls. More research is definitely needed to resolve questions of whether chaste tree would be harmful or might be helpful in cases of insufficient breast milk.

Menopause

Evidence confirming chaste tree's use in alleviating menopausal symptoms is lacking. Further research is needed. Nonetheless, traditional use and expert opinion support the inclusion of chaste tree in combination formulas to treat menopausal symptoms.

Menorrhagia

One study on chaste tree for menorrhagia compared it to mefenamic acid, a non-steroidal anti-inflammatory drug (NSAID). Both the women taking chaste tree and the women taking mefenamic acid showed decreased quantities of menstrual blood flow and increased hemoglobin, a marker of anemia, after four months of treatment. The authors of the study concluded that chaste tree was as effective as mefenamic acid but had significantly fewer side effects. Another randomized trial found that chaste tree reduced bleeding induced by an intrauterine device (IUD) as well as mefenamic acid after 4 months.

> **Did You Know?**
>
> **Patience Required**
> Chaste tree's beneficial effects may take several months to become apparent.

Polycystic Ovarian Syndrome

Research on the use of chaste tree in PCOS is very limited. Since chaste tree is believed to act through the pituitary to decrease prolactin release, it may indirectly increase follicle-stimulating hormone and estrogen production, which could benefit women with PCOS. It may also have antiandrogen effects, but these haven't been well studied.

Premenstrual Syndrome and Fibrocystic Breast Changes

In clinical studies, chaste tree has been found to be more effective than a placebo in treating premenstrual syndrome, especially where cyclic mastalgia (premenstrual breast tenderness and swelling) is one of the major complaints. Several systematic reviews have concluded that chaste tree is a safe and effective treatment for PMS.

Other studies have found that chaste tree results in a greater reduction in premenstrual symptoms than vitamin B_6 (pyridoxine) or magnesium oxide. Studies comparing the use of chaste tree to fluoxetine in premenstrual dysphoric disorder have reported mixed results.

Health Condition	Level of Scientific Evidence
Amenorrhea	Poor
Hyperprolactinemia	Good
Infertility	Good
Low milk supply	Poor
Menopause	Poor
Menorrhagia	Fair
Polycystic ovarian syndrome	Poor
Premenstrual syndrome/ fibrocystic breast changes	Good

Safety

Few adverse effects have been documented in studies on chaste tree. However, women who are taking birth control medications, women who may be pregnant and women who are breastfeeding should consult with a health-care provider before using chaste tree, as it affects hormone levels. Chaste tree should be used cautiously by people taking drugs that affect dopamine, such as most drugs used in the treatment of Parkinson's disease and some antipsychotics. Interactions may occur with both dopamine agonists and antagonists.

Further Reading

Bobab MZ, Farimani M, Nasr ESH. Efficacy of mefenamic acid and *Vitex* in reduction of menstrual blood loss and HB changes in patients with a complaint of menorrhagia. *Iranian Journal of Obstetrics, Gynecology and Infertility*, 2007; 10 (1): 79–86.

Carmichael AR. Can *Vitex agnus-castus* be used for the treatment of mastalgia? What is the current evidence? *Evidence-Based Complementary and Alternative Medicine*, 2008 Sep; 5 (3): 247–50.

Dugoua JJ, Seely D, Perri D, et al. Safety and efficacy of chastetree (*Vitex agnus-castus*) during pregnancy and lactation. *Canadian Journal of Clinical Pharmacology*, 2008 Winter; 15 (1): e74–79.

Schellenberg R, Zimmermann C, Drewe J, et al. Dose-dependent efficacy of the *Vitex agnus castus* extract Ze 440 in patients suffering from premenstrual syndrome. *Phytomedicine*, 2012 Nov 15; 19 (14): 1325–31.

van Die MD, Burger HG, Teede HJ, Bone KM. *Vitex agnus-castus* extracts for female reproductive disorders: A systematic review of clinical trials. *Planta Medica*, 2013 May; 79 (7): 562–75.

Wuttke W, Jarry H, Christoffel V, et al. Chaste tree (*Vitex agnus-castus*) — Pharmacology and clinical indications. *Phytomedicine*, 2003 May; 10 (4): 348–57.

Yavarikia P, Shahnazi M, Hadavand Mirzaie S, et al. Comparing the effect of mefenamic acid and *Vitex agnus* on intrauterine device induced bleeding. *Journal of Caring Sciences*, 2013 Aug 31; 2 (3): 245–54.

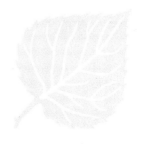

🍃 Cinnamon

Current Medicinal Uses

Thanks to its abilities to modulate blood sugar and improve insulin resistance, cinnamon is most commonly used to treat type 2 diabetes and other conditions, such as polycystic ovarian syndrome (PCOS), where blood sugar dysregulation is part of the picture. As an astringent, cinnamon is used for menorrhagia, fibroids and endometriosis. It also eases digestion and, like many aromatic herbs, has mild antimicrobial activity.

In Ayurvedic medicine, cinnamon is used to treat colds, diabetes, indigestion and high cholesterol. In traditional Chinese medicine, cinnamon is used to treat uterine fibroids and menorrhagia caused by blood stasis.

History and Energetics

Cinnamomum verum and *Cinnamomum cassia* are both mentioned in the Hebrew Bible and classic Greek texts, and each has been a valuable object of trade at different points in human history. Most of the cinnamon available in North American markets today is *Cinnamomum cassia*.

The word "cinnamon" is believed to derive from an Indonesian or Malay word meaning "sweet wood." Cinnamon sticks, or quills, reminded the Italians of cannons, so they called the herb *canela*, which became *cannelle* in French.

In ancient Egypt, cinnamon was burned as incense with myrrh and frankincense (also known as boswellia) and was used in embalming fluid, perfume and medicinal oils.

The Greeks believed that cinnamon originated from the home of Dionysus and that phoenix birds built their nests out of cinnamon bark. They used cinnamon to flavor wine.

The Ayurvedic understanding of cinnamon focuses on the herb's digestive effects. Cinnamon pacifies vata and kapha doshas and is used to warm the digestive system, increasing the absorption of nutrients from food. In traditional Chinese medicine (TCM), cinnamon is also viewed as a warming herb; however, its main medicinal actions are focused on the pelvic organs, where it works to warm the uterus, break up stagnant blood and relieve pain. It is also used to promote sweating in conditions such as early-stage colds.

Research Evidence

Diabetes and High Cholesterol

Multiple meta-analyses and systematic reviews have found that cinnamon significantly reduces fasting blood sugar, total cholesterol and triglycerides while increasing high-density lipoproteins (HDL) in people with diabetes mellitus. (However, one earlier review found the effects of cinnamon on blood sugar inconclusive.) Some reviews have concluded that cinnamon does not impact hemoglobin A1c (HgA1c); others have noted significant reductions.

One randomized controlled trial found significant reduction in both systolic and diastolic blood pressure in people with prediabetes and diabetes. Doses in trials on diabetes range from 1 to 6 grams daily and include both *Cinnamomum verum* and *Cinnamomum cassia*.

Fibroids and Menorrhagia

Cinnamon is one of the main ingredients in a traditional Chinese formula called *guizhi fuling*, used for fibroids and menorrhagia. In a recent systematic review, the authors found that *guizhi fuling*, given in conjunction with the drug mifepristone, resulted in a greater reduction in fibroid size than the drug alone. Unfortunately, the studies conducted to date have been poorly designed. High-quality research is needed to confirm these results.

Polycystic Ovarian Syndrome

Two small trials have studied the effects of cinnamon in women with PCOS. One trial found that cinnamon increased the regularity of menstrual cycles over six months of treatment. The other concluded that cinnamon improved blood sugar regulation compared to a placebo.

Did You Know?

Cassia Forest
In China, the city of Guilin was named "cassia forest" for the groves of cinnamon that once surrounded it.

Health Condition	Level of Scientific Evidence
Diabetes	Good
Fibroids	Fair
High cholesterol	Fair
Menorrhagia	Fair
Polycystic ovarian syndrome	Fair

Safety

Both *Cinnamomum verum* and *Cinnamomum cassia* are generally safe, but they should be avoided in large quantities during pregnancy, as they may stimulate the uterus to contract. When cinnamon is used topically, some people demonstrate an allergic sensitivity to cinnamic aldehyde, developing an itchy rash, swelling or hives on the skin. For people with ulcers or acid reflux, cinnamon may be overstimulating to the digestive system.

Further Reading

Akilen R, Pimlott Z, Tsiami A, Robinson N. Effect of short-term administration of cinnamon on blood pressure in patients with prediabetes and type 2 diabetes. *Nutrition*, 2013 Oct; 29 (10): 1192–96.

Akilen R, Tsiami A, Devendra D, Robinson N. Cinnamon in glycaemic control: Systematic review and meta analysis. *Clinical Nutrition*, 2012 Oct; 31 (5): 609–15.

Allen RW, Schwartzman E, Baker WL, et al. Cinnamon use in type 2 diabetes: An updated systematic review and meta-analysis. *Annals of Family Medicine*, 2013 Sep–Oct; 11 (5): 452–59.

Chen NN, Han M, Yang H, et al. Chinese herbal medicine guizhi fuling formula for treatment of uterine fibroids: A systematic review of randomised clinical trials. *BMC Complementary and Alternative Medicine*, 2014 Jan 2; 14: 2.

Kort DH, Lobo RA. Preliminary evidence that cinnamon improves menstrual cyclicity in women with polycystic ovary syndrome: A randomized controlled trial. *American Journal of Obstetrics & Gynecology*, 2014 Nov; 211 (5): 487.e1–6.

Leach MJ, Kumar S. Cinnamon for diabetes mellitus. *Cochrane Database of Systematic Reviews*, 2012 Sep 12; 9: CD007170.

Ranasinghe P, Jayawardana R, Galappaththy P, et al. Efficacy and safety of "true" cinnamon (*Cinnamomum zeylanicum*) as a pharmaceutical agent in diabetes: A systematic review and meta-analysis. *Diabetic Medicine*, 2012 Dec; 29 (12): 1480–92.

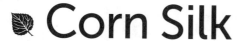# Corn Silk

Current Medicinal Uses

Corn silk is primarily used to treat urinary tract infections (UTIs), both for its diuretic effects and for its pain-relieving and sedating effects on the genitourinary system. It is also used in other conditions of the urinary tract, including cystitis, kidney stones, prostatitis and bedwetting in children.

History and Energetics

Corn silk was traditionally used by the Incas, Cherokee and others to treat kidney and bladder infections. Within Chinese herbal traditions, corn silk, known as *yi mi xu*, is used to drain dampness and heat from the bladder and to resolve painful urination.

Research Evidence

Urinary Tract Infections

Animal studies have shown that corn silk increases the flow and volume of urine. In one small open-label trial, an infusion of corn silk significantly decreased UTI symptoms after five, ten and twenty days of treatment. After five days, symptom scores decreased by 322%. Urine testing also revealed a significant decrease in the number of red blood cells, pus cells and crystals. More clinical trials are needed.

Health Condition	Level of Scientific Evidence
Urinary tract infections	Poor

Safety

In vitro and animal studies appear to show that corn silk is relatively safe in normal therapeutic doses.

Further Reading

Hasanudin K, Hashim P, Mustafa S. Corn silk (Stigma maydis) in healthcare: A phytochemical and pharmacological review. *Molecules*, 2012 Aug 13; 17 (8): 9697–715.

Sahib AS, Mohammed IH, Hamdan SJ. Use of aqueous extract of corn silk in the treatment of urinary tract infection. *Journal of Intercultural Ethnopharmacology*, 2012; 1 (2): 93–96.

Latin Name
• *Zea mays*

Parts Used
• Styles and stigmas (the silky hairs that surround a corn of cob, harvested from female plants before they are pollinated)

Common Combination
• **For UTIs:** Uva ursi and nettle

Did You Know?

Three Sisters
Corn — or, more accurately, maize — is part of the agricultural triad known as the three sisters, which also includes beans and squash. Maize is a staple part of the diets of North and South American indigenous peoples.

Did You Know?

Blood Pressure
Corn silk may theoretically decrease blood pressure through its diuretic effects.

Cramp Bark

Latin Name
• *Viburnum opulus*

Part Used
• Bark

Common Combination
• For dysmenorrhea: Valerian and ginger

Current Medicinal Uses

Cramp bark's traditional use is as an antispasmodic. Because it relaxes smooth muscles and has an affinity for the pelvic organs, it is used primarily for menstrual cramps (hence its common name). It has also been used in cases of threatened miscarriage due to uterine irritability and to help women prepare for childbirth.

History and Energetics

Cramp bark, also known as guelder rose, has a long history of use in Europe. The name "guelder rose" comes from the Dutch province of Gelderland, where formal cultivation of the plant may have originated. Cramp bark is most represented, however, in the folklore and history of Ukraine, where it is known as *kalyna* and respected for its symbolic meaning, medicinal qualities and aesthetics. Cramp bark features prominently in Ukrainian embroidery, songs and other art forms. The red of the berries symbolizes blood, including blood spilt in battle, and immortality. The berries have been used ceremonially to stop bleeding, as well as in rituals of brotherhood. The flowers represent a young woman's beauty and her coming of age, when she is said to be "blossoming like a *kalyna*."

In Ukrainian mythology, cramp bark is associated with the birth of the universe and is traditionally used at times of birth and death. It serves as an intermediary between worlds, helping ease the transition between childhood and adulthood and between life and death. Symbolically, cramp bark represents innocence, virginity, purity, fertility, love, joy, grief and sorrow. Ukrainian midwives used it in the ritual washing and purifying of infants and their mothers after birth. Newlyweds practiced a ritual called "breaking the *kalyna*," proving that they had consummated their marriage by showing off a blood-stained nightshirt or sheets. Cramp bark is also one of the most common plantings at Ukrainian gravesites.

Research Evidence

Dysmenorrhea

No clinical trials have been conducted to confirm the traditional use of cramp bark as an antispasmodic. However, evaluation of the constituents of cramp bark provides preliminary evidence supporting its role in spasmodic dysmenorrhea. In vitro studies show that cramp bark's main constituents, viburnin, viopudial and scopoletin, all demonstrate antispasmodic qualities.

Health Condition	Level of Scientific Evidence
Dysmenorrhea	Poor

Safety

The safety of cramp bark is difficult to determine because of a lack of clinical trials evaluating potential adverse effects. Although cramp bark has traditionally been used during pregnancy to prevent miscarriage and prepare for labor, research is needed to confirm its safety.

Further Reading

Jarboe CH, Zirvi KA, Nicholson JA, Schmidt CM. Scopoletin, an antispasmodic component of *Viburnum opulus* and *prunifolium*. *Journal of Medical Chemistry*, 1967 May 1; 10 (3): 488–89.

Nicholson JA, Darby TD, Jarboe CH. Viopudial, a hypotensive and smooth muscle antispasmodic from *Viburnum opulus*. *Proceedings of the Society for Experimental Biology and Medicine*, 1972 Jun; 140 (2): 457–61.

Yarnell E, Abascal K. Spasmolytic botanicals: Relaxing smooth muscle with herbs. *Alternative and Complementary Therapies*, 2011 Jun; 17 (3): 169–74.

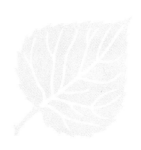

🍂 Cranberry

Latin Name
- *Vaccinium macrocarpon*

Part Used
- Berries

Common Combinations
- **To prevent UTIs:** Uva ursi
- **To treat UTIs:** Uva ursi, dandelion leaf and corn silk

Current Medicinal Uses

Cranberry is primarily used to prevent urinary tract infections (UTIs). The berries are high in antioxidant proanthocyanidins, which help maintain the overall health and resilience of the genitourinary tract.

History and Energetics

Cranberries are perhaps best known today in the form of a sauce paired with turkey and stuffing, but they have a long history of use as both food and medicine. Related to blueberries, bilberries and huckleberries, cranberries were used by indigenous peoples in North America for health promotion and prevention of a variety of infections. The berries were used as a poultice to draw out infected and poisonous wounds. The juice was used as a dye. Cranberries were mixed with meat and fat and made into pemmican, a preserved food eaten during cold winter months. Later the berries were used aboard ships to prevent scurvy, a deficiency of vitamin C.

Cranberry's English name is believed to derive from "crane berry," either because cranes like to eat the berries or because the position of the flowers on the stem looks like a crane's head and neck, depending on which historical source you believe.

Research Evidence
Urinary Tract Infections

Cranberry products have primarily been studied for the long-term prevention of UTIs. Reviews of the scientific literature often don't distinguish among unsweetened cranberry juice, sweetened cranberry juice, tablets and capsules, making amalgamation of results difficult, as cranberry products have been shown to vary considerably in their content of proanthocyanidins, the plant chemicals most likely to be responsible for the medicinal action. In addition, long-term treatment plans can be difficult for people to stick with, and in studies this has often meant the participants got sick of drinking up to 1 quart (1 L) daily of unconcentrated cranberry juice for months on end. Unfortunately, few studies on standardized cranberry powders or capsules exist.

The latest systematic reviews have shown mixed results. One review found no significant decrease in the occurrence of UTIs when cranberry products were taken preventatively. A previous review had found a small benefit, but the inclusion of a large trial on college women taking cranberry cocktail juice with negative results pushed the results toward the finding of no benefit.

A different meta-analysis concluded that cranberry products were significantly effective in reducing the occurrence of UTIs for women in general and especially for women with recurrent UTIs. The authors noted that the benefit appears to be dose-dependent. In other words, the greatest benefit comes from higher doses of cranberry products.

Overall, researchers tend to agree that cranberry is most effective for women with recurrent UTIs or elderly women. Cranberry products may need to be taken for up to a year before maximum benefits can be seen.

> **Did You Know?**
>
> **Take a Pass on Sugar**
> Since sugar suppresses immune functions and has been shown to increase infection by encouraging bacteria to replicate, unsweetened concentrated cranberry juices or powdered extracts are recommended.

Health Condition	Level of Scientific Evidence
Urinary tract infections	Fair/mixed

Safety

Cranberry products are quite safe, including during pregnancy.

Further Reading

Jepson RG, Williams G, Craig JC. Cranberries for preventing urinary tract infections. *Cochrane Database of Systematic Reviews*, 2012 Oct 17; 10: CD001321.

Shin CN. The effects of cranberries on preventing urinary tract infections. *Clinical Nursing Research*, 2014; 23 (1): 54–79.

Vasileiou I, Katsargyris A, Theocharis S, Giaginis C. Current clinical status on the preventive effects of cranberry consumption against urinary tract infections. *Nutrition Research*, 2013 Aug; 33 (8): 595–607.

Wang CH, Fang CC, Chen NC, et al. Cranberry-containing products for prevention of urinary tract infections in susceptible populations: A systematic review and meta-analysis of randomized controlled trials. *Archives of Internal Medicine*, 2012 Jul 9; 172 (13): 988–96.

Dandelion

Latin Name
- *Taraxacum officinale*

Parts Used
- Leaf
- Root

Common Combinations
- **For anemia:** Nettles and dang gui
- **For constipation:** Burdock
- **For high blood pressure:** Motherwort and hawthorn
- **For PMS:** Evening primrose oil and chaste tree
- **For UTIs:** Uva ursi, yarrow and corn silk

Current Medicinal Uses

The entire dandelion plant has food and medicinal uses. The leaf, slightly bitter, can be eaten to gently stimulate appetite and overall digestion. The leafy parts are also used in infusions or tinctures as a diuretic to help reduce water retention and edema during pregnancy and for premenstrual syndrome (PMS), urinary tract infections (UTIs), high blood pressure and many other conditions.

More bitter in flavor, the root contains inulin, a source of fiber. This part of the plant is used to gently induce laxation and improve the function of the liver and gallbladder. The root can be helpful in conditions such as constipation, acne, maldigestion of fats, gallstones, gallbladder inflammation and jaundice. Dandelion root is also used for anemia, as it is a good source of minerals. The root has even been used as a coffee substitute.

In traditional Chinese medicine (TCM), dandelion is called *pu gong ying*. The entire plant is used to clear heat and dampness from the liver and gallbladder. It is frequently used in herbal formulas for treating depression, breast nodules, hepatitis and kidney disease.

History and Energetics

Many North Americans recognize dandelion as a weed that they struggle to get out of their lawns and gardens before it spreads and takes over. Although it has a bad reputation, dandelion's prolific presence and ability to grow everywhere, even in cracks in the sidewalk, are reflected in its multitude of medicinal uses.

Dandelion's English name comes from the French *dent de lion*, meaning "lion's tooth," in reference to the shape of the leaves. The French also call it *pissenlit*, which literally translates as "urine in bed."

Dandelion is a great herb for overachievers. Working too hard may translate into an internal hardness, leading to constipation and muscle stiffness. In TCM, the liver and gallbladder are responsible for decision-making and willpower. They also control muscles, tendons and sinews. From a TCM perspective, when there is heat in the liver and gallbladder, the muscles become hard and tense. Dandelion energy supports softness within strength, allowing for relaxation within perseverance, endurance and busyness.

Research Evidence

Very little research has been conducted on dandelion despite its widespread traditional use in a variety of herbal medicine traditions around the world. However, animal studies have found decreases in cholesterol and blood sugar markers in animals on high-fat diets given dandelion leaf extract. Along with pharmacological and in vitro studies, these results are consistent with dandelion's traditional use in treating a variety of liver and gallbladder conditions.

Anemia

A study on mice found that dandelion significantly improved red blood cell markers compared to a placebo. Both total red blood cell count and hemoglobin increased, which supports the traditional use of dandelion for treating anemia.

Constipation

The use of dandelion for constipation has not been thoroughly studied. More research is needed.

High Blood Pressure

The traditional use of dandelion leaf in herbal formulas to address high blood pressure has been based on the herb's diuretic effects. While a small number of in vitro and animal trials have demonstrated its diuretic action, no human studies have yet investigated its specific use in lowering blood pressure. Nonetheless, dandelion's ability to lower cholesterol and blood sugar and act as a potassium-sparing diuretic make it useful in the treatment of hypertension, especially in the context of metabolic syndrome (a cluster of conditions that includes high blood pressure, abnormal cholesterol levels, obesity and diabetes).

Premenstrual Syndrome

Dandelion has traditionally been included in some formulas for PMS, especially where water retention, bloating and constipation are among the symptoms experienced. As a diuretic, dandelion leaf decreases fluid accumulation in the tissues. As a gentle laxative, dandelion relieves constipation, which may be associated with PMS. Some animal studies have shown dandelion to promote the release of bile from the gallbladder, which may help reduce PMS by encouraging the binding and excretion of excess hormones. More research is needed.

> **Did You Know?**
>
> **A Good Source of Iron**
> One hundred grams (about 3½ ounces) of cooked dandelion leaves provides 1.8 milligrams of iron, about 10% of the daily value (DV).

Urinary Tract Infections

The diuretic effects of dandelion have been demonstrated in pharmacological and animal trials. A small human study found that a tincture of dandelion leaf increased the frequency and amount of urination.

Health Condition	Level of Scientific Evidence
Anemia	Poor
Constipation	Poor
High blood pressure	Poor
Premenstrual syndrome	Poor
Urinary tract infections	Poor

Safety

Although dandelion has been used for years by herbalists, naturopaths and midwives, there is insufficient scientific evidence available to clearly state that it is safe in pregnancy. In small doses, dandelion may be considered in resistant cases of constipation. It may also be helpful to eat dandelion leaf in culinary amounts as a source of fiber with gentle laxation.

Although dandelion has long been used to treat liver and gallbladder conditions of all kinds, caution is advised when considering dandelion as a treatment for gallstones or other liver/gallbladder conditions.

Further Reading

Clare BA, Conroy RS, Spelman K. The diuretic effect in human subjects of an extract of *Taraxacum officinale* folium over a single day. *Journal of Alternative and Complementary Medicine*, 2009 Aug; 15 (8): 929–34.

Davaatseren M, Hur HJ, Yang HJ, et al. *Taraxacum officinale* (dandelion) leaf extract alleviates high-fat diet-induced nonalcoholic fatty liver. *Food and Chemical Toxicology*, 2013 Aug; 58: 30–36.

Modaresi M, Resalatpour N. The effect of *Taraxacum officinale* hydroalcoholic extract on blood cells in mice. *Advances in Hematology*, 2012; 2012: 653412.

Dang Gui

Current Medicinal Uses

Dang gui is traditionally used for amenorrhea, dysmenorrhea, irregular menses, infertility and menopause. Within traditional Chinese medicine (TCM), dang gui is considered a blood tonic and is used to support the normal production and circulation of blood, thus normalizing menstrual cycles and flow. As a yin tonic, it is added to formulas for sexual dysfunction to balance yang tonic herbs such as ginseng. In TCM it also moistens the intestines and resolves constipation.

History and Energetics

Dang gui, or dong quai, has a long history of use in China and Japan as a female tonic and is often called the "female ginseng." The name "dang gui" is commonly translated as "should come back" or "restore order." Chinese folklore tells of a husband who goes into the mountains to collect medicinal herbs. He instructs his wife to remarry if he does not return in three years. After three years, she remarries, only to have him return soon after. She is heartbroken and soon becomes weakened, until he gives her an herb that restores her strength and health. The herb was therefore named "dang gui" in honor of the faithful husband who should have come back sooner and who restored order by bringing his former wife back to health.

Research Evidence

Most of the research on dang gui has been conducted on TCM formulas containing many herbs. Researchers have noted that much of the therapeutic benefit of dang gui (as well as many other herbs with a long history of use in Asia) is likely lost in translation. Extracting a single herb from the TCM model takes the herb out of context in several ways: traditional processing, traditional medicinal use and cultural milieu. This same is often true of herbs from other traditions.

Latin Name
- *Angelica sinensis*

Part Used
- Root

Common Combinations
- **For infertility, menstrual irregularity and dysmenorrhea:** White peony

- **For menopausal symptoms:** Black cohosh, chaste tree and red clover

- **For tonifying blood and qi:** Astragalus (in a TCM formula)

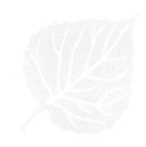

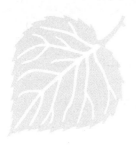

Amenorrhea

Research on dang gui for amenorrhea is limited. Several early case studies have noted that a fluid extract of dang gui induced menstrual flow in amenorrheic women. More research is needed.

Anemia

Recent clinical trials have supported the use of dang gui in the treatment of anemia. Several studies on iron-deficient animals have shown that the polysaccharides in dang gui improve the animals' hemoglobin, red blood cell and hematocrit levels. The same blood marker improvements were found in studies that used dang gui for anemia caused by drugs used to treat autoimmune disease or used as chemotherapy for cancer.

Menopause

Mixed results have been found in studies evaluating the TCM formula *danggui buxue tang* for hot flushes in postmenopausal women. Differences in preparation, dosage and research methodology make it difficult to assess the therapeutic benefit of this formula. None of the trials used TCM methods of diagnosis to determine whether or not this particular formula was appropriate. These results are an example of the challenges of taking an herb or a formula out of the context of the medical model in which it has been traditionally used.

Sexual Dysfunction

Because some studies on dang gui–containing formulas have seen positive results for their use in treating menopausal symptoms, and because pharmacological studies have shown possible estrogenic effects in animal models, it has been suggested that dang gui should be studied for its potential role in addressing sexual dysfunction. However, to date no such studies have been performed.

Health Condition	Level of Scientific Evidence
Amenorrhea	Poor
Anemia	Fair
Menopause	Poor
Sexual dysfunction	Poor

Safety

Dang gui may potentiate blood thinners. This caution is theoretical, based on the presence of coumarin in the plant. Although dang gui may be useful for regulating an abnormal menstrual cycle over time, it should not be used during menses in cases of menorrhagia, as it may increase bleeding.

Further Reading

Haines CJ, Lam PM, Chung TK, et al. A randomized, double-blind, placebo-controlled study of the effect of a Chinese herbal medicine preparation (Dang Gui Buxue Tang) on menopausal symptoms in Hong Kong Chinese women. *Climacteric*, 2008 Jun; 11 (3): 244–51.

Hook IL. Danggui to *Angelica sinensis* root: Are potential benefits to European women lost in translation? A review. *Journal of Ethnopharmacology*, 2014 Feb 27; 152 (1): 1–13.

Liu PJ, Hsieh WT, Huang SH, et al. Hematopoietic effect of water-soluble polysaccharides from *Angelica sinensis* on mice with acute blood loss. *Experimental Hematology*, 2010 Jun; 38 (6): 437–45.

Wang CC, Cheng KF, Lo WM, et al. A randomized, double-blind, multiple-dose escalation study of a Chinese herbal medicine preparation (Dang Gui Buxue Tang) for moderate to severe menopausal symptoms and quality of life in postmenopausal women. *Menopause*, 2013 Feb; 20 (2): 223–31.

Wang PP, Zhang Y, Dai LQ, Wang KP. Effect of *Angelica sinensis* polysaccharide-iron complex on iron deficiency anemia in rats. *Chinese Journal of Integrative Medicine*, 2007 Dec; 13 (4): 297–300.

Did You Know?

Dang Gui Preparations

Traditionally, dang gui is prepared as a decoction of the root. In traditional Chinese medicine, the typical daily dosage can be anywhere from 3 to 15 grams of the whole root when it is made into a decoction, depending on how the herb is used in combination with other herbs. Dang gui is also available as a tincture, an encapsulated extract and an herbal tablet.

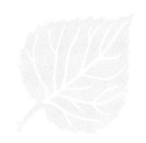

Devil's Claw

Latin Name
- *Harpagophytum procumbens*

Parts Used
- Root
- Tuber

Common Combinations
- **For osteoarthritis:** Turmeric, boswellia and ginger
- **For rheumatoid arthritis:** Evening primrose oil

Current Medicinal Uses

Devil's claw is used as an anti-inflammatory and pain reliever for arthritis, rheumatism and back pain, and to treat poor digestion, fever and painful conditions involving muscles and joints. Topically, it can be used as an ointment for sores and boils.

History and Energetics

Devil's claw has a long history of use in southern Africa. It is native to the Kalahari savannah and steppes from Namibia east through Botswana and into Madagascar. Devil's claw gained popularity in Europe after a German farmer who had been living in Namibia exported it in the 1950s. Much of the devil's claw supply in North America and Europe is still harvested in southern Africa.

The plant got its English name from the tiny hooks that cover its fruit, and its Latin genus name, *Harpagophytum*, means "hook plant." These hooks help devil's claw distribute its seeds: the fruit sticks to fur and clothing and is often carried far away from its original location before it is released for germination.

Called *kamangu* by many Namibian peoples, devil's claw has traditionally been used as a tonic for wasting, weakness, fatigue, urinary problems, fever, pain and digestive conditions. An infusion of the dried tuber in low doses has traditionally been used as a painkiller during pregnancy.

The climate devil's claw grows in — deserts and other dry, arid places — can serve to remind us of its medicinal qualities: it is helpful in degenerative osteoarthritis and joint pain where there is a decrease in cartilage in the joints and a lack of lubrication.

From an energetic perspective, devil's claw is most appropriate for people who "dig in their heels" and push beyond their own physical or emotional limits, leading to pain. The flower essence is used to encourage confidence in and comfort with one's essential identity, rather than feeling the need to conform to others' expectations. It is also helpful for those who use charisma, charm or physical attractiveness to manipulate others, hiding their true self in the process.

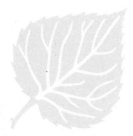

Research Evidence
Osteoarthritis and Low Back Pain

A review of the clinical research into the use of devil's claw for osteoarthritis of the knee, hip and spine found that it effectively reduces pain compared to a placebo and appears to have fewer side effects than non-steroidal anti-inflammatory drugs (NSAIDs), although it may cause digestive upset.

Other studies have shown that devil's claw is just as effective as diacerein in its ability to reduce pain. In one study, people taking devil's claw took fewer NSAIDs and other pain-relieving medications than the control group taking diacerein.

Similar reductions in pain ratings and improvements in quality of life have been shown in trials looking at the use of devil's claw for chronic low back pain and general rheumatism.

Health Condition	Level of Scientific Evidence
Low back pain	Good
Osteoarthritis	Good

Safety

Because it is bitter and stimulates the gastrointestinal system, devil's claw can irritate the stomach and may cause digestive upset or aggravate conditions such as ulcers and acid reflux. It may also interfere with blood-thinning medications. There is no research to confirm the safety of devil's claw during pregnancy or breastfeeding.

Further Reading

[No authors listed]. *Harpagophytum procumbens* (devil's claw). Monograph. *Alternative Medicine Review*, 2008 Sep; 13 (3): 248–52.

Brien S, Lewith GT, McGregor G. Devil's claw (*Harpagophytum procumbens*) as a treatment for osteoarthritis: A review of efficacy and safety. *Journal of Alternative and Complementary Medicine*, 2006 Dec; 12 (10): 981–93.

Gagnier JJ, Chrubasik S, Manheimer E. *Harpagophytum procumbens* for osteoarthritis and low back pain: A systematic review. *BMC Complementary and Alternative Medicine*, 2004 Sep 15; 4: 13.

Vlachojannis J, Roufogalis BD, Chrubasik S. Systematic review on the safety of *Harpagophytum* preparations for osteoarthritic and low back pain. *Phytotherapy Research*, 2008 Feb; 22 (2): 149–52.

Echinacea

- *Echinacea pallida* (pale purple coneflower)
- *Echinacea purpurea* (purple coneflower)
- *Echinacea angustifolia* (narrow-leaved coneflower)

Parts Used
- Root
- Seeds
- Whole plant

Common Combinations
- **For bacterial vaginosis and vaginal candidiasis:** Garlic, goldenseal and oregano
- **For herpes prevention and treatment:** Lemon balm, licorice and St. John's wort

Current Medicinal Uses

Echinacea is primarily used to boost immune system responsiveness in bacterial and viral infections. It is used both preventatively and for acute treatment of colds and flus. Echinacea's antibacterial and antiviral effects have supported its use in treating vaginitis, chronic upper respiratory tract infections and other viral and bacterial infections. Topically, echinacea is used to prevent infection of skin conditions, as well as for boils, cuts and poorly healing wounds.

As useful as it is for stimulating the immune system to ward off an acute infection, herbalists have recently begun to understand that echinacea may also be useful for calming an overactive immune system in autoimmune diseases.

History and Energetics

The name "echinacea" comes from the Greek word *echinos*, meaning spiny or pointed, in reference to the seed head, which looks like a sea urchin or hedgehog.

Echinacea has a long history of use for bacterial infections. The Lakota used it for snakebites and sepsis; the Blackfoot used it for toothaches; the Delaware used it for venereal disease; the Comanche and Choctaw used it for coughs and sore throats; and the Dakota used it for eye infections. Echinacea's immune-stimulating and antibacterial actions were later confirmed by eclectic pharmacists and hundreds of scientific trials. It is one of the most well-studied herbs in the world.

Native to the Great Plains of North America, echinacea grows tall and strong in the wind and open sky. Its bright, purple-pink flower petals stand out among the other wildflowers of the prairies, while its rigid stem holds fast when the wind blows. Similarly, echinacea helps the person taking it stay strong and healthy even as others get sick.

Echinacea's immune-boosting effects are also paralleled in the action of the flower essence, which helps the user connect to and maintain a strong sense of identity. The immune system creates a boundary between self and non-self, defining what is unique about each individual and enabling interaction with others without confusion or self-doubt. By strengthening the immune system, echinacea encourages a healthy sense of self and confident interaction with the external environment. Because of its robustness and certainty of self, echinacea is most helpful when the wind blows — in other words, when the immune system is challenged by an external force such as a bacterial infection.

Research Evidence

Cervical Dysplasia

To date, there are no clinical studies looking at the use of echinacea in the treatment or prevention of cervical dysplasia.

Common Cold

In general, pharmacological and animal research on echinacea's effects on immune system responsiveness shows a weak ability to counter bacterial infections and a better ability to inhibit viral infections. Research on the use of echinacea for treating or preventing the common cold is mixed. Although some trials have found benefits, the results cannot be easily compared because the preparation and dosage of echinacea vary among the studies. Nevertheless, a recent systematic review found that echinacea used preventatively may reduce by a small amount the likelihood of getting a cold.

Genital Warts

Little research has been conducted on echinacea specifically for the treatment of genital warts. One study compared the use of an herbal product that included echinacea to no treatment after surgical removal of genital warts, to see if herbs were effective in preventing the recurrence of warts. For patients who used the herbal formula for one month after surgery, recurrence rates six months later were significantly lower than for those who had no treatment after surgery.

Herpes

In vitro and animal studies show that *Echinacea purpurea* and *Echinacea pallida* have antiviral activity against both types of herpes simplex virus, HSV-1 and HSV-2. Best evidence supports the use of echinacea to prevent recurrent herpes outbreaks. A single human study found that echinacea did not significantly decrease the recurrence of genital herpes compared to a placebo. More research in this area is needed.

Health Condition	Level of Scientific Evidence
Cervical dysplasia	Poor
Common cold	Poor
Genital warts	Poor
Herpes	Poor

Safety

There is some controversy over the safety of echinacea in autoimmune conditions and HIV, but no clinical evidence exists to either support or deny the supposed risks.

One study on the use of echinacea during the first trimester of pregnancy showed no risk of major malformations. Echinacea is likely safe during pregnancy; however, caution is still advised pending further evidence.

Further Reading

Ghaemi A, Soleimanjahi H, Gill P, et al. *Echinacea purpurea* polysaccharide reduces the latency rate in herpes simplex virus type-1 infections. *Intervirology*, 2009; 52 (1): 29–34.

Holst L, Havnen GC, Nordeng H. Echinacea and elderberry — Should they be used against upper respiratory tract infections during pregnancy? *Frontiers in Pharmacology*, 2014 Mar 4; 5: 31.

Karsch-Völk M, Barrett B, Kiefer D, et al. Echinacea for preventing and treating the common cold. *Cochrane Database of Systematic Reviews*, 2014 Feb 20; 2: CD000530.

Mistrangelo M, Cornaglia S, Pizzio M, et al. Immunostimulation to reduce recurrence after surgery for anal condyloma acuminata: A prospective randomized controlled trial. *Colorectal Disease*, 2010 Aug; 12 (8): 799–803.

Schneider S, Reichling J, Stintzing FC, et al. Anti-herpetic properties of hydroalcoholic extracts and pressed juice from *Echinacea pallida*. *Planta Medica*, 2010 Feb; 76 (3): 265–72.

Sharma M, Anderson SA, Schoop R, Hudson JB. Induction of multiple pro-inflammatory cytokines by respiratory viruses and reversal by standardized *Echinacea*, a potent antiviral herbal extract. *Antiviral Research*, 2009 Aug; 83 (2): 165–70.

Vonau B, Chard S, Mandalia S, et al. Does the extract of the plant *Echinacea purpurea* influence the clinical course of recurrent genital herpes? *International Journal of STD & AIDS*, 2001 Mar; 12 (3): 154–58.

Eleuthero

Current Medicinal Uses

Eleuthero is used as an adaptogen, to help one adapt to stressful situations and conditions, especially when stress is long-term, as in chronic fatigue syndrome. Because it helps people perform better under stress, it is also used for sleep-deprived parents and shift workers, endurance athletes, astronauts and others working or living in stressful conditions.

History and Energetics

Eleuthero, also known as Siberian ginseng, has a long history of use in northern Russia, China, Korea and Japan. Like other herbs used for stress, such as rhodiola, eleuthero grows in a cold climate and has traditionally been used to increase resistance to the environmental and physical stresses of living in a harsh environment.

In traditional Chinese medicine, eleuthero is known as *ci wu jia* and is used to tonify and warm the spleen, stomach and kidney channels. It was historically used to treat weakness, low energy, insomnia, poor concentration, mild depression and pain in the low back and knees.

Research Evidence

Stress

In clinical studies, eleuthero has been shown to significantly improve memory, fatigue, stamina, mood and other cognitive functions. In patients with chronic fatigue, eleuthero substantially reduced physical and mental fatigue compared to a placebo. These effects were more pronounced in a sub-group of people with mild to moderate fatigue.

A small study on people over sixty-five with high blood pressure showed that taking eleuthero for eight weeks improved social functioning when compared to a placebo. Taking eleuthero did not appear to have any effects on blood pressure or medication taken for hypertension.

Latin Name
- *Eleutherococcus senticosus*

Part Used
- Root

Common Combination
- **For stress-related fatigue:** Rhodiola, schisandra and ginseng

Several studies have noted that the positive effects of eleuthero appear to diminish over time. This is consistent with what herbalists and naturopathic doctors have observed: for sustained effects, adaptogens must be changed every six to eight weeks or discontinued for a couple of weeks and then restarted.

Health Condition	Level of Scientific Evidence
Stress	Fair

Safety

Overall, eleuthero, like many other general tonic herbs, is relatively safe. There is some concern that it may raise blood pressure, but a study on people with hypertension observed no change in blood pressure over an eight-week period.

The safety of eleuthero during pregnancy or breast-feeding has not been established.

Further Reading

Cicero AF, Derosa G, Brillante R, et al. Effects of Siberian ginseng (*Eleutherococcus senticosus* maxim.) on elderly quality of life: A randomized clinical trial. *Archives of Gerontology and Geriatrics*, Supplement, 2004; (9): 69–73.

Hartz AJ, Bentler S, Noyes R, et al. Randomized controlled trial of Siberian ginseng for chronic fatigue. *Psychological Medicine*, 2004 Jan; 34 (1): 51–61.

Kuo J, Chen KW, Cheng IS, et al. The effect of eight weeks of supplementation with *Eleutherococcus senticosus* on endurance capacity and metabolism in human. *Chinese Journal of Physiology*, 2010 Apr 30; 53 (2): 105–11.

Panossian AG. Adaptogens in mental and behavioral disorders. *Psychiatric Clinics of North America*, 2013 Mar; 36 (1): 49–64.

Evening Primrose

Current Medicinal Uses

Evening primrose oil is used to treat premenstrual symptoms (especially breast pain and tenderness), acne, eczema and rheumatoid arthritis. Late in pregnancy, it may be used to encourage cervical ripening and the gentle induction of labor.

History and Energetics

The seed oil of evening primrose is what is primarily used today, but the flowers and roots of the plant were traditionally used as physical and spiritual medicine. The roots were eaten to decrease the effects of drinking too much wine, allowing one to drink more without negative consequences. Considered a cure-all in the early 1600s, the whole plant was used to treat asthma, whooping cough and gastrointestinal disorders and to reduce pain. Traditional herbalists still use the whole plant for many of these uses today.

Because its flowers bloom at night, evening primrose was historically considered a moon plant, associated with women and the feminine aspects of health. It is said to stimulate the solar plexus and heart, allowing the user to experience love without fear of rejection or betrayal.

Research Evidence
Cervical Ripening

Although evening primrose oil has been used by midwives to encourage cervical ripening, few studies have investigated these effects. One observational study showed no difference in either length of pregnancy or length of labor when comparing women who took oral evening primrose oil to those who did not. The authors expressed concern over possible increases in prolonged rupture of membranes and the need for medical interventions (such as oxytocin or a vacuum) during labor.

Vaginal use of evening primrose oil has not been studied. Nonetheless, a national survey of certified nurse-midwives in the United States indicated that 60% used evening primrose oil to stimulate labor.

Latin Name
- *Oenothera biennis*

Part Used
- Seed oil

Common Combinations
- Evening primrose oil is rarely mixed with other herbs for internal use. In the case of sexual function, the oil can be infused with medicinal herbs and used topically as a medicinal lubricant.

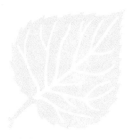

Cyclic Mastalgia and Premenstrual Syndrome

A limited number of research studies have shown that evening primrose oil may be effective in reducing cyclic mastalgia (premenstrual breast pain) compared to a placebo or standard pharmaceutical treatment. One recent study showed that evening primrose oil, both on its own and when taken with vitamin E, significantly lessened pain scores for women with cyclic mastalgia when compared to a placebo.

A placebo-controlled trial on a proprietary formula containing evening primrose oil, vitamin B_6 and vitamin E found significant changes in premenstrual symptom scores in the areas of mood, behavior and physical symptoms. Other studies, however, do not consistently yield positive results. Negative findings may be due to the fact that some studies look at only a few months' worth of data. Clinical experience and research studies suggest that evening primrose oil must be taken for a long period of time (over six months) before beneficial results can be seen.

Rheumatoid Arthritis

Clinical studies using gamma-linolenic acid (an omega-6 fatty acid) from evening primrose and other plant sources have consistently shown significant decreases in overall pain, joint tenderness, swelling and duration of morning stiffness in people diagnosed with rheumatoid arthritis.

Sexual Dysfunction

Evening primrose oil makes a great lubricant for sexual function. Two clinical studies on a topical product containing evening primrose oil, borage oil and medicinal herbs demonstrated significant improvements in arousal, satisfaction, sensation and ability to orgasm compared to a placebo. Women with sexual dysfunction noted greater improvements than women who were already satisfied with their sexual health. More studies are needed to confirm these results.

Did You Know?

GLA

Gamma-linolenic acid (GLA), an omega-6 fatty acid, is considered conditionally essential, which means the body can't easily make it on its own and relies on diet to ensure amounts adequate for good health. GLA is important in treating rheumatoid arthritis because it can help the body transition from a pro-inflammatory response to a non-inflammatory response.

Health Condition	Level of Scientific Evidence
Cervical ripening	Poor
Cyclic mastalgia	Fair/mixed
Premenstrual syndrome	Fair/mixed
Rheumatoid arthritis	Good
Sexual dysfunction	Fair

Safety

Evening primrose oil is generally safe, with minor gastro-intestinal side effects. Discuss its use with your health-care provider if you have a history of mania or epilepsy, or if you are taking antipsychotic medications or blood thinners.

Further Reading

Dante G, Facchinetti F. Herbal treatments for alleviating premenstrual symptoms: A systematic review. *Journal of Psychosomatic Obstetrics and Gynaecology*, 2011 Mar; 32 (1): 42–51.

Dove D, Johnson P. Oral evening primrose oil: Its effect on length of pregnancy and selected intrapartum outcomes in low-risk nulliparous women. *Journal of Nurse-Midwifery*, 1999 May–Jun; 44 (3): 320–24.

Ferguson DM, Hosmane B, Heiman JR. Randomized, placebo-controlled, double-blind, parallel design trial of the efficacy and safety of Zestra in women with mixed desire/interest/arousal/orgasm disorders. *Journal of Sex & Marital Therapy*, 2010; 36 (1): 66–86.

Ferguson DM, Steidle CP, Singh GS, et al. Randomized, placebo-controlled, double blind, crossover design trial of the efficacy and safety of Zestra for Women in women with and without female sexual arousal disorder. *Journal of Sex & Marital Therapy*, 2003; 29 Suppl 1: 33–44.

Kashani L, Saedi N, Akhondzadeh S. Femicomfort in the treatment of premenstrual syndromes: A double-blind, randomized and placebo controlled trial. *Iranian Journal of Psychiatry*, 2010 Spring; 5 (2): 47–50.

McFarlin BL, Gibson MH, O'Rear J, Harman P. A national survey of herbal preparation use by nurse-midwives for labor stimulation: Review of the literature and recommendations for practice. *Journal of Nurse-Midwifery*, 1999 May–Jun; 44 (3): 205–16.

Pruthi S, Wahner-Roedler DL, Torkelson CJ, et al. Vitamin E and evening primrose oil for management of cyclical mastalgia: A randomized pilot study. *Alternative Medicine Review*, 2010 Apr; 15 (1): 59–67.

Srivastava A, Mansel RE, Arvind N, et al. Evidence-based management of mastalgia: A meta-analysis of randomised trials. *Breast*, 2007 Oct; 16 (5): 503–12. Epub 2007 May 16.

Did You Know?

Latex Condoms

When used during sexual activity, evening primrose oil (like all other oils) is not appropriate for use with latex condoms, as the oil will degrade the latex, making the condom ineffective.

Fennel

Latin Name
- *Foeniculum vulgare*

Part Used
- Seeds

Common Combinations
- **For dysmenorrhea:** Ginger, cramp bark and valerian
- **For indigestion with gas and bloating:** Chamomile and peppermint
- **To promote lactation:** Fenugreek, milk thistle and blessed thistle

Current Medicinal Uses

Fennel improves digestion, thereby potentially decreasing blood sugar and cholesterol levels, and relieves gas, bloating and cramping (spasmodic pain in smooth muscle organs such as the intestines and uterus). It is also used to increase breast milk production.

History and Energetics

Fennel has a long history of use in the Mediterranean basin and is mentioned in several Greek myths. Prometheus, the bringer of fire, was said to have concealed the fire within a stalk of fennel. Fennel's hollow stalk was also used as a wand by the followers of Dionysus and was carried by Pheidippides during his two-day run to Sparta to get more soldiers for the battle of Marathon.

Medicinally, fennel was best known for its use as an appetite suppressant during periods of fasting, and was also used to ease digestion and to promote lactation.

Research Evidence

Thanks to fennel's distinctive smell and taste, many studies have failed to adequately blind participants to whether they are receiving the fennel extract or the placebo. In studies where liquid fennel extracts were used, some women dropped out because of the taste.

Dysmenorrhea

Several studies have looked at the use of fennel for the treatment of primary dysmenorrhea (where no cause for the pain can be found), most with positive results. One recent randomized trial found that 30 milligrams of fennel taken every four hours during menses significantly reduced nausea and feelings of weakness and increased quality of life and well-being. After three months, the length of the participants' menses was also significantly shorter. An earlier randomized trial using a similar treatment protocol showed similar results.

Another study showed that a combination of fennel and vitamin E was more effective than ibuprofen in decreasing the intensity of menstrual pain, especially in the first two hours after the onset of pain. Compared to mefenamic acid, fennel was found to be equally effective in addressing menstrual pain. These results were consistent with two earlier studies.

Low Milk Supply

Although fennel has traditionally been used as part of formulas to improve breast milk supply, no human studies have yet been conducted.

Health Condition	Level of Scientific Evidence
Dysmenorrhea	Fair
Low milk supply	Poor

Did You Know?

Absinthe
Along with anise and wormwood, fennel is an ingredient in absinthe, a spirit that was popular in Europe in the late nineteenth century, especially among artists.

Safety

As a culinary spice, fennel is a relatively safe herb for most people. Fennel is not recommended in concentrated forms in pregnancy.

Further Reading

Ghodsi Z, Asltoghiri M. The effect of fennel on pain quality, symptoms, and menstrual duration in primary dysmenorrhea. *Journal of Pediatric and Adolescent Gynecology*, 2014 Oct; 27 (5): 283–86.

Nasehi M, Sehhatie F, Zamanzadeh V, et al. Comparison of the effectiveness of combination of fennel extract/vitamin E with ibuprofen on the pain intensity in students with primary dysmenorrhea. *Iranian Journal of Nursing and Midwifery Research*, 2013 Sep; 18 (5): 355–59.

Omidvar S, Esmailzadeh S, Baradaran M, Basirat Z. Effect of fennel on pain intensity in dysmenorrhoea: A placebo-controlled trial. *Ayu*, 2012 Apr; 33 (2): 311–13.

❧ Fenugreek

Latin Name
- *Trigonella foenum-graecum* L.

Part Used
- Seeds

Common Combinations
- **For diabetes:** Milk thistle, cinnamon and gymnema
- **To promote lactation:** Blessed thistle, milk thistle and fennel

Current Medicinal Uses

Fenugreek is used to promote breast milk production, ensure healthy digestion and treat fevers. Recent use also includes the treatment of diabetes, high cholesterol and gastritis.

History and Energetics

Fenugreek — or methi, as it is called in several languages in India — is one of the oldest documented herbal medicines in the world. A description of fenugreek is found in the Ebers Papyrus, a medical text from Egypt, circa 1550 BCE. It was also used in Ancient Egypt as incense and for embalming. The tomb of Tutankhamun is said to have contained fenugreek to ensure he would not go hungry in the afterlife. Egyptian women may have also used fenugreek to ease menstrual pain.

When soaked in water, fenugreek seeds produce a mucilaginous liquid a lot like egg whites. During the first Jewish-Roman war (66–73 CE), Josephus was said to have ordered his troops to boil and pour fenugreek seeds over the siege ramps to literally slip up the Romans.

Greeks and Romans grew and used fenugreek as cattle fodder. Its Latin species name, *foenum-graecum*, means "Greek hay." It is still fed to dairy cows today to increase their milk production. This galactagogue effect also works in humans, and in some regions of India, a porridge made of fenugreek seeds and rice is given to new mothers to promote lactation.

From an Ayurvedic perspective, fenugreek reduces vata (ether) and kapha (phlegm).

Research Evidence
Diabetes

In a recent meta-analysis, fenugreek was found to significantly decrease fasting blood sugar, blood sugar after eating and HbA1c, a measure of average blood sugar level over the previous three months, in people with type 2 diabetes.

Low Milk Supply

A systematic review on the use of herbal galactagogues, including fenugreek, concluded that there isn't enough evidence because the trials are small and poorly designed. The studies that do exist, however, show positive effects. One small study found that infants whose mothers drank fenugreek tea lost significantly less weight and returned to their birth weight more quickly than infants in either a placebo group or a control group. Most important, the women who drank fenugreek tea had a significantly greater volume of breast milk than the women in the other two groups.

Health Condition	Level of Scientific Evidence
Diabetes	Good
Low milk supply	Poor

Safety

Fenugreek may cause hypoglycemia. Women with diabetes who are taking hypoglycemic medications should be cautious about also taking this herb. Fenugreek should not be used by people with allergies to peanuts or chickpeas, as it is from the same family of plants. Fenugreek should be avoided in large doses during pregnancy, as it can act as an emmenagogue.

Further Reading

Mortel M, Mehta SD. Systematic review of the efficacy of herbal galactogogues. *Journal of Human Lactation*, 2013 May; 29 (2): 154–62.

Neelakantan N, Narayanan M, de Souza RJ, van Dam RM. Effect of fenugreek (*Trigonella foenum-graecum* L.) intake on glycemia: A meta-analysis of clinical trials. *Nutrition Journal*, 2014 Jan 18; 13: 7.

Suksomboon N, Poolsup N, Boonkaew S, Suthisisang CC. Meta-analysis of the effect of herbal supplement on glycemic control in type 2 diabetes. *Journal of Ethnopharmacology*, 2011 Oct 11; 137 (3): 1328–33.

Turkyilmaz C, Onal E, Hirfanoglu IM, et al. The effect of galactagogue herbal tea on breast milk production and short-term catch-up of birth weight in the first week of life. *Journal of Alternative and Complementary Medicine*, 2011 Feb; 17 (2): 139–42.

Zapantis A, Steinberg JG, Schilit L. Use of herbals as galactagogues. *Journal of Pharmacy Practice*, 2012 Apr; 25 (2): 222–31.

🌿 Garlic

Latin Name
- *Allium sativum*

Part Used
- Bulb/cloves

Common Combinations
- **For bacterial vaginosis or vaginal yeast infections:** Tea tree oil or goldenseal
- **For high blood pressure:** Hawthorn and motherwort

Current Medicinal Uses

Garlic has many medicinal functions, from treating infections, thanks to its strong antimicrobial action, to lowering blood pressure and cholesterol.

History and Energetics

One of the earliest domesticated plants, garlic has been used for thousands of years, and not just to ward off vampires: there are few health conditions people *haven't* tried to treat with garlic. It is touted for its healing properties in Ancient Egyptian, Indian, Chinese and Greek writings. Garlic bulbs were found in the tomb of Tutankhamun. In Ayurvedic medicine, garlic was used for sinus problems and ear infections. Unani healers used it to regulate menses and treat fevers. It has also been used to treat parasites, colic, high blood pressure, lung infections and scabies.

The Ancient Greeks and Romans ate garlic to build up their strength for athletic competitions and battles. Midwives hung garlic in birthing rooms to keep away the evil eye. Palestinian bridegrooms wore garlic in a buttonhole, as it was considered an aphrodisiac.

Religious Hindus, Jains and Buddhists avoid eating garlic (and onions) because its physically stimulating and aphrodisiac qualities detract from their spiritual practices. The Ancient Greeks held similar views: garlic was great for athletes, workers and soldiers but was not welcome in temples.

Research Evidence
High Blood Pressure

Recent meta-analyses of clinical trials on the use of garlic for hypertension show that garlic may reduce blood pressure compared to a placebo. In the trials, systolic blood pressure decreased by 10 to 15 mmHg and diastolic blood pressure decreased by 6 to 10 mmHg. It is difficult to definitively say that garlic lowers blood pressure, as these reductions fall within the normal potential variations; however, the reductions are consistent with those achieved by standard blood pressure medications.

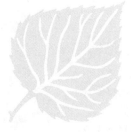

When taken during pregnancy, garlic does not appear to affect the likelihood of developing high blood pressure or pre-eclampsia. In studies on garlic compared to a placebo, there were no increases in side effects or effects on rates of Caesarean section or infant death.

High Cholesterol

Two recent meta-analyses showed that garlic is effective in reducing total cholesterol and low-density lipoprotein (LDL), or "bad," cholesterol when taken for longer than two months.

Vaginitis

In a trial of women with bacterial vaginosis, garlic was shown to be as effective as metronidazole. In another study, garlic-thyme cream inserted vaginally was as effective as clotrimazole for yeast infections, with fewer side effects. Garlic may also be an effective treatment for other causes of vaginitis. More research is needed.

Health Condition	Level of Scientific Evidence
High blood pressure	Good
High cholesterol	Good
Vaginitis	Fair

Did You Know?

Garlic Safeguards

For those who don't want to smell like garlic, odorless garlic is available in supplement form. Alternatively, chewing fresh parsley leaves gets rid of garlic breath. If taking raw garlic, eat the cloves or oil with food, as garlic can cause stomach upset.

Safety

Large amounts of garlic can cause nausea and stomach upset. Garlic may also cause colic in breastfed infants when eaten by the lactating parent. Since garlic can dilate blood vessels, it may increase the risk of bleeding in people taking blood-thinning medications. Garlic appears to be relatively safe in pregnancy.

Further Reading

Aalami-Harandi R, Karamali M, Asemi Z. The favorable effects of garlic intake on metabolic profiles, hs-CRP, biomarkers of oxidative stress and pregnancy outcomes in pregnant women at risk for pre-eclampsia: Randomized, double-blind, placebo-controlled trial. *Journal of Maternal-Fetal & Neonatal Medicine*, 2014 Nov 7: 1–8.

Bahadoran P, Rokni FK, Fahami F. Investigating the therapeutic effect of vaginal cream containing garlic and thyme compared to clotrimazole cream for the treatment of mycotic vaginitis. *Iranian Journal of Nursing and Midwifery Research*, 2010 Dec; 15 (Suppl 1): 343–49.

Kwak JS, Kim JY, Paek JE, et al. Garlic powder intake and cardiovascular risk factors: A meta-analysis of randomized controlled clinical trials. *Nutrition Research and Practice*, 2014 Dec; 8 (6): 644–54.

Meher S, Duley L. Garlic for preventing pre-eclampsia and its complications. *Cochrane Database of Systematic Reviews*, 2006 Jul 19; (3): CD006065.

Mohammadzadeh F, Dolatian M, Jorjani M, et al. Comparing the therapeutic effects of garlic tablet and oral metronidazole on bacterial vaginosis: A randomized controlled clinical trial. *Iranian Red Crescent Medical Journal*, 2014 Jul; 16 (7): e19118.

Ried K, Fakler P. Potential of garlic (*Allium sativum*) in lowering high blood pressure: Mechanisms of action and clinical relevance. *Integrated Blood Pressure Control*, 2014 Dec 9; 7: 71–82.

Ried K, Toben C, Fakler P. Effect of garlic on serum lipids: An updated meta-analysis. *Nutrition Reviews*, 2013 May; 71 (5): 282–99.

Stabler SN, Tejani AM, Huynh F, Fowkes C. Garlic for the prevention of cardiovascular morbidity and mortality in hypertensive patients. *Cochrane Database of Systematic Reviews*, 2012 Aug 15; 8: CD007653.

Geranium

Current Medicinal Uses

Geranium is used as an astringent for the abdominal and pelvic organs, to help stop bleeding, and for conditions with passive hemorrhaging, such as stomach ulcers, inflammatory bowel disease, irritable bowel syndrome, chronic diarrhea, menorrhagia and leukorrhea (vaginal discharge). It is also used to treat canker sores and ulcerated gums. Externally, geranium can be used on wounds and sores.

History and Energetics

Geranium is also called cranesbill because the long seed pods resemble a crane's long beak, and indeed, the word "geranium" comes from the Greek word for "crane." Another story about geranium suggests that it is related to mallow, which has similar leaves. In this story, the prophet Mohammed lay his shirt on a bed of mallow to dry. The mallow, honored at the opportunity to serve, blushed pink and was renamed geranium.

Native Americans used geranium for sore throats and gums, canker sores, oral candida infections, hemorrhoids and gonorrhea. The Iroquois used it to counteract a love medicine. Various geranium species have also been used to treat diarrhea in North America, Africa and China.

A related species, *Geranium wilfordii*, known in traditional Chinese medicine (TCM) as *lao guan cao*, is used for diarrhea, open sores in the digestive tract, rheumatic conditions and muscular pain. From the TCM perspective, *lao guan cao* dispels wind dampness, clears heat and toxicity from the blood and stops diarrhea. *Geranium thunbergii* is used in Kampo (traditional Japanese medicine). Other geranium species are used in medical traditions around the world. Almost all species of geranium contain high concentrations of tannins and are used as astringent and antihemorrhagic herbs with an affinity for the digestive tract.

Research Evidence

Animal studies on geranium species have confirmed the antidiarrheal effects of the plant. Mexican species have shown the ability to inhibit protozoal infections, such as

Latin Name
- *Geranium maculatum*

Part Used
- Root

Common Combination
- For menorrhagia: Yarrow and shepherd's purse

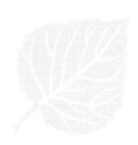

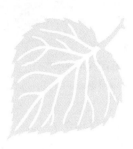

giardia, in vitro. The Chinese species may inhibit *H. pylori* bacteria, which cause stomach ulcers, according to some in vitro studies.

Menorrhagia

Geranium contains gallotannins, which act as powerful astringents and hemostatics. Although research has been done on the use of tannins to stop bleeding in a variety of health conditions, no research has been done specifically on the use of geranium for menorrhagia.

Health Condition	Level of Scientific Evidence
Menorrhagia	Poor

Safety

In high doses or if given for long periods of time, geranium may cause constipation. The tannins in geranium may reduce the absorption of minerals, so geranium should not be taken at the same time as iron, zinc or other minerals. Likewise, geranium may interact with many drugs, altering the rate of drug metabolism as the bowel slows down.

Further Reading

Amabeoku GJ. Antidiarrhoeal activity of *Geranium incanum* Burm. f. (Geraniaceae) leaf aqueous extract in mice. *Journal of Ethnopharmacology*, 2009 May 4; 123 (1): 190–93.

Calzada F, Cervantes-Martínez JA, Yépez-Mulia L. In vitro antiprotozoal activity from the roots of *Geranium mexicanum* and its constituents on *Entamoeba histolytica* and *Giardia lamblia*. *Journal of Ethnopharmacology*, 2005 Apr 8; 98 (1–2): 191–93.

Zhang XQ, Gu HM, Li XZ, et al. Anti-*Helicobacter pylori* compounds from the ethanol extracts of *Geranium wilfordii*. *Journal of Ethnopharmacology*, 2013 May 2; 147 (1): 204–7.

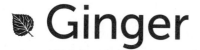 Ginger

Current Medicinal Uses

As a medicinal herb, ginger is anti-inflammatory, carminative, antinausea, antispasmodic, warming and a circulatory stimulant. It can be used for nausea of any kind: motion sickness, morning sickness or even drug-induced nausea, such as postoperative and post-chemotherapy nausea. It is also used to treat arthritis, indigestion and dysmenorrhea.

History and Energetics

Revered since ancient times, ginger's historical uses were much the same as they are today. The earliest records of the medicinal use of ginger come from India and China. Ginger later spread to Europe and then to the Americas, becoming popular everywhere it traveled.

From a traditional Chinese medicine perspective, fresh ginger, known as *sheng jiang*, warms the body from the inside and encourages perspiration. It is used for acute colds and flus, for nausea and vomiting when the stomach is "cold," and in combination formulas to help lessen the toxicity of other herbs.

In Ayurvedic medicine, ginger is used to warm the digestive system and improve circulation, especially for people with vata constitutions.

Research Evidence
Chemotherapy-Induced Nausea and Vomiting

Reviews of the scientific literature and clinical trials on the use of ginger to treat chemotherapy-induced nausea and vomiting have noted mixed results. Two 2013 reviews concluded that they could not support the use of ginger for this purpose. However, in one randomized, open-label trial on women with advanced breast cancer, the addition of ginger to standard antiemetic drug therapy significantly reduced nausea up to twenty-four hours after chemotherapy treatments.

Latin Name
- *Zingiber officinale*

Part Used
- Rhizome

Common Combinations
- **For dysmenorrhea:** Fennel and valerian
- **For rheumatoid arthritis:** Boswellia, turmeric and willow

Dysmenorrhea

Several studies have looked at the use of ginger in alleviating the pain of primary dysmenorrhea (where no cause for the pain can be found). One randomized, controlled trial showed that ginger was just as effective as mefenamic acid, a pharmaceutical drug commonly prescribed in some countries. Other trials have found that ginger decreased menstrual pain as effectively as zinc sulfate or ibuprofen, better than progressive muscle relaxation and significantly better than a placebo. Studies on the use of ginger for dysmenorrhea have primarily been conducted on young women taking doses up to 2 grams total daily.

Morning Sickness

A recent randomized clinical trial studied 120 women who were less than sixteen weeks pregnant and were experiencing mild to moderate morning sickness. The study compared 250-milligram ginger capsules taken three times daily to a placebo and control. The women who took ginger experienced significantly less nausea and vomiting than the women in the placebo and control groups. Vomiting decreased by 51% and nausea by 46%.

Other studies have shown that ginger is more effective than either acupressure or placebo and just as effective as vitamin B6 in reducing mild to moderate morning sickness.

Systematic reviews and meta-analyses have generally been positive. One meta-analysis of twelve trials including 1,278 pregnant women found that ginger significantly reduced nausea but not vomiting. Another meta-analysis of six studies concluded that ginger significantly reduced both nausea and vomiting of pregnancy.

Rheumatoid Arthritis

The phytochemicals in ginger have been studied for their anti-inflammatory properties. In animal studies, ginger has been shown to reduce prostaglandins and leukotrienes, inflammatory markers associated with rheumatoid arthritis. A combination of ginger and turmeric was shown to protect rats from systemic inflammation, joint degeneration, anemia, kidney and cardiovascular impairments and other physiological changes associated with rheumatoid arthritis.

In one clinical trial, a combination Ayurvedic formula with ginger and guduchi was found to be as effective as a disease-modifying antirheumatic drug (DMARD)

Did You Know?

A Powerful Family

Ginger is a member of the same family as turmeric and cardamom, other medicinal herbs used for their anti-inflammatory and digestive properties.

in reducing pain. Unfortunately, the study was poorly designed. Another small, open study found that ginger significantly reduced both pain and swelling in rheumatoid arthritis. More high-quality research is needed.

Health Condition	Level of Scientific Evidence
Chemotherapy-induced nausea and vomiting	Mixed
Dysmenorrhea	Good
Morning sickness	Good
Rheumatoid arthritis	Poor

Safety

Ginger is relatively safe, even during the first trimester of pregnancy, though some clinical studies have noted a slight increase in heartburn. Trials on ginger in doses up to 2 grams daily during pregnancy have found no adverse outcomes, and ginger does not appear to increase the risk of spontaneous abortion.

Further Reading

Al-Nahain A, Jahan R, Rahmatullah M. *Zingiber officinale*: A potential plant against rheumatoid arthritis. *Arthritis*, 2014; 2014: 159089.

Ding M, Leach M, Bradley H. The effectiveness and safety of ginger for pregnancy-induced nausea and vomiting: A systematic review. *Women and Birth*, 2013 Mar; 26 (1): e26–30.

Haji Seid Javadi E, Salehi F, Mashrabi O. Comparing the effectiveness of vitamin B_6 and ginger in treatment of pregnancy-induced nausea and vomiting. *Obstetrics and Gynecology International*, 2013; 2013: 927834.

Kashefi F, Khajehei M, Tabatabaeichehr M, et al. Comparison of the effect of ginger and zinc sulfate on primary dysmenorrhea: A placebo-controlled randomized trial. *Pain Management Nursing*, 2014 Dec; 15 (4): 826–33.

Lee J, Oh H. Ginger as an antiemetic modality for chemotherapy-induced nausea and vomiting: A systematic review and meta-analysis. *Oncology Nursing Forum*, 2013 Mar; 40 (2): 163–70.

Marx WM, Teleni L, McCarthy AL, et al. Ginger (*Zingiber officinale*) and chemotherapy-induced nausea and vomiting: A systematic literature review. *Nutrition Reviews*, 2013 Apr; 71 (4): 245–54.

Matthews A, Haas DM, O'Mathúna DP, et al. Interventions for nausea and vomiting in early pregnancy. *Cochrane Database of Systematic Reviews*, 2014 Mar 21; 3: CD007575.

Panahi Y, Saadat A, Sahebkar A, et al. Effect of ginger on acute and delayed chemotherapy-induced nausea and vomiting: A pilot, randomized, open-label clinical trial. *Integrative Cancer Therapies*, 2012 Sep; 11 (3): 204–11.

Rahnama P, Montazeri A, Huseini HF, et al. Effect of *Zingiber officinale* R. rhizomes (ginger) on pain relief in primary dysmenorrhea: A placebo randomized trial. *BMC Complementary and Alternative Medicine*, 2012 Jul 10; 12: 92.

Ramadan G, El-Menshawy O. Protective effects of ginger-turmeric rhizomes mixture on joint inflammation, atherogenesis, kidney dysfunction and other complications in a rat model of human rheumatoid arthritis. *International Journal of Rheumatic Diseases*, 2013 Apr; 16 (2): 219–29.

Saberi F, Sadat Z, Abedzadeh-Kalahroudi M, Taebi M. Effect of ginger on relieving nausea and vomiting in pregnancy: A randomized, placebo-controlled trial. *Nursing and Midwifery Studies*, 2014 Apr; 3 (1): e11841.

Shirvani MA, Motahari-Tabari N, Alipour A. The effect of mefenamic acid and ginger on pain relief in primary dysmenorrhea: A randomized clinical trial. *Archives of Gynecology and Obstetrics*, 2014 Nov 16. [Epub ahead of print.]

Thomson M, Corbin R, Leung L. Effects of ginger for nausea and vomiting in early pregnancy: A meta-analysis. *Journal of the American Board of Family Medicine*, 2014 Jan–Feb; 27 (1): 115–22.

Viljoen E, Visser J, Koen N, Musekiwa A. A systematic review and meta-analysis of the effect and safety of ginger in the treatment of pregnancy-associated nausea and vomiting. *Nutrition Journal*, 2014 Mar 19; 13: 20.

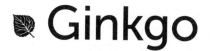 Ginkgo

Current Medicinal Uses

Gingko supports blood circulation throughout the body, but particularly to the brain. It can improve cognition, focus and concentration when these have decreased because of poor circulation. Ginkgo is used therapeutically for cerebral vascular insufficiency, hemorrhoids, varicosities, Raynaud's syndrome, post-traumatic brain injury, stroke recovery, tinnitus, age-related macular degeneration and asthma. Since ginkgo works by dilating small to medium-sized arteries, it is also useful in conditions like premenstrual syndrome (PMS) and sexual dysfunction where circulation in smaller vessels may be a factor in the development of symptoms.

History and Energetics

Ginkgo is a truly ancient tree, around since the time of the dinosaurs. It has likely been used medicinally for as long as there have been humans.

The shape of the leaves resembles the outline of a brain, which contributed to the belief that ginkgo was good for brain health, memory and concentration. Ginkgo's association with healthy aging and longevity may relate to how long individual trees can live: some trees in Taoist temple courtyards in Asia are said to be over 2,500 years old. Gingko trees are also seen as resilient. Many sources claim that the first living things to thrive after the atomic bombings in Hiroshima and Nagasaki were cockroaches and ginkgos.

Traditional Chinese medicine (TCM) uses the seeds of the ginkgo tree as well as the leaves. Known as *bai guo*, or white nut, the seeds are slightly toxic and are thus used only in small amounts. As an astringent, ginkgo seeds are used for asthma, chronic cough, leukorrhea (vaginal discharge) and incontinence.

Research Evidence

As mentioned earlier, women's health conditions are not the primary health issues that ginkgo is known for. Two recent systematic reviews found that ginkgo may help improve cognitive and behavioral symptoms in people with Alzheimer's disease but does not slow the disease's progression.

Latin Name
- *Ginkgo biloba*

Parts Used
- Leaf
- Seeds (in TCM)

Common Combinations
- **For PMS with breast tenderness and fluid retention:** Chaste tree and dandelion leaf

- **For sexual dysfunction due to poor circulation to sexual organs:** Ginseng

- **For hemorrhoids and varicose veins:** Horse chestnut, witch hazel and calendula

Did You Know?

Ornamentals
Although ginkgo trees are now endangered in the wild, they are widely planted as ornamentals in urban areas in Asia, Europe and North America.

Hemorrhoids and Varicose Veins

The main plant constituents in ginkgo are flavonoids, which promote the integrity and strength of blood vessel walls and are known to decrease inflammation. One small open-label study investigating a combination herbal product containing ginkgo for the treatment of hemorrhoids found improvements in bleeding, pain and discharge after one week of use. Several other open-label trials on the use of the same product for varicose veins and chronic venous insufficiency also reported decreased symptoms. More research is needed.

Premenstrual Syndrome

Since ginkgo has been found to decrease the frequency and duration of migraines when given prophylactically in some studies, it may also be helpful for preventing PMS-related headaches and migraines. Few studies have looked at using ginkgo specifically for PMS symptoms. One randomized, controlled study found that ginkgo significantly reduced the congestive symptoms of PMS, in particular breast tenderness and fluid retention. A similar study found that ginkgo significantly reduced physical, psychological and overall PMS symptoms compared to a placebo.

Sexual Dysfunction

Preclinical studies on ginkgo demonstrated the herb's ability to dilate small blood vessels, relax smooth muscles and influence the release of nitric oxide. Because all three of these actions are involved in sexual arousal and responses, ginkgo has since been studied for its potential use in addressing both male and female sexual dysfunction. Additionally, in some trials that looked at the use of ginkgo in relieving the decreased sexual function commonly experienced by people taking antidepressant medication, women experienced greater improvements than men.

A few trials have been conducted on ginkgo specifically for female sexual dysfunction. The results are tentative but promising. One small trial found that ginkgo improved physiological sexual arousal but failed to change the women's sense of whether they were aroused. Another trial, on postmenopausal women, found significant improvements in sexual desire in the women taking ginkgo compared to those taking a placebo. An open-label study on a combination product with ginkgo and muira puama also had positive results, as have two studies on a product containing ginkgo, ginseng, damiana and other nutrients.

Health Condition	Level of Scientific Evidence
Hemorrhoids/varicose veins	Poor
Premenstrual syndrome	Poor
Sexual dysfunction	Fair

Safety

Ginkgo should be avoided or used cautiously by people with bleeding disorders or those taking blood thinners, as the herb can increase the risk of bleeding. It should be avoided up to one week before surgery for the same reason.

Caution is advised during the later stages of pregnancy, as ginkgo's blood-thinning effects may prolong bleeding in labor and delivery. There is insufficient evidence to confirm the safety of ginkgo during breastfeeding.

Further Reading

Allais G, Castagnoli Gabellari I, Burzio C, et al. Premenstrual syndrome and migraine. *Neurological Sciences*, 2012 May; 33 Suppl 1: S111–15.

Meston CM, Rellini AH, Telch MJ. Short- and long-term effects of *Ginkgo biloba* extract on sexual dysfunction in women. *Archives of Sexual Behavior*, 2008 Aug; 37 (4): 530–47.

Ozgoli G, Selselei EA, Mojab F, Majd HA. A randomized, placebo-controlled trial of *Ginkgo biloba* L. in treatment of premenstrual syndrome. *Journal of Alternative and Complementary Medicine*, 2009 Aug; 15 (8): 845–51.

Pebdani MA, Taavoni S, Seyedfatemi N, Haghani H. Triple-blind, placebo-controlled trial of *Ginkgo biloba* extract on sexual desire in postmenopausal women in Tehran. *Iranian Journal of Nursing and Midwifery Research*, 2014 May; 19 (3): 262–65.

Sumboonnanonda K, Lertsithichai P. Clinical study of the *Ginkgo biloba* — Troxerutin-heptaminol Hce in the treatment of acute hemorrhoidal attacks. *Journal of the Medical Association of Thailand*, 2004 Feb; 87 (2): 137–42.

Yang M, Xu DD, Zhang Y, et al. A systematic review on natural medicines for the prevention and treatment of Alzheimer's disease with meta-analyses of intervention effect of ginkgo. *American Journal of Chinese Medicine*, 2014; 42 (3): 505–21.

Zhukov BN, Kukol'nikova EL. [Clinical response to Ginkor-Fort in the treatment of chronic venous insufficiency in varicosity]. [Article in Russian]. *Terapevticheskiĭ arkhiv*, 2004; 76 (12): 48–50.

Ginseng

Latin Name
- *Panax ginseng*

Part Used
- Root

Common Combination
- **For sexual function:** Ginkgo, rehmannia and damiana

Current Medicinal Uses

As a general tonic and adaptogen, ginseng improves responses to stress. It restores vitality in the elderly and in those who have been depleted by chronic illness. Ginseng is also used to improve sexual function in both women and men.

In traditional Chinese medicine (TCM) terms, ginseng tonifies yuan qi (source energy). It is used for weakness, shortness of breath, low appetite, diarrhea, fatigue, organ prolapse, profuse sweating and poor memory.

History and Energetics

Ginseng's Chinese name, *ren shen*, translates as "person roots." This name refers to the shape of the plant's roots, which are forked in a way that looks like a human body, complete with head, arms and legs. Ginseng looks like a whole person and is used as a tonic, or panacea, to treat the whole person. In fact, the plant's Latin name, *Panax*, comes from the same Greek root as "panacea," which means "all-healing."

Research Evidence
Sexual Dysfunction

Although research on ginseng in regard to sexual function has primarily been related to improving erectile function, researchers have begun exploring the potential of ginseng in enhancing sexual function in women as well. Animal studies have found that ginseng relaxes clitoral and vaginal smooth muscle tissue in rats and rabbits. One small placebo-controlled, randomized, crossover study in postmenopausal women found that ginseng significantly improved subjective assessments of sexual arousal compared to a placebo. Two women in the study experienced vaginal bleeding while taking ginseng, but otherwise no adverse effects were noted.

Two older randomized, controlled studies on combination herbal products containing ginseng, ginkgo, damiana and other nutrients found that the combination product significantly increased sexual desire and satisfaction in premenopausal women. In perimenopausal women, the product substantially improved desire, satisfaction, frequency of intercourse and vaginal dryness compared to a placebo, while postmenopausal women showed improvement only in sexual desire.

Health Condition	Level of Scientific Evidence
Sexual dysfunction	Fair

Safety

Ginseng is a stimulating herb and can lead to insomnia, headaches, nausea, high blood pressure and heart palpitations when taken in large amounts. Use ginseng cautiously if you have high blood pressure, in particular if taking the herb in large doses, long-term and concurrently with caffeine. Avoid ginseng in the early stages of pregnancy, as there is some evidence that it may lead to negative outcomes.

Further Reading

Ito TY, Polan ML, Whipple B, Trant AS. The enhancement of female sexual function with ArginMax, a nutritional supplement, among women differing in menopausal status. *Journal of Sex & Marital Therapy*, 2006; Oct–Dec; 32 (5): 369–78.

Ito TY, Trant AS, Polan ML. A double-blind placebo-controlled study of ArginMax, a nutritional supplement for enhancement of female sexual function. *Journal of Sex & Marital Therapy*, 2001 Oct–Dec; 27 (5): 541–49.

Kim MS, Lim HJ, Yang HJ, et al. Ginseng for managing menopause symptoms: A systematic review of randomized clinical trials. *Journal of Ginseng Research*, 2013 Mar; 37 (1): 30–36.

Oh KJ, Chae MJ, Lee HS, et al. Effects of Korean red ginseng on sexual arousal in menopausal women: Placebo-controlled, double-blind crossover clinical study. *Journal of Sexual Medicine*, 2010 Apr; 7 (4 Pt 1): 1469–77.

Did You Know?

Herbal Viagra

In vitro and animal studies show that ginseng may work in a similar way to sildenafil — better known as Viagra — as both increase nitric oxide, which dilates blood vessels and allows for better blood flow through the sexual organs.

Goldenseal

Latin Name
- *Hydrastis canadensis*

Part Used
- Root

Common Combinations
- **For infectious vaginitis:** Garlic and thyme
- **For UTIs:** Uva ursi and corn silk

Did You Know?

Fictional Fancy
Pharmacist and eclecticist John Uri Lloyd used goldenseal as part of the plot in his novel *Stringtown on the Pike*. In the book, an expert testifying in a murder trial claims the victim had strychnine in his stomach when it was actually goldenseal. This story likely contributed to the development of a myth that goldenseal can mask the presence of morphine, marijuana and cocaine.

Current Medicinal Uses

Goldenseal is a mucous membrane tonic that helps restore health to tissues such as the nose, mouth and vagina. It is used in a variety of conditions where there is excess mucus, such as allergic rhinitis, upper respiratory tract infections, ulcers, urinary tract infections (UTIs) and vaginitis.

At some point goldenseal became popular as an "herbal antibiotic" even though it was not used that way traditionally. The assumption behind this use seems to be that goldenseal's tonifying and astringent effect on mucous membranes is due to a direct antimicrobial action that creates an unfavorable environment for bacteria. Although berberine and other constituents of goldenseal have indeed shown antimicrobial action in vitro, "herbal antibiotic" effects have not yet been reproduced in human studies.

History and Energetics

Goldenseal is named for the color of its root: a deep, golden yellow. Historically, in addition to its use for healing mucous membranes, goldenseal was used to treat jaundice, eczema, ringworm, postpartum hemorrhage, gonorrhea, leukorrhea (vaginal discharge), ulcers and loss of appetite. The Cherokee used it as a wash for eye infections, to improve the appetite and to treat cancer. The Iroquois used it for diarrhea, liver disease, ear infections and indigestion.

Research Evidence
Urinary Tract Infections

In vitro, goldenseal — and, in particular, the plant chemical berberine — has been shown to prevent bacteria such as *E. coli* from sticking to the walls of the bladder and the intestines, and even to have an antibacterial effect against resistant strains of bacteria. More research in humans is needed to support this use.

Vaginitis

In vitro studies show some promise in confirming goldenseal's traditional use to help reduce secretions and excess mucus in cases of vaginitis. The yeast *Candida albicans* and the protozoa *Trichomonas vaginalis*, common causes of vaginitis, are both inhibited by berberine in vitro.

Health Condition	Level of Scientific Evidence
Urinary tract infections	Poor
Vaginitis	Poor

Safety

Goldenseal should not be used during pregnancy, as some of its plant constituents are known to cause uterine contractions. It should be avoided during the first few weeks of breastfeeding because it can become toxic in a newborn with jaundice. The alkaloid chemicals in goldenseal may strain kidney function in those with kidney disease or kidney failure. Like all bitter-tasting herbs, goldenseal may irritate the stomach in sensitive people.

Further Reading

Dhamgaye S, Devaux F, Vandeputte P, et al. Molecular mechanisms of action of herbal antifungal alkaloid berberine, in *Candida albicans*. *PLoS One*, 2014 Aug 8; 9 (8): e104554.

Head KA. Natural approaches to prevention and treatment of infections of the lower urinary tract. *Alternative Medicine Review*, 2008 Sep; 13 (3): 227–44.

Soffar SA, Metwali DM, Abdel-Aziz SS, et al. Evaluation of the effect of a plant alkaloid (berberine derived from *Berberis aristata*) on *Trichomonas vaginalis* in vitro. *Journal of the Egyptian Society of Parasitology*, 2001 Dec; 31 (3): 893–904.

Did You Know?

Endangered Species

Goldenseal is at risk of becoming endangered in the wild in North America, a result of deforestation and overharvesting. Be certain to look for cultivated rather than wildcrafted sources.

🍃 Green Tea

Latin Name
- *Camellia sinensis*

Parts Used
- Leaf
- Extract of EGCG

Common Combinations
- **For androgen excess in PCOS:** Licorice and spearmint
- **For breast cancer prevention:** Soy
- **For high blood pressure:** Hawthorn and motherwort

Current Medicinal Uses

Green tea and its most abundant and powerful catechin, epigallocatechin gallate (EGCG), are perhaps best known for breast cancer prevention. Green tea consumption is associated with lower rates of breast cancer, heart disease and stroke. Research suggests that green tea may also be useful for regulating metabolism in promoting weight loss and treating metabolic conditions such as diabetes.

Although it is less researched for other uses, green tea is also used clinically in the treatment of endometriosis and autoimmune causes of infertility. Topically, green tea is used in the treatment of acne, cervical dysplasia and genital warts.

History and Energetics

People have been drinking green tea for over 4,000 years. It is said to have been discovered by the emperor Shen Nong, who accidentally dropped the leaves into boiled water in 2737 BCE. He drank the water anyway and afterward felt more vital and alert.

For thousands of years, tea was primarily used medicinally by monks and emperors, and very little was documented about its use. In 59 BCE, Wang Bao wrote the first known book with detailed instructions about buying and preparing tea. In the eighth century, Lu Yu wrote *Tea Classic*, a book about the joy of green tea. Around the same time, tea drinking spread to Japan. In both China and Japan, elaborate tea ceremonies developed. The sharing and drinking of tea became a sacred spiritual experience.

Tea was first imported to Europe during the sixteenth century through Portuguese merchants. Soon thereafter, it was planted for cultivation on the Azores. Tea drinking in England spread by way of Catherine of Braganza, wife of King Charles II, who brought tea from Portugal to England. By the eighteenth century, tea could be found in coffee houses and became so popular that the government decided to charge heavy taxes on it. Heavy taxes, and the resultant smuggling of tea to avoid taxes, became commonplace in both the United Kingdom and the British colonies in the Americas. The Tea Act of 1773 was created to reduce the surplus of tea held by the British East India Company and to undercut smugglers' prices while continuing to collect taxes from the colonies.

Opposition and resistance to the Tea Act solidified and became a turning point in history. On December 16, 1773, protestors in Boston boarded ships docked in the harbor and then dumped their tea cargo. The ensuing reactions to the "Boston Tea Party" raised tensions, eventually leading to the American Revolution in April 1775 and the creation of the United States of America.

In the 1800s, the British attempted to cultivate tea in India to avoid the Chinese monopoly on the tea trade. Although their attempts to grow Chinese varietals in India were unsuccessful, they began large-scale cultivation of the local varietal of tea in Assam, a state in northeastern India, for export to England.

Research Evidence

Acne

In vitro studies have demonstrated green tea's potential to inhibit *Propionibacterium acnes* and encourage anti-inflammatory effects. In one open-label study, a 2% green tea extract applied to skin twice a day for six weeks decreased the number of acne lesions by 58% and the overall severity of the acne by 39%. A second, uncontrolled human study observed decreased sebum production in healthy men who used green tea cream topically for eight weeks. Additional high-quality research is needed.

Breast Cancer

Overall, reviews of the studies conducted suggest that green tea may reduce the risk of breast, endometrial, ovarian and cervical cancers. In vitro and animal studies support the cancer-preventative effects of green tea, suggesting that EGCG alters cancer cell regulation, increasing the death and decreasing the spread of cancer cells. Some of the studies also indicate that EGCG may enhance the effects of tamoxifen, a drug commonly used in the treatment and prevention of estrogen-receptor-positive breast cancer.

Epidemiological research on green tea consumption and breast cancer has been mixed. No association has been found between drinking green tea and the risk of developing breast cancer in Japanese women. In Asian-American women, however, the risk of breast cancer is significantly lower in those who regularly drink green tea.

Did You Know?

Polyphenols

At the root of green tea's health benefits are its antioxidant polyphenols, which are understood to be the main constituent responsible for prolonging life and preventing heart disease and cancer.

Cervical Dysplasia

One study investigated the use of a caffeine-free green tea catechin extract (Polyphenon E) as treatment for cervical dysplasia. After four months of oral supplementation, the dysplasia had completely cleared in 17% of women in the green tea group and 14% of women in the placebo group. This study failed to show a statistically significant difference between the treatment and placebo groups, despite in vitro research supporting the theory that green tea has chemopreventive activity. Another study demonstrated positive effects using both oral and topical formulations, but the quality of the study was poor.

Diabetes

Studies evaluating the effects of green tea on insulin resistance and blood sugar have shown inconsistent but promising results. A recent systematic review concluded that green tea did not significantly decrease fasting glucose, fasting insulin, oral glucose tolerance test results, hemoglobin A1c or insulin resistance in people at risk of type 2 diabetes when compared to a placebo. However, several individual high-quality studies have found positive effects on blood sugar, insulin and other measures in people who already have type 2 diabetes.

Endometriosis

A few recent in vitro and animal studies have demonstrated the ability of the green tea extract epigallocatechin gallate (EGCG) to slow, and even reverse, the growth of endometrial lesions. More studies are needed.

Genital Warts

Several well-designed trials found that a proprietary topical green tea cream resolved genital warts significantly better than a placebo. Over 75% of the study participants saw significant improvements after four months of using the cream; for 50% of them, the warts had completely disappeared. The cream is officially approved for use in the United States and Europe under different brand names.

Heart Disease and Obesity

Green tea catechins may protect against the risk of heart disease and stroke. Several recent systematic reviews concluded that green tea significantly lowers total cholesterol, low-density lipoprotein (LDL), or "bad," cholesterol and blood pressure. Another, earlier systematic review reported similar effects on cholesterol and LDL.

One systematic review found a small, non-significant weight loss among overweight adults taking green tea. Animal and in vitro studies support the theory that green tea catechins have anti-obesity effects.

Polycystic Ovarian Syndrome

Green tea may act as an antiandrogen by inhibiting the enzyme 5-alpha reductase, which reduces the impact of testosterone on the body. Green tea has also been investigated for its role in weight loss and cardiovascular effects. In one meta-analysis, including a study specifically on women with PCOS, green tea was shown to induce a small but non-significant weight loss.

Did You Know?

Green Tea and Soy

Green tea and soy have much in common. They are both native to Asia, where they are an important part of the diet of many cultures. Both have inspired large-scale population studies that have triggered many other clinical trials. One could say that green tea is to heart disease and cancer as soy is to menopause.

Health Condition	Level of Scientific Evidence
Acne	Fair
Breast cancer	Mixed
Cervical dysplasia	Poor
Diabetes	Fair
Endometriosis	Poor
Genital warts	Good
Heart disease	Good
Polycystic ovarian syndrome	Poor

Safety

Excessive consumption of green tea can result in excessive caffeine intake, which should be avoided in pregnancy and by people with heart disorders. EGCG supplements are typically standardized to contain only small amounts of caffeine.

Further Reading

Ahn WS, Yoo J, Huh SW, et al. Protective effects of green tea extracts (Polyphenon E and EGCG) on human cervical lesions. *European Journal of Cancer Prevention*, 2003 Oct; 12 (5): 383–90.

Chan CC, Koo MW, Ng EH, et al. Effects of Chinese green tea on weight, and hormonal and biochemical profiles in obese patients with polycystic ovary syndrome — A randomized placebo-controlled trial. *Journal of the Society for Gynecologic Investigation*, 2006 Jan; 13 (1): 63–68.

Elsaie ML, Abdelhamid MF, Elsaaiee LT, Emam HM. The efficacy of topical 2% green tea lotion in mild-to-moderate acne vulgaris. *Journal of Drugs in Dermatology*, 2009 Apr; 8 (4): 358–64.

Garcia FA, Cornelison T, Nuño T, et al. Results of a phase II randomized, double-blind, placebo-controlled trial of Polyphenon E in women with persistent high-risk HPV infection and low-grade cervical intraepithelial neoplasia. *Gynecologic Oncology*, 2014 Feb; 132 (2): 377–82.

Hartley L, Flowers N, Holmes J, et al. Green and black tea for the primary prevention of cardiovascular disease. *Cochrane Database of Systematic Reviews*, 2013 Jun 18; 6: CD009934.

Johnson R, Bryant S, Huntley AL. Green tea and green tea catechin extracts: An overview of the clinical evidence. *Maturitas*, 2012 Dec; 73 (4): 280–87.

Jurgens TM, Whelan AM, Killian L, et al. Green tea for weight loss and weight maintenance in overweight or obese adults. *Cochrane Database of Systematic Reviews*, 2012 Dec 12; 12: CD008650.

Khalesi S, Sun J, Buys N, et al. Green tea catechins and blood pressure: A systematic review and meta-analysis of randomised controlled trials. *European Journal of Nutrition*, 2014 Sep; 53 (6): 1299–311.

Kim A, Chiu A, Barone MK, et al. Green tea catechins decrease total and low-density lipoprotein cholesterol: A systematic review and meta-analysis. *Journal of the American Dietetic Association*, 2011 Nov; 111 (11): 1720–29.

Liu CY, Huang CJ, Huang LH, et al. Effects of green tea extract on insulin resistance and glucagon-like peptide 1 in patients with type 2 diabetes and lipid abnormalities: A randomized, double-blinded, and placebo-controlled trial. *PLoS One*, 2014 Mar 10; 9 (3): e91163.

Onakpoya I, Spencer E, Heneghan C, Thompson M. The effect of green tea on blood pressure and lipid profile: A systematic review and meta-analysis of randomized clinical trials. *Nutrition, Metabolism and Cardiovascular Diseases*, 2014 Aug; 24 (8): 823–36.

Tzellos TG, Sardeli C, Lallas A, et al. Efficacy, safety and tolerability of green tea catechins in the treatment of external anogenital warts: A systematic review and meta-analysis. *Journal of the European Academy of Dermatology and Venereology*. 2011 Mar; 25 (3): 345–53.

Wang CC, Xu H, Man GC, et al. Prodrug of green tea epigallocatechin-3-gallate (Pro-EGCG) as a potent anti-angiogenesis agent for endometriosis in mice. *Angiogenesis*, 2013 Jan; 16 (1): 59–69.

Wang X, Tian J, Jiang J, et al. Effects of green tea or green tea extract on insulin sensitivity and glycaemic control in populations at risk of type 2 diabetes mellitus: A systematic review and meta-analysis of randomised controlled trials. *Journal of Human Nutrition and Dietetics*, 2014 Oct; 27 (5): 501–12.

Xu H, Becker CM, Lui WT, et al. Green tea epigallocatechin-3-gallate inhibits angiogenesis and suppresses vascular endothelial growth factor C/vascular endothelial growth factor receptor 2 expression and signaling in experimental endometriosis in vivo. *Fertility and Sterility*, 2011 Oct; 96 (4): 1021–28.

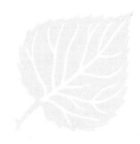

Gymnema

Latin Name
- *Gymnema sylvestre*

Part Used
- Leaf

Common Combination
- For diabetes: Cinnamon and fenugreek

Current Medicinal Uses

Gymnema, an herb from the Ayurvedic herbal tradition, is used primarily for diabetes mellitus. It decreases sugar cravings and alters the taste of sweet foods on the tongue, making them seem less desirable, and has been touted as a potential anti-obesity herb, thanks to its effects on blood sugar and cholesterol.

History and Energetics

Gymnema's Sanskrit name is *madhunashini*, which means "that which kills sugar," a reference to the fact that chewing the leaves of gymnema blocks sweet receptors on the tongue for a short time (fifteen minutes to a few hours). This property provides a clue to the herb's role in treating diabetes: gymnema suppresses the body's reaction to excess sugar just as it suppresses the taste of sugar on the tongue. In India, gymnema has been used to treat diabetes for almost 2,000 years, balancing kapha constitutions, which are associated with obesity.

Gymnema leaf's other traditional medical uses include asthma, eye complaints, inflammation, prevention of dental cavities and snakebites. The roots have been used to treat stomach pain, snakebites, hemorrhoids and insect bites.

Research Evidence
Diabetes

Based on phytopharmacological research, gymnema works by stimulating insulin secretion from the pancreas, delaying absorption of sugar into the intestines and, therefore, the blood. Several in vitro and non-human animal studies have shown that gymnema improves glucose tolerance and insulin secretion. In animal models of obesity and diabetes mellitus, gymnema decreased blood lipids, glucose and leptin while increasing insulin secretion. Significant body weight reductions were also reported.

Open-label trials in humans have been promising. In one small trial, participants with type 2 diabetes who took gymnema had significant improvements in fasting blood sugar and hemoglobin A1c levels compared to the control group. Another, uncontrolled trial found that gymnema

reduced fasting blood sugar and hemoglobin A1c in people with either type 1 or type 2 diabetes. Randomized clinical trials are needed to confirm these positive preliminary findings.

Health Condition	Level of Scientific Evidence
Diabetes	Fair

Safety
People with diabetes who take gymnema alongside diabetic medications may need to adjust their dose of hypoglycemic drugs because of gymnema's additive herb–drug effects. Overall, gymnema appears to be safe, with few other noted side effects.

Further Reading

Nahas R, Moher M. Complementary and alternative medicine for the treatment of type 2 diabetes. *Canadian Family Physician*, 2009 Jun; 55 (6): 591–96.

Pothuraju R, Sharma RK, Chagalamarri J, et al. A systematic review of *Gymnema sylvestre* in obesity and diabetes management. *Journal of the Science of Food and Agriculture*, 2014 Mar 30; 94 (5): 834–40.

Tiwari P, Mishra BN, Sangwan NS. Phytochemical and pharmacological properties of *Gymnema sylvestre*: An important medicinal plant. *BioMed Research International*, 2014; 2014: 830285.

Ulbricht C, Abrams TR, Basch E, et al. An evidence-based systematic review of gymnema (*Gymnema sylvestre* R. Br.) by the Natural Standard Research Collaboration. *Journal of Dietary Supplements*, 2011 Sep; 8 (3): 311–30.

Hawthorn

Latin Names

- *Crataegus laevigata* (Midland hawthorn)
- *Crataegus monogyna* (common hawthorn)

Parts Used

- Berries, flowers and leaves

Common Combination

- For high blood pressure: Motherwort and garlic

Did You Know?

A Sacred Stand

Westminster Abbey was built on grounds once called Thorney Island, so called because a sacred stand of hawthorn once stood there.

Current Medicinal Uses

Hawthorn is a cardiovascular tonic for high blood pressure, coronary artery disease (the most common type of heart disease) and congestive heart failure. It is also used as a general tonic and antioxidant, with an affinity for the heart, after illnesses such as pneumonia, scarlet fever or influenza.

History and Energetics

Hawthorn has a long history of use in Europe, for both physical and spiritual purposes. Maypoles were originally made of hawthorn because the tree's white flowers bloom near the beginning of May. As a symbol of courtship, love and sexuality, hawthorn branches were also used to make wedding crowns.

However, in apparent opposition to its connection with spring fever, hawthorn was also associated with misfortune and the wrath of powerful witches and fairies. Hedges of hawthorn were seen as gateways to other worlds and magical beings — but were grown to protect towns from thieves. Hawthorn was often used as decoration outside a house, as a means of protection, but it was considered an invitation to illness or death to bring it inside the home.

Because of these contradictions and others, hawthorn has come to be associated with balance and duality and the open-heartedness required to play with fairies. As a medicine, hawthorn can be used to open the heart to new experiences and deeper love, while also providing protection from harm and calming fears of vulnerability.

Research Evidence

Most of the clinical trials on hawthorn have been conducted using a patented extract of the leaves and flowers called WS 1442.

Heart Disease

Studies on hawthorn consistently show that people with New York Heart Association functional classifications I to III (from mild heart disease with no limitations on activity to more severe heart disease with marked limitations on activity and comfort only during rest) have better

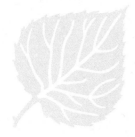

clinical outcomes compared to controls. A meta-analysis of fourteen studies published in 2008 concluded that hawthorn significantly increases maximum workload and exercise tolerance and significantly decreases weakness, fatigue, heart palpitations and shortness of breath.

High Blood Pressure

Because of the positive outcomes found in studies on heart disease, hawthorn has also been studied for use in high blood pressure. In several randomized, controlled trials, including one on people with diabetes, hawthorn significantly reduced diastolic blood pressure compared to a placebo. One of the trials additionally noted a decrease in anxiety symptoms among participants taking hawthorn.

Health Condition	Level of Scientific Evidence
Heart disease	Good
High blood pressure	Good

Safety

Hawthorn is generally safe and well tolerated. In clinical trials, hawthorn has sometimes caused nausea, dizziness, headaches and mild gastrointestinal upset.

Further Reading

Asgary S, Naderi GH, Sadeghi M, et al. Antihypertensive effect of Iranian *Crataegus curvisepala* Lind.: A randomized, double-blind study. *Drugs under Experimental and Clinical Research*, 2004; 30 (5–6): 221–25.

Pittler MH, Guo R, Ernst E. Hawthorn extract for treating chronic heart failure. *Cochrane Database of Systematic Reviews*, 2008 Jan 23; (1): CD005312.

Walker AF, Marakis G, Morris AP, Robinson PA. Promising hypotensive effect of hawthorn extract: A randomized double-blind pilot study of mild, essential hypertension. *Phytotherapy Research*, 2002 Feb; 16 (1): 48–54.

Walker AF, Marakis G, Simpson E, et al. Hypotensive effects of hawthorn for patients with diabetes taking prescription drugs: A randomised controlled trial. *British Journal of General Practice*, 2006 Jun; 56 (527): 437–43.

Wang J, Xiong X, Feng B. Effect of *Crataegus* usage in cardiovascular disease prevention: An evidence-based approach. *Evidence-Based Complementary and Alternative Medicine*, 2013; 2013: 149363.

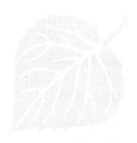

Folklore

Christian Legend

Hawthorn trees are also connected to the Holy Grail. According to legend, when Joseph of Arimathea arrived at Glastonbury in England, he thrust his staff into the ground. From this place, a hawthorn tree grew that bloomed at Christmas in celebration of Jesus' birth. (Some people suggest that Christian monks may have invented this story to disassociate hawthorn from the pagan sexuality of spring festivals.)

Did You Know?

Delayed Action

Hawthorn works slowly and needs to be used for at least four to eight weeks before its benefits can be observed.

Horse Chestnut

Latin Name
- *Aesculus hippocastanum*

Part Used
- Outer seed coat

Common Combination
- For hemorrhoids or varicose veins: Yarrow and witch hazel (both topically and internally)

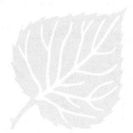

Did You Know?

Conkers

Horse chestnut seeds are used to play conkers, a traditional children's game in Britain and Ireland.

Current Medicinal Uses

Horse chestnut is used as an astringent and vascular tonic for the treatment of varicose veins, hemorrhoids, chronic venous insufficiency, swelling and pain in the legs or feet due to fragility of the vein walls.

History and Energetics

Originally from the Balkan Peninsula, horse chestnut is said to have gotten its name from the shape of the leaf scar (the mark left on a branch or twig after the leaf falls off), which looks like a horseshoe, complete with nail holes. However, that's just one explanation for the origin of its name. Others include the theory that horse chestnuts were ground up and fed to horses to treat coughs, or that the name refers to the hardness of the large seed, said to have the strength of a horse.

From a homeopathic perspective, horse chestnut is specific for hemorrhoids where the rectum feels as though it were full of sticks, with sharp pains radiating to the back and hips and feelings of fullness and pain that are worse with standing. On the emotional side, the Bach flower essence of horse chestnut is used for people who feel bogged down, are unable to find rest or peace and are subject to obsessive thoughts. Overall, someone needing horse chestnut has a feeling of heaviness and spillage of thoughts and/or blood.

Research Evidence
Hemorrhoids

Studies on the use of horse chestnut for hemorrhoids are limited in spite of long-term traditional use. Nonetheless, the results of these trials are positive. One randomized, controlled trial showed that horse chestnut seed extract significantly reduced hemorrhoid symptoms, including bleeding, itching, burning and swelling, compared to a placebo. A physician who visually examined the hemorrhoids also noted significant improvements in the horse chestnut group.

Varicose Veins

Horse chestnut seed extract has been well studied for its use in the treatment of chronic venous insufficiency. Research has shown it to be safe and effective at resolving swelling and pain. A 2012 meta-analysis of seventeen clinical trials concluded that horse chestnut seed extract significantly reduces leg volume, leg circumference, pain, edema and itching in people with chronic venous insufficiency. One trial found that horse chestnut seed extract was as effective as compression stockings.

Health Condition	Level of Scientific Evidence
Hemorrhoids	Fair
Varicose veins	Good

Safety

Horse chestnut seed extract appears to pose minimal risk during pregnancy and has been used internally for pregnancy-induced venous insufficiency. One randomized trial on the use of horse chestnut seed extract in pregnant women found no serious adverse effects after two weeks of use.

In higher doses, horse chestnut seed extract may lead to minor gastrointestinal symptoms, headaches, itching and dizziness. As with many herbs used topically, some people may experience redness and irritation.

Folklore

Spiders Away!
Folklore suggests that leaving horse chestnut seeds on your windowsill will deter spiders from entering your house.

Further Reading

[No authors listed]. *Aesculus hippocastanum* (Horse chestnut). Monograph. *Alternative Medicine Review*, 2009 Sep; 14 (3): 278–83.

Mills E, Duguoa JJ, Koren G. *Herbal Medicines in Pregnancy and Lactation: An Evidence-Based Approach*. London: Taylor & Francis, 2006.

Pittler MH, Ernst E. Horse chestnut seed extract for chronic venous insufficiency. *Cochrane Database of Systematic Reviews*, 2012 Nov 14; 11: CD003230.

Kava

Part Used
- Root

Common Combinations
- **For anxiety:** Lavender and passionflower
- **For depression and anxiety:** St. John's wort

Did You Know?

Intoxicating Pepper

Kava's Latin name, *Piper methysticum*, means "intoxicating pepper," referring to the plant's perceived psychoactive properties.

Current Medicinal Uses

Kava, or kava-kava, has been used ceremoniously and medicinally by people in the South Pacific for thousands of years. It is calming and relaxing, yet keeps mental focus and alertness intact. Kava is used for anxiety, restlessness, stress and insomnia. As an antispasmodic for the musculoskeletal system, it is also used for nerve pain, migraines and painful urinary tract infections.

History and Energetics

Traditionally, the fresh or dried root of kava is chewed or ground into a powder, mixed with cold water and drunk as a thick, starchy milk. Kava roots and drinks were often given to or by visitors as part of formal ceremonies. Kava was also traditionally used as an important part of religious ceremonies, coronations, political ceremonies, weddings, funerals, naming ceremonies and initiation ceremonies. In the South Pacific today, kava is primarily a social drink, used much like alcohol.

Kava became popular in Europe in the 1990s but was later banned in many countries because of reports of liver toxicity associated with its use. However, liver toxicity has not been reproduced in recent clinical trials on whole kava extracts. Researchers have now determined that adulteration or contamination by certain molds during the preparation process are the most likely causes of the reported liver toxicity.

Research Evidence
Anxiety and Depression

Kava has been well researched for its use in generalized anxiety. A 2003 meta-analysis concluded that kava was an effective treatment for anxiety — significantly better than a placebo at reducing symptoms. Since the publication of that review, several new randomized, controlled trials have been conducted. One study of people with generalized anxiety disorder found that kava significantly reduced symptoms of anxiety compared to a placebo, with no effects

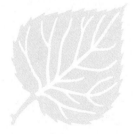

on liver function. Neither withdrawal nor addiction was observed with short-term kava use. Another study found that kava substantially lessened symptoms of both anxiety and depression. In a different study on patients with both depression and anxiety, a combination of kava and St. John's wort was found to significantly reduce symptoms of depression compared to a placebo.

Health Condition	Level of Scientific Evidence
Anxiety	Good
Anxiety and depression together	Fair

Safety

Because of concerns about potential liver toxicity, many countries have issued warnings about possible risks associated with using kava. In 2002, the U.S. Food and Drug Administration (FDA) issued a consumer advisory and a letter to health-care professionals outlining the potential risk of severe liver toxicity associated with using kava, and encouraging consumers to consult with a physician before using any supplements that contain kava. In Canada, kava-containing products are approved for sale only if they are whole-root or water-based extracts containing no more than 125 milligrams of kavalactones (the active medicinal component) per dosage unit and no more than 250 milligrams of kavalactones per recommended daily dosage. To err on the side of caution, avoid kava if you have a liver disorder or are taking drugs that affect the liver.

Do not use kava if you are taking drugs for Parkinson's disease or other dopamine-agonist drugs, as kava has been shown to antagonize dopamine and may worsen tremors. Likewise, avoid using kava in combination with alcohol or other sedative herbs or drugs, as the sedative effects may be increased.

Headaches have been noted as a possible side effect of kava use in some studies.

Kava should not be used during pregnancy or breastfeeding. Kavalactones have been shown to enter breast milk.

Further Reading

Cairney S, Maruff P, Clough AR, et al. Saccade and cognitive impairment associated with kava intoxication. *Human Psychopharmacology*, 2003 Oct; 18 (7): 525–33.

Pittler MH, Ernst E. Kava extract for treating anxiety. *Cochrane Database of Systematic Reviews*, 2003; (1): CD003383.

Sarris J, Kavanagh DJ, Byrne G, et al. The Kava Anxiety Depression Spectrum Study (KADSS): A randomized, placebo-controlled crossover trial using an aqueous extract of *Piper methysticum*. *Psychopharmacology* (Berlin), 2009 Aug; 205 (3): 399–407.

Sarris J, Kavanagh DJ, Deed G, Bone KM. St. John's wort and kava in treating major depressive disorder with comorbid anxiety: A randomised double-blind placebo-controlled pilot trial. *Human Psychopharmacology*, 2009 Jan; 24 (1): 41–48.

Sarris J, Stough C, Bousman CA, et al. Kava in the treatment of generalized anxiety disorder: A double-blind, randomized, placebo-controlled study. *Journal of Clinical Psychopharmacology*, 2013 Oct; 33 (5): 643–48.

Sarris J, Stough C, Teschke R, et al. Kava for the treatment of generalized anxiety disorder RCT: Analysis of adverse reactions, liver function, addiction, and sexual effects. *Phytotherapy Research*, 2013 Nov; 27 (11): 1723–28.

❧ Lavender

Current Medicinal Uses

Lavender is most frequently used to relieve anxiety and insomnia. It is also relaxing to the digestive tract when taken internally, relieving stomach queasiness. Applied topically, lavender is good for headaches and sore muscles. Like many plants high in volatile oils (the constituents that give plants their smell), lavender is also known to be a mild antiseptic and antibacterial.

History and Energetics

Lavender has a long history of use in food, medicine and cosmetics. It was used by the Egyptians as perfume and during the process of mummification. Jars of lavender perfume were found in the tomb of Tutankhamun ("King Tut"), sealed for 3,000 years before they were discovered in the 1920s. Lavender was said to be used by Cleopatra to seduce Julius Caesar and Mark Anthony.

   The Ancient Greeks and Romans used lavender for bathing, anointing and medicinal purposes. Some of the earliest Greek medical texts note the use of lavender for headaches, indigestion and sore throat.

Research Evidence
Anxiety and Depression

Lavender oil capsules have been reasonably well studied for their use in treating generalized anxiety disorder. In a recent review of seven clinical trials, researchers concluded that lavender significantly decreased anxiety symptoms, better than a placebo and as well as lorazepam, a benzodiazepine drug commonly prescribed for anxiety. A more recent trial has confirmed these results and added that lavender oil capsules may reduce concomitant symptoms of depression as well. Lavender has also been shown to be effective for other anxiety disorders, such as post-traumatic stress disorder and somatization disorder.

   In an open-label study on depressed patients taking the drug citalopram, lavender infusion significantly decreased symptoms of depression compared to the control group. A series of case studies also reported that the concurrent use of lavender oil capsules with antidepressant medication resulted in improvements in depression symptoms, anxiety,

Latin Name
- *Lavandula angustifolia*

Part Used
- Flower

Common Combination
- **For anxiety:** Passionflower and lemon balm

Did You Know?

Household Uses

Lavender prevents moth damage in closets and discourages insects from crawling into beds. It can be used to flavor baked goods and sweets, made into wine or infused into cosmetic products. I often keep a bouquet of dried lavender in my office for the flowers' delicate aroma and aesthetic beauty.

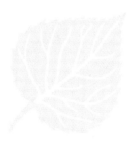

agitation and insomnia. More placebo-controlled research on the use of lavender for depression is needed.

In two separate studies, lavender essential oil aromatherapy was found to significantly decrease anxiety in patients who had recently experienced a heart attack and to decrease anxiety and depression in women at high risk after childbirth. Another study found that lavender aromatherapy decreased the anxiety experienced during intrauterine device (IUD) insertion when inhaled prophylactically.

Safety

Lavender is a generally safe herb with very few side effects. A recent study confirmed that oral lavender oil capsules are safe to take concurrently with oral contraceptive drugs. No herb–drug interactions have been reported.

Health Condition	Level of Scientific Evidence
Anxiety	Good
Depression	Poor

Further Reading

Heger-Mahn D, Pabst G, Dienel A, et al. No interacting influence of lavender oil preparation Silexan on oral contraception using an ethinyl estradiol/levonorgestrel combination. *Drugs in R&D*, 2014 Dec; 14 (4): 265–72.

Kasper S. An orally administered lavandula oil preparation (Silexan) for anxiety disorder and related conditions: An evidence based review. *International Journal of Psychiatry in Clinical Practice*, 2013 Nov; 17 Suppl 1: 15–22.

Kasper S, Gastpar M, Müller WE, et al. Lavender oil preparation Silexan is effective in generalized anxiety disorder — A randomized, double-blind comparison to a placebo and paroxetine. *International Journal of Neuropsychopharmacology*, 2014 Jun; 17 (6): 859–69.

Nikfarjam M, Parvin N, Assarzadegan N, Asghari S. The effects of *Lavandula angustifolia* mill infusion on depression in patients using citalopram: A comparison study. *Iranian Red Crescent Medical Journal*, 2013 Aug; 15 (8): 734–39.

Uehleke B, Schaper S, Dienel A, et al. Phase II trial on the effects of Silexan in patients with neurasthenia, post-traumatic stress disorder or somatization disorder. *Phytomedicine*, 2012 Jun 15; 19 (8–9): 665–71.

Lemon Balm

Current Medicinal Uses

Lemon balm is used as a relaxing herb for the nervous and digestive systems. It has been used for anxiety, irritable bowel syndrome, colic, nervous indigestion, headaches and heart palpitations due to anxiety. Since lemon balm contains volatile oils that work against certain viruses, it is also used for herpes simplex virus (HSV) and other viruses, especially those that are triggered by stress or otherwise related to the nervous system.

History and Energetics

Lemon balm, a member of the mint family, has long been used to calm the nerves. Avicenna, the famous Persian physician, used it to treat depression and melancholy. Paracelsus associated lemon balm with happiness and longevity. French kings and Holy Roman Emperors were said to drink lemon balm to promote health and a long life. Lemon balm was included as the foremost ingredient in Carmelite water, developed by friars of the Carmelite religious order to improve nervous headaches and brighten moods.

Lemon balm's Latin genus name, *Melissa*, comes from the Greek word for "bee," and indeed the plant is a favorite of honeybees, encouraging swarms to return year after year. Grown near the temple of Artemis, lemon balm was also associated with Diana, the Roman goddess of the hunt, the moon and fertility.

Research Evidence
Anxiety and Insomnia

Several animal studies and one open-label human study support the traditional use of lemon balm for anxiety and insomnia. The open-label study found that lemon balm decreased anxiety by 18% and insomnia by over 40%. Almost all of the study's participants responded to treatment. In another study, a combination of lemon balm and valerian was shown to improve restlessness and sleep in children.

Genital Warts

Lemon balm has not yet been studied for use in the treatment of HPV.

Latin Name
- *Melissa officinalis*

Parts Used
- Leaf
- Whole plant before flowering

Common Combinations
- **For generalized anxiety:** Passionflower and lavender
- **For herpes:** St. John's wort
- **To promote restful sleep:** Lavender (in an eye pillow)

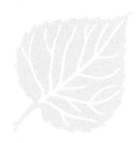

Herpes

In vitro studies have demonstrated that lemon balm has strong antiviral activity against both HSV-1 and HSV-2, even in cases where the virus has become resistant and standard pharmaceutical drugs fail to work. A few randomized, controlled trials have studied the use of topical lemon balm for the treatment of oral and genital herpes. A 1% lemon balm cream, applied four times a day, significantly reduced both the size and severity of herpes sores after forty-eight hours compared to a placebo.

Health Condition	Level of Scientific Evidence
Anxiety and insomnia	Fair
Genital warts	Poor
Herpes	Good

Safety

Lemon balm should be avoided by people with hypothyroidism, as it may decrease the amount of active thyroid hormone (triiodothyronine, or T3). Because of its potential impact on thyroid metabolism and potential emmenagogue effects, lemon balm is best avoided during pregnancy.

Further Reading

Cases J, Ibarra A, Feuillère N, et al. Pilot trial of *Melissa officinalis* L. leaf extract in the treatment of volunteers suffering from mild-to-moderate anxiety disorders and sleep disturbances. *Mediterranean Journal of Nutrition and Metabolism*, 2011 Dec; 4 (3): 211–18. Epub 2010 Dec 17.

Koytchev R, Alken RG, Dundarov S. Balm mint extract (Lo-701) for topical treatment of recurring herpes labialis. *Phytomedicine*, 1999 Oct; 6 (4): 225–30.

Sarris J, McIntyre E, Camfield DA. Plant-based medicines for anxiety disorders, part 2: A review of clinical studies with supporting preclinical evidence. *CNS Drugs*, 2013 Apr; 27 (4): 301–19.

Wölbling RH, Leonhardt K. Local therapy of herpes simplex with dried extract from *Melissa officinalis*. *Phytomedicine*, 1994 Jun; 1 (1): 25–31.

🍃 Licorice

Current Medicinal Uses

Licorice has seemingly endless medicinal uses. As a demulcent, it is great for sore throat and easing heartburn, canker sores and stomach ulcers. As an anti-inflammatory, it can treat gastritis, coughs, upper respiratory tract infections and asthma. As an antiviral, it is found in formulas for viral infections of all kinds, including hepatitis. Licorice is also used for conditions of androgen excess, as in some cases of polycystic ovarian syndrome (PCOS).

History and Energetics

Licorice's English and Latin names both come from the Greek words for "sweet root," and many people today think of candy when they think of licorice. Although licorice candies aren't always made from actual licorice root anymore, licorice has long been used as a flavoring to disguise the taste of medicine, and as a medicine in its own right.

Like many of the herbs in this book, licorice was found in Tutankhamun's tomb. The Egyptians chewed licorice to prevent thirst. Avicenna prescribed it for sore throats and laryngitis. Licorice was used in much the same way in Ayurvedic medicine (where it is known as *yashtimadhu*) and traditional Chinese medicine (where it is known as *gan cao*).

In traditional Chinese medicine, licorice is added to almost all formulas for its ability to harmonize the herbs in the formula and lead them into the appropriate channels (also known as meridians).

Research Evidence

Amenorrhea

In several small open-label studies, a combination of licorice and white peony root lowered testosterone and induced ovulation in the majority of study participants. This classic formula has also been shown in a randomized controlled trial to have comparable effects to the drug bromocriptine in addressing drug-induced high prolactin levels and resulting amenorrhea caused by risperidone, a commonly used antipsychotic medication. More research is needed to confirm these results.

Latin Names
- *Glycyrrhiza glabra* (licorice)
- *Glycyrrhiza uralensis* (Chinese licorice)

Part Used
- Root

Common Combinations
- **For androgen excess or PCOS causing amenorrhea:** Peony
- **For cervical dysplasia:** Green tea
- **For heartburn:** Slippery elm and chamomile

Cervical Dysplasia

Phytopharmacology and in vitro studies have shown that licorice has strong antiviral properties, including against some strains of HPV, but no randomized human clinical studies have yet been conducted on licorice for the treatment of cervical dysplasia. In an open-label, poorly reported trial, glycyrrhizinic acid was given orally and topically to women with cervical dysplasia. Resolution of the dysplasia was achieved in 74% of women after twelve weeks. More research is needed to confirm these results and determine whether these cases of dysplasia would have resolved on their own without treatment.

Heartburn

A chewing gum containing licorice extract was found to alleviate heartburn and reflux better than a placebo in a recent small study. In earlier preliminary studies, a combination product containing licorice, chamomile and peppermint was shown to relieve the symptoms of reflux and indigestion.

Research on deglycyrrhizinated licorice (DGL) for heartburn, peptic ulcer disease and reflux was conducted mostly in the 1970s, with mixed results. Since then, little research has been performed in this area. While some researchers thought that DGL helped manage only the symptoms of heartburn, it appears that it may also address potential causes, such as Aspirin-induced ulcers and *Helicobacter pylori* infection. In a recent study on *H. pylori* infection, treatment with triple antibiotic therapy plus DGL was just as effective as triple antibiotic therapy plus bismuth, the standard drug treatment. A second trial found that DGL on its own was better than a placebo in eradicating *H. pylori*. Another randomized trial on DGL found that the licorice extract significantly improved digestion, including symptoms related to heartburn, regurgitation, nausea and bloating, compared to a placebo.

Polycystic Ovarian Syndrome

In vitro studies have shown that licorice can prevent the conversion of certain hormones into testosterone. Several clinical studies have demonstrated positive results that support this use of licorice to treat androgen excess. One study found that women without PCOS who took licorice had lower testosterone levels in their blood. Several studies on a Chinese formula containing licorice and peony showed decreased testosterone levels in women with PCOS. In a study of women with PCOS who were taking the drug spironolactone, licorice decreased the negative side effects of the drug, including breakthrough bleeding.

Health Condition	Level of Scientific Evidence
Amenorrhea	Fair
Cervical dysplasia	Poor
Heartburn	Fair
Polycystic ovarian syndrome	Fair

Safety

Licorice, specifically its constituent glycyrrhizin, can raise blood pressure by acting in a similar way to aldosterone, an adrenal hormone that acts on the kidneys to increase blood pressure. The pseudoaldosteronism effects of licorice aren't concerning in people with low blood pressure and healthy kidneys. People who have high blood pressure, who are taking anti-hypertensive medications or who have kidney disease should avoid taking licorice. Increased blood pressure and pseudoaldosteronism may worsen kidney disease. Anyone taking licorice long-term should routinely monitor their blood pressure.

Whole licorice root and extracts should be avoided during pregnancy and breastfeeding. High doses of glycyrrhizin (500 milligrams per week or more) have been associated with an increased risk of preterm delivery, as well as potential long-term cognitive and behavioral effects in children.

The glycyrrhizin constituent of licorice causes the majority of the adverse effects, especially those related to the kidneys and blood pressure. Deglycyrrhizinated licorice is available and can be used for heartburn, reflux and gastric ulcers.

Further Reading

Arentz S, Abbott JA, Smith CA, Bensoussan A. Herbal medicine for the management of polycystic ovary syndrome (PCOS) and associated oligo/amenorrhoea and hyperandrogenism: A review of the laboratory evidence for effects with corroborative clinical findings. *BMC Complementary and Alternative Medicine*, 2014 Dec 18; 14 (1): 511.

Armanini D, Castello R, Scaroni C, et al. Treatment of polycystic ovary syndrome with spironolactone plus licorice. *European Journal of Obstetrics, Gynecology, and Reproductive Biology*, 2007 Mar; 131 (1): 61–67.

Brown R, Sam CH, Green T, Wood S. Effect of GutsyGum™, a novel gum, on subjective ratings of gastroesophageal reflux following a refluxogenic meal. *Journal of Dietary Supplements*, 2014 Aug 21.

Momeni A, Rahimian G, Kiasi A, et al. Effect of licorice versus bismuth on eradication of *Helicobacter pylori* in patients with peptic ulcer disease. *Pharmacognosy Research*, 2014 Oct; 6 (4): 341–44.

Puram S, Suh HC, Kim SU, et al. Effect of GutGard in the management of *Helicobacter pylori*: A randomized double blind placebo controlled study. *Evidence-Based Complementary and Alternative Medicine*, 2013; 2013: 263805.

Raveendra KR, Jayachandra, Srinivasa V, et al. An extract of *Glycyrrhiza glabra* (GutGard) alleviates symptoms of functional dyspepsia: A randomized, double-blind, placebo-controlled study. *Evidence-Based Complementary and Alternative Medicine*, 2012; 2012: 216970.

Valencia MH, Pacheco AC, Quijano TH, et al. Clinical response to glycyrrhizinic acid in genital infection due to human papillomavirus and low-grade squamous intraepithelial lesion. *Clinics and Practice*, 2011 Nov; 1 (4): e93.

Yuan HN, Wang CY, Sze CW, et al. A randomized, crossover comparison of herbal medicine and bromocriptine against risperidone-induced hyperprolactinemia in patients with schizophrenia. *Journal of Clinical Psychopharmacology*, 2008 Jun; 28 (3): 264–370.

Milk Thistle

Current Medicinal Uses

Milk thistle is primarily used to protect the liver from damage caused by alcohol, acetaminophen, toxic mushrooms, chemotherapeutics or other drugs. It is also used to treat a variety of liver conditions, including gallstones, hepatitis and cirrhosis. Like its cousin blessed thistle, milk thistle is used to increase breast milk production.

History and Energetics

Milk thistle got its name from the milky white veins in the leaves and the sap that runs out when the leaves are crushed. Legends say this sap is the breast milk of the Virgin Mary — a reminder of the herb's use in supporting lactation.

Early physicians in Ancient Greece and Rome used milk thistle for liver conditions, gallstones and jaundice. The leaves and stalks were eaten as a leafy green vegetable in soups and salads. The seeds have been used as a coffee substitute.

Research Evidence
Diabetes

One high-quality randomized, controlled trial found that milk thistle significantly reduced fasting blood sugar, hemoglobin A1c, total cholesterol, low-density lipoprotein (LDL), or "bad," cholesterol and triglycerides in people with type 2 diabetes compared to a placebo. Another recent study concluded that barberry plus milk thistle was more effective than barberry alone in decreasing levels of hemoglobin A1c, a marker of long-term blood sugar management, in people with poorly controlled diabetes. Several preliminary studies indicate that milk thistle may also help to prevent kidney damage in diabetes.

Low Milk Supply

Milk thistle, like other galactagogues, has been used to increase milk production in dairy cows. In human research, one small placebo-controlled trial found that milk thistle extract increased daily breast milk production by 85%, while a placebo increased it by 32%.

Latin Name
- *Silybum marianum*

Part Used
- Seeds

Common Combinations
- **For diabetes:** Barberry
- **For low milk supply:** Fennel and fenugreek
- **For osteoporosis:** Black cohosh and red clover

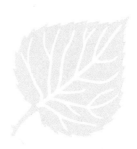

Osteoporosis

Researchers don't know yet whether milk thistle can slow down or prevent the progression of osteoporosis, but early research is hopeful. A small number of in vitro and animal studies suggest that milk thistle may decrease bone loss and increase calcium and phosphorus. More research is needed.

Health Condition	Level of Scientific Evidence
Diabetes	Fair
Low milk supply	Poor
Osteoporosis	Poor

Safety

Overall, milk thistle is a relatively safe herb but it is not known whether it is safe during pregnancy. Most of its herb–drug interactions reflect the herb's ability to prevent liver and kidney damage due to alcohol and various pharmaceutical drugs. Avoid taking milk thistle if you have a known allergy to the Asteraceae family of plants.

Further Reading

Di Pierro F, Callegari A, Carotenuto D, Tapia MM. Clinical efficacy, safety and tolerability of BIO-C (micronized *Silymarin*) as a galactagogue. *Acta BioMedica*, 2008 Dec; 79 (3): 205–10.

Di Pierro F, Putignano P, Villanova N, et al. Preliminary study about the possible glycemic clinical advantage in using a fixed combination of *Berberis aristata* and *Silybum marianum* standardized extracts versus only *Berberis aristata* in patients with type 2 diabetes. *Clinical Pharmacology*, 2013 Nov 19; 5: 167–74.

Huseini HF, Larijani B, Heshmat R, et al. The efficacy of *Silybum marianum* (L.) Gaertn. (silymarin) in the treatment of type II diabetes: A randomized, double-blind, placebo-controlled, clinical trial. *Phytotherapy Research*, 2006 Dec; 20 (12): 1036–39.

Rafieian-Kopaie M, Nasri H. Silymarin and diabetic nephropathy. *Journal of Renal Injury Prevention*, 2012 Jan 1; 1 (1): 3–5.

Motherwort

Current Medicinal Uses

Motherwort is used for high blood pressure, especially in those who also experience anxiety. It is especially useful when stress and/or worry lead to an increase in blood pressure and heart palpitations. It is also used to treat amenorrhea, nervous excitability or unrest and hyperthyroidism.

History and Energetics

Motherwort was first used by the Greeks to soothe anxiety in pregnant women. It has a long history of use in anxiety, palpitations, tachycardia (fast heart rate) and high blood pressure.

Energetically, motherwort gives strength and support to those who focus on taking care of other people, especially when doing so leaves them with little energy to care for themselves. It also bolsters courage and confidence while calming an overactive mind. Motherwort's Latin name, *Leonurus cardiaca*, translates as "lion heart," referring to the strength and power it restores to the spirit.

Overall, motherwort is an herb to mother mothers.

Research Evidence
High Blood Pressure

Despite its long-term use, little clinical research has been conducted on motherwort. Overall, phytochemical and in vitro research confirms its hypotensive and sedative effects. One open-label trial investigating the use of motherwort oil extract by patients with stage 1 and 2 hypertension noted significant improvements in blood pressure, symptoms of anxiety and symptoms of depression.

Latin Name
- *Leonurus cardiaca*

Parts Used
- Whole plant

Common Combination
- **For high blood pressure with anxiety:** Hawthorn and linden

---

Did You Know?

Yi Mu Cao
A related species, *Leonurus japonicus*, is known in traditional Chinese medicine as *yi mu cao*, meaning "benefit mother herb." *Yi mu cao* promotes menstruation and urination and clears heat and toxicity. It is used for amenorrhea, dysmenorrhea and postpartum abdominal pain.

Health Condition	Level of Scientific Evidence
High blood pressure	Poor

Safety

Although motherwort was used by Ancient Greek physicians to calm anxiety during pregnancy, it should be avoided during pregnancy, especially in the first trimester, as it can act as an emmenagogue.

Further Reading

Shang X, Pan H, Wang X, et al. *Leonurus japonicus* Houtt.: Ethnopharmacology, phytochemistry and pharmacology of an important traditional Chinese medicine. *Journal of Ethnopharmacology*, 2014 Feb 27; 152 (1): 14–32.

Shikov AN, Pozharitskaya ON, Makarov VG, et al. Effect of *Leonurus cardiaca* oil extract in patients with arterial hypertension accompanied by anxiety and sleep disorders. *Phytotherapy Research*, 2011 Apr; 25 (4): 540–43.

Wojtyniak K, Szymański M, Matławska I. *Leonurus cardiaca* L. (motherwort): A review of its phytochemistry and pharmacology. *Phytotherapy Research*, 2013 Aug; 27 (8): 1115–20.

Nettle

Current Medicinal Uses

Nettle is best known as a nutritive skin tonic and gentle detoxifier, but it also has diuretic, galactagogue and rubefacient actions. It is used in a wide variety of health conditions, including anemia, acne, eczema, hair loss, arthritis, allergies, urinary tract infections (UTIs), gout, low breast milk production and benign prostatic hyperplasia.

History and Energetics

Nettles grow wild all over Europe and North America. They are often called stinging nettles because of the small hairs on the leaves and stems, which release formic acid, histamine and other compounds, causing a local rash. Nettle stings were used medicinally for rheumatic muscle and joint pains by many Native peoples in North America. The release of histamine and formic acid increases blood circulation locally, which helps to relieve swelling and inflammation.

The Cree believed that nettle (called *masan* in Cree) was once a golden plant with a beautiful shimmering aura, but that humans took it for granted and didn't show reverence or offer tobacco to the plant spirit. Over time, the plant took on a green color, blending in with other plants, and grew stinging hairs to surprise and sting humans passing by, commanding respect. Similarly, the flower essence of nettle is used for those who feel angry and powerless to change a stressful situation, especially when they feel a lack of respect or appreciation in close relationships.

Rudolph Steiner, the originator of Waldorf education and biodynamic farming, believed that planting nettles beside plants high in volatile oils (such as rosemary, peppermint or sage) would increase their potency. In fact, nettles concentrate minerals from the soil into their roots and leaves, which explains why they are so nutritious and make a great addition to your compost pile.

Research Evidence

Most of the research on nettle has been conducted on its use in treating benign prostatic hyperplasia. Several randomized clinical trials have shown that nettle root

Latin Name
- *Urtica dioica*

Parts Used
- Leaf
- Root

Common Combinations
- **For acne and/or anemia:** Dandelion root and burdock
- **For low milk supply:** Fenugreek, milk thistle and fennel
- **For male-pattern hair loss:** Saw palmetto
- **To prevent UTIs:** Dandelion leaf and cranberry

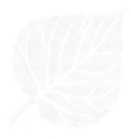

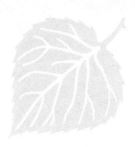

reduces prostate size, prostate-specific antigen and prostate-related symptoms. In vitro research has identified nettle root's ability to inhibit 5-alpha reductase, an enzyme implicated in both benign prostatic hyperplasia and male-pattern hair loss. Although there is a lack of research on the potential use of nettle root for women with male-pattern hair loss or polycystic ovarian syndrome, it may also be considered for these conditions.

Anemia

The use of nettles for anemia is largely based on its nutritive qualities and use in agriculture as a dynamic accumulator, a plant that draws minerals up from the soil into the plant. In animal studies, nettle has been shown to improve red blood cell and hemoglobin levels. Human trials are needed to confirm nettle's use in anemia.

Low Milk Supply

The increased need for calories and nutrients during lactation has led traditional herbalists to prescribe nutritive herbs such as nettles. Because of their mineral content, dried nettles have been used to boost milk production in dairy cows. Human studies are needed to confirm the traditional use of nettle to support lactation.

Osteoarthritis

A handful of trials have studied the topical use of nettle for osteoarthritis. In one trial, fresh nettle leaf decreased pain significantly better than the dead nettle used as a placebo. A second, open-label trial that used a 13% nettle cream also noted improved function and decreased pain. Unsurprisingly, side effects of mild discomfort and tingling were noted in both studies.

One problem limiting further research is the fact that it is challenging to create a placebo that mimics nettle's stinging effect.

Urinary Tract Infections

Animal and in vitro studies support the traditional use of nettle as a diuretic for UTIs, but human trials are lacking.

Safety

Nettles are very safe overall; however, caution is advised when purchasing them. Because nettles draw minerals

---

Did You Know?

Stinging away Frostbite

During the First World War, soldiers were said to have intentionally stung their hands or feet as treatment for frostbite.

Health Condition	Level of Scientific Evidence
Anemia	Poor
Low milk supply	Poor
Osteoarthritis	Fair
Urinary tract infections	Poor

and even heavy metals out of the soil, nettles grown in contaminated soils should be avoided. Humans can be exposed to toxic metals, such as arsenic and lead, through contaminated nettle. It is always important to know the source of your herbal products, but it is crucial when it comes to herbs that accumulate minerals from soil.

Large doses of nettle should be avoided in pregnancy, as it can act as an emmenagogue.

Fresh nettle applied topically may cause stinging pain, rash and other signs of allergic hypersensitivity in some people.

Folklore

Fishing Nets

In Norse mythology, Loki created fishing nets out of nettle. The Makah and Nitinaht peoples rubbed nettle leaves on their fishing lines, which were also made of nettle.

Further Reading

Ghorbanibirgani A, Khalili A, Zamani L. The efficacy of stinging nettle (*Urtica dioica*) in patients with benign prostatic hyperplasia: A randomized double-blind study in 100 patients. *Iranian Red Crescent Medical Journal*, 2013 Jan; 15 (1): 9–10.

Meral I, Kanter M. Effects of *Nigella sativa* L. and *Urtica dioica* L. on selected mineral status and hematological values in CCl4-treated rats. *Biological Trace Element Research*, 2003 Winter; 96 (1–3): 263–70.

Nahata A, Dixit VK. Evaluation of 5α-reductase inhibitory activity of certain herbs useful as antiandrogens. *Andrologia*, 2014 Aug; 46 (6): 592–601.

Randall C, Randall H, Dobbs F, et al. Randomized controlled trial of nettle sting for treatment of base-of-thumb pain. *Journal of the Royal Society of Medicine*, 2000 Jun; 93 (6): 305–9.

Rayburn K, Fleischbein E, Song J, et al. Stinging nettle cream for osteoarthritis. *Alternative Therapies in Health and Medicine*, 2009 Jul–Aug; 15 (4): 60–1.

Safarinejad MR. *Urtica dioica* for treatment of benign prostatic hyperplasia: A prospective, randomized, double-blind, placebo-controlled, crossover study. *Journal of Herbal Pharmacotherapy*, 2005; 5 (4): 1–11.

Passionflower

Latin Name
- *Passiflora incarnata*

Parts Used
- Leaf
- Flower

Common Combinations
- **For anxiety and insomnia:** Valerian
- **For anxiety with depression:** St. John's wort
- **For anxiety with nervous stomach:** Lemon balm and chamomile

Current Medicinal Uses

Passionflower is used as a nervous system sedative for anxiety, insomnia and related conditions, as well as for neuralgia, dysmenorrhea and the alleviation of symptoms during opiate withdrawal.

History and Energetics

The Aztecs, Incas and other indigenous peoples of Central and South America used passionflower to relieve anxiety and ease the passage to sleep. Passionflower has large, impressive flowers that look as hypnotic as they act medicinally. The radiating circular shape of the flower was associated with the sun in Inca, Maya and Aztec cultures.

The plant was given its Latin name by European Christians who saw the Passion of Christ within the plant. *Passiflora incarnata* means "suffering flower, made of flesh." One Spanish historian believed he had discovered the fruit of temptation from the Garden of Eden.

Did You Know?

Edible Fruit

Certain species of passionflower yield an edible fruit, which looks like an egg.

Research Evidence
Anxiety

Studies have shown that passionflower may reduce anxiety in people undergoing medical procedures, including dental/periodontal work and spinal anesthesia. Passionflower has also been studied for its use in alleviating symptoms associated with withdrawal from drugs, including opiates, benzodiazepines, alcohol, marijuana and nicotine. One clinical trial on ADHD found that passionflower may alleviate anxiety associated with this condition.

A small randomized, placebo-controlled trial found that passionflower tea improved overall sleep quality (but not anxiety) in healthy adults. Another trial found passionflower to be as effective as the antianxiety drug oxazepam in people diagnosed with generalized anxiety disorder, after one month of treatment. An earlier trial of 162 people with neurosis/anxiety concluded that passionflower was as effective as a different benzodiazepine, mexazolam.

The authors of a 2007 systematic review stated that passionflower may be effective for generalized anxiety but too few studies had been conducted at that time to draw conclusions. The majority of the participants in clinical trials have been women.

Depression

Although passionflower alone has not been studied for use in treating depression, one pharmacological study suggests that passionflower combined with low-dose St. John's wort may be more effective than St. John's wort alone.

Health Condition	Level of Scientific Evidence
Anxiety	Good
Depression	Poor

Safety

Passionflower is best avoided during pregnancy, as some of its constituents may have emmenagogue effects. Phytopharmacological research suggests that passionflower may increase the sedative action of benzodiazepines and other sedative drugs.

Further Reading

Aslanargun P, Cuvas O, Dikmen B, et al. *Passiflora incarnata* Linnaeus as an anxiolytic before spinal anesthesia. *Journal of Anesthesia*, 2012 Feb; 26 (1): 39–44.

Fiebich BL, Knörle R, Appel K, et al. Pharmacological studies in an herbal drug combination of St. John's wort (*Hypericum perforatum*) and passion flower (*Passiflora incarnata*): In vitro and in vivo evidence of synergy between *Hypericum* and *Passiflora* in antidepressant pharmacological models. *Fitoterapia*, 2011 Apr; 82 (3): 474–80.

Kaviani N, Tavakoli M, Tabanmehr M, Havaei R. The efficacy of *Passiflora incarnata* Linnaeus in reducing dental anxiety in patients undergoing periodontal treatment. *Journal of Dentistry* (Shiraz, Iran), 2013 Jun; 14 (2): 68–72.

Miyasaka LS, Atallah AN, Soares BG. *Passiflora* for anxiety disorder. *Cochrane Database of Systematic Reviews*, 2007 Jan 24; (1): CD004518.

Movafegh A, Alizadeh R, Hajimohamadi F, et al. Preoperative oral *Passiflora incarnata* reduces anxiety in ambulatory surgery patients: A double-blind, placebo-controlled study. *Anesthesia and Analgesia*, 2008 Jun; 106 (6): 1728–32.

Ngan A, Conduit R. A double-blind, placebo-controlled investigation of the effects of *Passiflora incarnata* (passionflower) herbal tea on subjective sleep quality. *Phytotherapy Research*, 2011 Aug; 25 (8): 1153–59.

Did You Know?

Clock Flower

In non-Christian parts of the world, passionflower is frequently called "clock flower," another reference to its circular shape.

Did You Know?

State Flower

Passionflower, known to the Cherokee as *ocoee*, is the state wildflower of Tennessee. A river and valley in Tennessee and a city in Florida are all named Ocoee after this strikingly beautiful flower.

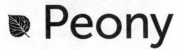# Peony

Latin Name
- *Paeonia lactiflora*

Part Used
- Root

Common Combinations
- For amenorrhea due to blood deficiency (from a TCM perspective): Dang gui and rehmannia
- For amenorrhea due to hyper-androgenism and/or PCOS: Licorice

Current Medicinal Uses

Peony is used in several traditional Chinese herbal formulas for a variety of menstrual conditions, including amenorrhea and oligomenorrhea, for polycystic ovarian syndrome (PCOS) and to prevent miscarriage. Peony is also used to treat anemia, muscle spasms and abdominal pain, including dysmenorrhea.

History and Energetics

In traditional Chinese medicine (TCM), peony, or *shao yao*, is divided into two different herbal preparations, *bai shao* and *chi shao*. (A third Chinese herb called *mu dan pi* is made from *Paeonia suffruticosa*.) To make *bai shao*, known as white peony, the bark is peeled off the root, then the root is steamed and dried. To make *chi shao*, or red peony, on the other hand, the whole root is dried. Although they come from the same plant, the two preparations have slightly different properties: in TCM terms, white peony is best at building and nourishing the blood, while red peony is best at invigorating the circulation of blood.

Peony's name comes from a Greek myth about Paeon, physician to the gods. After Asclepias, the god of medicine, threatened to kill Paeon out of jealousy, Zeus transformed Paeon into a flower in order to save him.

Research Evidence
Amenorrhea/Oligomenorrhea

Pharmacological and animal studies show that peony increases luteinizing hormone and decreases testosterone, hormones involved in amenorrhea and oligomenorrhea caused by hyperandrogenism. Two very small open-label trials on women with either hyperandrogenism or PCOS confirmed these findings, showing that an herbal combination of peony and licorice reduced free and total testosterone, increased sex hormone–binding globulin and decreased the ratio of luteinizing hormone to follicle-stimulating hormone. One of the trials found a significant improvement in ovulation. Another open-label trial of a combination of peony and cinnamon improved ovulation rates in 50% of women with PCOS and 60% of women without PCOS. Placebo-controlled trials are needed.

Health Condition	Level of Scientific Evidence
Amenorrhea/ oligomenorrhea	Fair

Safety

Peony should be avoided in pregnancy.

Further Reading

Arentz S, Abbott JA, Smith CA, Bensoussan A. Herbal medicine for the management of polycystic ovary syndrome (PCOS) and associated oligo/amenorrhoea and hyperandrogenism: A review of the laboratory evidence for effects with corroborative clinical findings. *BMC Complementary and Alternative Medicine*, 2014 Dec 18; 14 (1): 511.

Ushiroyama T, Ikeda A, Sakai M, et al. Effects of unkei-to, an herbal medicine, on endocrine function and ovulation in women with high basal levels of luteinizing hormone secretion. *Journal of Reproductive Medicine*, 2001 May; 46 (5): 451–56.

Did You Know?

Fragrant Flowers
A peony bush yields large, fragrant flowers that are a favorite of gardeners and florists. Prolific bloomers, peony bushes have been cultivated for use as an ornamental, with flowers ranging from white to red. Peonies are frequently given as a twelfth wedding anniversary gift, to symbolize a long and happy marriage. In China, the flowers represent prosperity and honor.

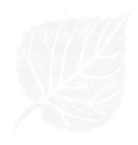

🍃 Peppermint

Latin Name
- *Mentha x piperita*

Parts Used
- Aerial parts (everything above the ground)

Common Combinations
- For indigestion, gas and bloating: Chamomile
- For morning sickness: Ginger
- For weaning from breastfeeding: Sage

Current Medicinal Uses

Peppermint is used primarily for digestive upset, including nausea, vomiting, indigestion, gas, bloating and abdominal pain. It is also a cooling diaphoretic, used to relieve fever in colds and flus. Peppermint oil contains a high concentration of menthol, which is used topically for muscle pain, rheumatism and neuralgia. Peppermint oil also opens the sinuses and breaks up congestion in the lungs. Taken internally, peppermint oil is used to treat irritable bowel syndrome (IBS).

History and Energetics

Peppermint is a hybrid, a cross between spearmint and watermint. (The "x" in its Latin name indicates that the plant is a hybrid.) Peppermint has an extremely long history of use for nausea and vomiting in many contexts. Its digestive uses were recorded by traditional physicians from Egypt, India, China, Greece and Rome.

Energetically, peppermint is associated with money, protection and lust. In Greek mythology, Minthe, a beautiful nymph, was pursued by Pluto, god of the dead. Pluto's wife, Persephone, grew so jealous of his interest in Minthe that she turned the nymph into a plant so that people would step on her as they walked. Pluto couldn't return Minthe to her nymph form, so he made the plant fragrant instead.

Research Evidence

A recent meta-analysis of trials for the treatment of IBS concluded that peppermint oil significantly improved overall symptoms compared to a placebo. Peppermint oil was also shown to be more effective than a placebo at reducing abdominal pain associated with IBS.

Nausea

Most of the clinical research on peppermint for nausea has centered on its use in preventing and alleviating postoperative nausea. Results on using peppermint oil

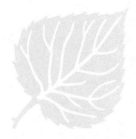

aromatherapy for postoperative and chemotherapy-induced nausea have been mixed, though they trend toward showing some benefit.

One trial investigating the use of peppermint oil aromatherapy before bed by pregnant women found the peppermint treatment no more effective than a placebo in decreasing the severity of nausea or the frequency of vomiting. Nonetheless, the authors noted a trend toward reduced nausea in the peppermint group.

Nipple Cracks

In a randomized clinical trial, peppermint oil applied topically to nipple fissures on breastfeeding women was significantly more effective than breast milk alone in alleviating pain and reducing nipple discharge. A previous study found that peppermint water applied topically was more effective than breast milk at preventing the development of nipple cracks. A similar study found a peppermint gel more effective than lanolin at preventing and healing nipple cracks.

Weaning

Peppermint oil administered as a tea, in capsules or through inhalation has traditionally been used to decrease milk supply, but no clinical research has been conducted in this area.

Did You Know?

Breath Freshener
Many people use peppermint-flavored products to freshen their breath and ease digestion. It is one of the most popular herbal teas on the market, and the most common mint flavor for candies, toothpaste, chewing gum, tobacco and foods.

Health Condition	Level of Scientific Evidence
Nausea	Mixed
Nipple cracks	Good
Weaning	Poor

Safety

Overall, peppermint is a safe herb, especially in culinary doses. However, it can relax the lower esophageal sphincter leading into the stomach and aggravate heartburn and acid reflux in some people. Excessive use of peppermint should be avoided in early pregnancy, as it may act as an emmenagogue.

Further Reading

Akbari SA, Alamolhoda SH, Baghban AA, Mirabi P. Effects of menthol essence and breast milk on the improvement of nipple fissures in breastfeeding women. *Journal of Research in Medical Sciences*, 2014 Jul; 19 (7): 629–33. .

Ferruggiari L, Ragione B, Rich ER, Lock K. The effect of aromatherapy on postoperative nausea in women undergoing surgical procedures. *Journal of Perianesthesia Nursing*, 2012 Aug; 27 (4): 246–51.

Khanna R, MacDonald JK, Levesque BG. Peppermint oil for the treatment of irritable bowel syndrome: A systematic review and meta-analysis. *Journal of Clinical Gastroenterology*, 2014 Jul; 48 (6): 505–12.

Pasha H, Behmanesh F, Mohsenzadeh F, et al. Study of the effect of mint oil on nausea and vomiting during pregnancy. *Iranian Red Crescent Medical Journal*, 2012 Nov; 14 (11): 727–30.

Sayyah Melli M, Rashidi MR, Delazar A, et al. Effect of peppermint water on prevention of nipple cracks in lactating primiparous women: A randomized controlled trial. *International Breastfeeding Journal*, 2007 Apr 19; 2: 7.

Tayarani-Najaran Z, Talasaz-Firoozi E, Nasiri R, et al. Antiemetic activity of volatile oil from *Mentha spicata* and *Mentha* x *piperita* in chemotherapy-induced nausea and vomiting. *Ecancermedicalscience*, 2013; 7: 290.

🍃 Propolis

Current Medicinal Uses

Propolis, like honey, has strong antimicrobial properties. It is used for wound healing, burns and topical skin infections such as the herpes simplex viruses (HSV), as well as canker sores and post-chemotherapy oral mucositis (mouth pain and inflammation).

History and Energetics

The word "propolis" derives from Greek words meaning "at the entrance of the city," a reference to the way bees defend their hive with propolis, using it to seal cracks and to encase any dead animals or other bugs that have gotten into the hive.

The Egyptians used propolis as an embalming ingredient. Greek and Roman doctors used it for mouth sores and infections. In other parts of Europe, propolis was used to treat sore throats, burns and wounds. The Incas used it for fevers.

Research Evidence

Herpes

In vitro studies have shown that propolis has strong antiviral properties against HSV-1 and HSV-2. In animal studies, propolis has been shown to reduce the size of vaginal herpes lesions.

One small randomized, controlled trial on people with genital HSV-2 compared propolis with acyclovir and a placebo. The group that used propolis had lesions that healed significantly faster than the other two groups. More people in the propolis group had completely healed lesions after ten days than in either the acyclovir or the placebo group. Of the women in the study, 66% had additional vaginal infections at the start of the trial. These infections were improved in the women using propolis, whereas there was no change in those taking either acyclovir or the placebo.

Latin Name
- Not applicable; propolis is a bee product made of sap, tree buds and other plant materials that bees use to seal up small holes and cracks in the hive

Parts Used
- Not applicable

Common Combination
- **For acute herpes lesions:** Lemon balm

Health Condition	Level of Scientific Evidence
Herpes	Fair

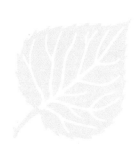

Safety

Propolis is generally safe and non-toxic when applied topically or taken orally. However, allergies to bee products, including propolis, are quite common.

Further Reading

Huleihel M, Isanu V. Anti-herpes simplex virus effect of an aqueous extract of propolis. *Israel Medical Association Journal*, 2002 Nov; 4 (11 Suppl): 923–27.

Sartori G, Pesarico AP, Pinton S, et al. Protective effect of brown Brazilian propolis against acute vaginal lesions caused by herpes simplex virus type 2 in mice: Involvement of antioxidant and anti-inflammatory mechanisms. *Cell Biochemistry and Function*, 2012 Jan; 30 (1): 1–10.

Vynograd N, Vynograd I, Sosnowski Z. A comparative multi-centre study of the efficacy of propolis, acyclovir and placebo in the treatment of genital herpes (HSV). *Phytomedicine*, 2000 Mar; 7 (1): 1–6.

Did You Know?

Variable Constituents

Much like honey, propolis changes according to the bees that make it and the climate they live in. Different plants are used as sources, depending on the bees' location. As a result, constituents also vary from one source of propolis to the next, although the main active compounds are very similar.

Raspberry

Current Medicinal Uses

Raspberry leaf is a tonifying herb for the uterus. It is used for many different conditions involving the uterus, including dysmenorrhea, menorrhagia, infertility and irregular menses.

History and Energetics

Associated with uterine health and fertility, raspberry was historically used as a partus preparator, an herb used to prepare the uterus for labor. It has also been used for centuries by midwives and traditional aboriginal healers to help speed labor and to prepare the uterus for conception and implantation.

Raspberry was also associated with protection in many cultures. The thorny canes were hung outside houses in the Philippines to prevent uninvited souls from entering. Raspberries may also symbolize kindness and fragility.

North American indigenous peoples relied on the astringent quality of raspberry leaves to treat diarrhea, menstrual bleeding and postpartum bleeding, and also used the leaves in a wash for eye infections.

Research Evidence

Infertility

Although raspberry has long been used as a nutritive herb and gentle tonic to help prepare the uterus for implantation and pregnancy, there is currently no research to support this use. Clinical studies are needed to confirm the use of raspberry to help improve the thickness and quality of the uterine lining in supporting implantation and pregnancy, either as a stand-alone treatment or in conjunction with assisted reproductive technologies such as ovarian stimulation drugs or embryo transfer after in vitro fertilization (IVF).

Labor and Delivery

Research results on raspberry leaf in pregnancy are quite mixed. One study found that raspberry leaf use was associated with a shorter second stage of labor and less frequent use of forceps during delivery. Another found an association between raspberry leaf use during pregnancy and decreased incidence of early and post-due-date labor. This study suggested that those taking raspberry leaf also

Latin Name
- *Rubus idaeus*

Part Used
- Leaf

Common Combination
- To prepare for conception and implantation: Black cohosh

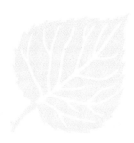

had less need for interventions during labor, including artificial rupture of membranes, forceps or vacuum use and Caesarean sections. A different study, however, noted an association between the use of raspberry leaf during pregnancy and increased rates of Caesarean delivery.

Animal studies are also inconclusive in supporting the use of raspberry to increase the efficiency or strength of uterine contractions during labor. In one study, rats given raspberry leaf throughout pregnancy had a longer gestation period, and their female offspring demonstrated faster reproductive development.

Health Condition	Level of Scientific Evidence
Infertility	Poor
Labor and delivery	Mixed

Safety

Raspberry leaf is generally safe. No consistent safety issues have been noted in human studies of raspberry use during pregnancy.

Further Reading

Dante G, Pedrielli G, Annessi E, Facchinetti F. Herb remedies during pregnancy: A systematic review of controlled clinical trials. *Journal of Maternal-Fetal & Neonatal Medicine*, 2013 Feb; 26 (3): 306–12.

Holst L, Haavik S, Nordeng H. Raspberry leaf — Should it be recommended to pregnant women? *Complementary Therapies in Clinical Practice*, 2009 Nov; 15 (4): 204–8.

Johnson JR, Makaji E, Ho S, et al. Effect of maternal raspberry leaf consumption in rats on pregnancy outcome and the fertility of the female offspring. *Reproductive Sciences* (Thousand Oaks, CA), 2009 Jun; 16 (6): 605–9.

Nordeng H, Bayne K, Havnen GC, Paulsen BS. Use of herbal drugs during pregnancy among 600 Norwegian women in relation to concurrent use of conventional drugs and pregnancy outcome. *Complementary Therapies in Clinical Practice*, 2011 Aug; 17 (3): 147–51.

Parsons M, Simpson M, Ponton T. Raspberry leaf and its effect on labour: Safety and efficacy. *Australian College of Midwives Incorporated Journal*, 1999 Sep; 12 (3): 20–25.

Simpson M, Parsons M, Greenwood J, Wade K. Raspberry leaf in pregnancy: Its safety and efficacy in labor. *Journal of Midwifery & Women's Health*, 2001 Mar–Apr; 46 (2): 51–59.

Red Clover

Current Medicinal Uses

Red clover is a nutritive tonic and alterative. It is used as a skin cleanser for conditions such as eczema, and as an anticancer agent. Because of its content of a class of phytoestrogens known as isoflavones, red clover is also used for amenorrhea, menopausal symptoms, including hot flushes, and other menstrual complaints.

History and Energetics

Red clover was historically used as a blood cleanser or alterative for skin conditions such as eczema and psoriasis and for fevers, infections and cancer. The Iroquois used red clover as a "blood medicine"; the Algonquin used it to treat whooping cough. The Iroquois and Cherokee used it as a gynecological aid, both for vaginal infections and during life-cycle changes such as menopause.

Red clover is one of the main ingredients in Hoxsey's formula and Essiac, two classic anticancer herbal combinations.

Red clover is the first herbal remedy I can remember clearly from my childhood (although I had no idea of its medicinal uses back then). I have fond memories of lying in the grass, looking at the blossoms. These days, my children like to suck on the flowers, extracting their sweetness much like the bees who collect nectar from red clover to make a rich, delicious honey.

Red clover's relationship to bees is also seen in the energetics of the plant. Red clover flower essence is used to separate someone from a panicked or hysterical "hive mentality" during a family crisis, public emergency or other crowded situation. Red clover users maintain individuality and avoid the influence of a strong group energy. Red clover is best suited for someone with menopausal symptoms or a skin condition who is easily carried away by the emotions of a crowd and feels the need for protection. In some cases of eczema or psoriasis, the scales and plaques that develop create a thicker barrier or boundary between the person and the rest of the world. The skin condition may itself be a form of protection, but it can be let go of with the help of red clover.

Latin Name
- *Trifolium pratense*

Parts Used
- Flowers
- Aerial parts (everything above the ground)

Common Combinations
- **For acne and other skin conditions:** Burdock and nettles
- **For menopausal symptoms including hot flushes:** Sage and black cohosh
- **For osteoporosis:** Soy and black cohosh

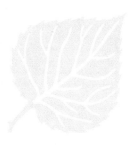

Research Evidence

Amenorrhea/Oligomenorrhea

Red clover's phytoestrogens could potentially be helpful in cases of amenorrhea related to inadequate estrogen or primary ovarian insufficiency (loss of normal ovarian function before the age of forty), but at this point in time, there is a lack of research evidence to support this use.

Breast Cancer

Theoretical concerns have been raised about the possibility that phytoestrogens may help estrogen-receptor-positive (ER-positive) breast cancers grow faster. However, a recent systematic review found that the existing studies failed to show that red clover had any breast cancer–promoting effects in menopausal women. In the studies reviewed, red clover extracts did not adversely affect breast density, bone strength, endometrial thickness or cardiovascular health. On the contrary, one in vitro study found that formononetin, a constituent in red clover, induced the death of cancerous ER-positive breast cancer cells.

Menopause and Osteoporosis

Some studies on red clover isoflavones have shown improvements in menopausal symptoms; others have not. A 2012 Iranian study noted no difference in menopausal symptoms when comparing red clover and a placebo. A separate crossover study conducted the same year found significant improvements in hot flushes and overall menopausal scores with red clover compared to a placebo. The dosage of isoflavones in the second study was almost double that of the former study.

In a 2012 study of breast cancer survivors, red clover users were less likely to report night sweats, weight gain and difficulty concentrating, though these results were not statistically significant. A single study investigating the impacts of red clover on mood found a significant decrease in depression and anxiety compared to a placebo among postmenopausal women.

A review published in 2013 concluded that red clover did not decrease the incidence of hot flushes in menopausal women as compared to a placebo; however, an earlier review found a small but significant decrease in the frequency of hot flushes.

Experimental animal research has begun to investigate the potential use of red clover in preventing fractures and osteoporosis in postmenopausal women. Several studies indicate that red clover may inhibit bone resorption and thus reduce bone turnover.

It is important to note that all these clinical trials use red clover isoflavone extracts rather than whole plant preparations. This focus on isoflavones is based on epidemiological research that shows decreased incidence and intensity of menopausal symptoms in populations that eat a higher amount of food-based isoflavones, such as those found in soy. Traditional preparations of red clover are whole plant infusions, which may have different clinical outcomes than isoflavone extracts. A few authors note that some of red clover's effects may be attributable, at least in part, to other plant constituents, such as flavonoids and phenolic acids, rather than simply to isoflavones. They also note that the effects of red clover may be variable because of individual differences in intestinal flora and the role of bacteria in increasing the bioavailability of plant constituents.

These issues are an important reminder that the whole is greater than the sum of its parts. Whole plant preparations may have different effects than standardized extracts. Likewise, absorption and activation of herbal extracts depend in part on the function of an individual's digestive system, liver and bacterial flora.

Health Condition	Level of Scientific Evidence
Amenorrhea/ oligomenorrhea	Poor
Breast cancer	Fair
Menopause	Mixed
Osteoporosis	Poor

Safety

Cautions against the use of red clover during pregnancy and breastfeeding are based on the theoretical impact of phytoestrogens. Similar cautions are advised in hormonally dependent conditions such as fibroids, endometriosis and estrogen-positive cancers. However, phytoestrogens are better understood as amphoteric, or balancing. In other words, they may appear to increase estrogen effects when biological estrogen is low, but they decrease it when biological estrogen is high.

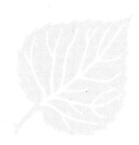

Further Reading

Cegieła U, Folwarczna J, Pytlik M, Zgórka G. Effects of extracts from *Trifolium medium* L. and *Trifolium pratense* L. on development of estrogen deficiency–induced osteoporosis in rats. *Evidence-Based Complementary and Alternative Medicine*, 2012; 2012: 921684.

Chen J, Sun L. Formononetin-induced apoptosis by activation of Ras/p38 mitogen-activated protein kinase in estrogen receptor–positive human breast cancer cells. *Hormone and Metabolic Research*, 2012 Dec; 44 (13): 943–48.

Ehsanpour S, Salehi K, Zolfaghari B, Bakhtiari S. The effects of red clover on quality of life in post-menopausal women. *Iranian Journal of Nursing and Midwifery Research*, 2012 Jan; 17 (1): 34–40.

Fritz H, Seely D, Flower G, et al. Soy, red clover, and isoflavones and breast cancer: A systematic review. *PLoS One*, 2013 Nov 28; 8 (11): e81968.

Lethaby A, Marjoribanks J, Kronenberg F, et al. Phytoestrogens for menopausal vasomotor symptoms. *Cochrane Database of Systematic Reviews*, 2013 Dec 10; 12: CD001395.

Lipovac M, Chedraui P, Gruenhut C, et al. The effect of red clover isoflavone supplementation over vasomotor and menopausal symptoms in postmenopausal women. *Gynecological Endocrinology*, 2012 Mar; 28 (3): 203–7.

Ma H, Sullivan-Halley J, Smith AW, et al. Estrogenic botanical supplements, health-related quality of life, fatigue, and hormone-related symptoms in breast cancer survivors: A HEAL study report. *BMC Complementary and Alternative Medicine*, 2011 Nov 8; 11: 109.

Rhodiola

Current Medicinal Uses

Rhodiola is used to improve the body's physical responses to chronic stress and to reduce fatigue. It may also increase cognitive performance and memory, especially when these are impaired by long-term stress. Recently rhodiola has been acknowledged for its potential in helping ease depression.

Known in traditional Chinese medicine as *hong jing tian*, rhodiola is considered a qi and yin tonic, used to stop coughs.

History and Energetics

Rhodiola is native to parts of China, including Tibet, and northern areas of Europe and Asia. In the Himalayas, rhodiola has been used to help alleviate mild symptoms of altitude sickness. In Mongolia, it has been used to treat lung diseases and infections such as tuberculosis. In Russia, it has been used to improve the stamina of athletes and the performance of cosmonauts in space. In Siberia, it was given to newlyweds as a symbol of fertility and longevity. Rhodiola has also been used to improve sexual function.

From an energetic perspective, rhodiola helps people adjust to challenges of all kinds, from high altitude to cold temperatures during long winters and from athletic competitions to space missions.

Research Evidence

Depression

Pharmacodynamic research suggests that rhodiola enhances the action of neurotransmitters such as serotonin and dopamine, which are involved in depression. In one study on sixty people with mild to moderate depression, rhodiola significantly improved the symptoms of depression compared to a placebo.

Stress

Rhodiola may decrease cortisol and catecholamines, hormones released in response to stress. It has also been shown to decrease fatigue and measured symptoms of "burnout" compared to a placebo. A study on students taking an exam found that rhodiola significantly increased

Latin Name
- *Rhodiola rosea*

Part Used
- Root

Common Combinations
- **For depression:** St. John's wort and/or saffron

- **For stress:** Eleuthero and ashwagandha

> **Did You Know?**
>
> **Culinary Use**
> In many countries, the stems and leaves of rhodiola are eaten raw or cooked as vegetables.

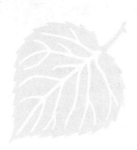

their feeling of well-being, reduced fatigue and improved neurological fitness testing compared to a placebo. Additional studies have shown that rhodiola improves hand–eye coordination and mental fatigue in students during examination periods, and heightens the visual perception, short-term memory and perception of order in night-shift workers.

In a placebo-controlled clinical trial on strenuous physical exercise, rhodiola delayed the time to exhaustion and increased oxygen intake. In another study, it improved muscle recovery after exercise.

Overall, research on rhodiola has been very positive, but no two trials have had a similar methodology, making it difficult to come to clear conclusions on its effectiveness.

Health Condition	Level of Scientific Evidence
Depression	Fair
Stress	Fair

Safety

Very few side effects have been reported in clinical trials on rhodiola. Because it is a stimulating adaptogen, some people may find that it interferes with sleep or aggravates anxiety. Rhodiola has not been investigated for its safety in pregnancy or breastfeeding.

Further Reading

Darbinyan V, Aslanyan G, Amroyan E, et al. Clinical trial of *Rhodiola rosea* L. extract SHR-5 in the treatment of mild to moderate depression. *Nordic Journal of Psychiatry*, 2007; 61 (5): 343–48.

Hung SK, Perry R, Ernst E. The effectiveness and efficacy of *Rhodiola rosea* L.: A systematic review of randomized clinical trials. *Phytomedicine*, 2011 Feb 15; 18 (4): 235–44.

Ishaque S, Shamseer L, Bukutu C, Vohra S. *Rhodiola rosea* for physical and mental fatigue: A systematic review. *BMC Complementary and Alternative Medicine*, 2012 May 29; 12: 70.

Olsson EM, von Schéele B, Panossian AG. A randomised, double-blind, placebo-controlled, parallel-group study of the standardised extract SHR-5 of the roots of *Rhodiola rosea* in the treatment of subjects with stress-related fatigue. *Planta Medica*, 2009 Feb; 75 (2): 105–12.

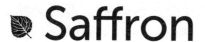 Saffron

Current Medicinal Uses

Saffron is currently used primarily for depression, sexual dysfunction and age-related macular degeneration. It may also help improve digestion, reduce menstrual cramps and bring on menses in cases of amenorrhea.

History and Energetics

Written records indicate that saffron has been used for over 4,000 years. The bright red stigmas — or threads, as they are often called — are extremely valuable. They have been woven into fabrics and used to alleviate melancholy. Persian physicians may have used saffron for sexual dysfunction. Saffron was also used as perfume and has long been considered an aphrodisiac.

Research Evidence
Depression

Clinical research supports the use of saffron in the treatment of mild to moderate depression. A recent systematic review of six studies concluded that saffron has significant antidepressant effects comparable to standard antidepressant medications. An earlier review of five studies came to a similar conclusion.

Saffron not only appears to be as effective as anti-depressant medications but also enhances the effects of those medications when taken alongside them. One placebo-controlled trial found that selective serotonin reuptake inhibitors (SSRIs) taken along with the saffron constituent crocin were more effective than the SSRIs alone.

Saffron has also been shown to improve the sexual side effects of antidepressant medications. In one study on women taking fluoxetine, saffron improved sexual function, arousal, lubrication and pain compared to a placebo.

In another placebo-controlled trial, saffron was found to be effective in relieving the symptoms of premenstrual depression.

Latin Name
- *Crocus sativus*

Part Used
- Stigma

Common Combination
- For depression: Rhodiola and/or St. John's wort

Health Condition	Level of Scientific Evidence
Depression	Good

Safety

Saffron should be avoided in pregnancy, as it may act as an emmenagogue.

Further Reading

Agha-Hosseini M, Kashani L, Aleyaseen A, et al. *Crocus sativus* L. (saffron) in the treatment of premenstrual syndrome: A double-blind, randomised and placebo-controlled trial. *BJOG: An International Journal of Obstetrics and Gynaecology*, 2008 Mar; 115 (4): 515–19.

Hausenblas HA, Saha D, Dubyak PJ, Anton SD. Saffron (*Crocus sativus* L.) and major depressive disorder: A meta-analysis of randomized clinical trials. *Journal of Integrative Medicine*, 2013 Nov; 11 (6): 377–83.

Kashani L, Raisi F, Saroukhani S, et al. Saffron for treatment of fluoxetine-induced sexual dysfunction in women: Randomized double-blind placebo-controlled study. *Human Psychopharmacology*, 2013 Jan; 28 (1): 54–60.

Lopresti AL, Drummond PD. Saffron (*Crocus sativus*) for depression: A systematic review of clinical studies and examination of underlying antidepressant mechanisms of action. *Human Psychopharmacology*, 2014 Nov; 29 (6): 517–27.

Talaei A, Hassanpour Moghadam M, Sajadi Tabassi SA, Mohajeri SA. Crocin, the main active saffron constituent, as an adjunctive treatment in major depressive disorder: A randomized, double-blind, placebo-controlled, pilot clinical trial. *Journal of Affective Disorders*, 2014 Nov 26; 174C: 51–56.

Did You Know?

Saffron Robes

Buddhist monks are said to wear saffron-colored robes, even though the fabric is almost always dyed with gamboge or turmeric, much cheaper alternatives.

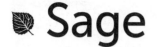 # Sage

Current Medicinal Uses

Thanks to its astringent properties, sage is most frequently used for sore throats and gum disease, and also to reduce hot flushes during menopause and to support weaning from breastfeeding or after a perinatal loss.

History and Energetics

Sage was once considered a cure-all, used to treat everything from coughs to snakebites, to increase a woman's fertility and to prevent infectious diseases. The name *Salvia* comes from the Latin word *salvere*, which means "to be in good health." It was reputed to impart wisdom and longevity, even immortality, to those who used it regularly.

White sage is one of the four main herbs (the others are tobacco, sweetgrass and cedar) used by indigenous peoples in North America during smudging ceremonies. It is bundled and burned to protect, cleanse and heal.

Research Evidence

Menopause

A pilot study looked at the effects of a combination of sage and alfalfa for reducing hot flushes in menopausal women. Out of thirty women in the study, twenty reported a complete disappearance of hot flushes and night sweats after three months of treatment. The other ten women reported improvements as well. There was no control group in this study.

In a more recent study, sage significantly reduced both the frequency and intensity of hot flushes in menopausal women after four weeks of treatment. Further improvements were seen after eight weeks. Menopause Rating Scale scores also decreased significantly over the course of this study.

Weaning

Lactation consultants and midwives have long warned that large amounts of sage will decrease milk supply. They have suggested sage infusions to ease the transition to weaning, especially in cases where weaning is abrupt. Research is lacking to confirm this traditional use.

Latin Name
- *Salvia officinalis*

Part Used
- Leaf

Common Combination
- For menopausal symptoms with anxiety or nervousness: Motherwort

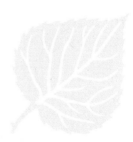

Health Condition	Level of Scientific Evidence
Menopause	Fair
Weaning	Poor

Safety

Like many other herbs, sage should be avoided in therapeutic doses during pregnancy. Regular culinary use is generally regarded as safe. Caution is advised during breastfeeding, as sage may decrease breast milk production.

Further Reading

Bommer S, Klein P, Suter A. First time proof of sage's tolerability and efficacy in menopausal women with hot flushes. *Advances in Therapy*, 2011 Jun; 28 (6): 490–500.

De Leo V, Lanzetta D, Cazzavacca R, Morgante G. [Treatment of neurovegetative menopausal symptoms with a phytotherapeutic agent]. [Article in Italian]. *Minerva ginecologica*, 1998 May; 50 (5): 207–11.

St. John's Wort

Current Medicinal Uses

St. John's wort is best used for depression and in combination with other herbs when depression occurs as a premenstrual or menopausal symptom, in conjunction with anxiety or because of a concussion. It is also used for its antiviral and vulnerary actions in cases of herpes, genital warts and other viral infections that affect the skin. Topically, St. John's wort is used for neuralgia, sunburns, muscle pain, wounds, hemorrhoids and varicose veins.

History and Energetics

St. John's wort has a long history of magical and religious uses. Its Latin genus name, *Hypericum*, comes from the Greek word *hyperikon*, meaning "above a picture," as St. John's wort was hung over religious images and windows to ward off evil spirits on St. John's Eve, the night before the feast day of St. John the Baptist — a celebration coinciding with the midsummer solstice, when the flowers are in full bloom.

The plant's bright yellow flowers carry the happiness and brightness of the sun into the herbal medicine and then to the user. Making a tincture of the flowers harvested in midsummer is like bottling sunshine. St. John's wort illuminates and brightens the spirit of the user from the inside out, lifting depression and filling the person with solar power. The plant is particularly useful in seasonal affective disorder, where feelings of depression are related to the diminished sunshine during winter months. Ingesting this plant literally makes the user more receptive to sunshine — it may lead to photosensitivity, which could cause skin rashes with overexposure to the sun.

Research Evidence
Depression

St. John's wort is primarily known for its use as a natural antidepressant. In systematic reviews of randomized, double-blind, controlled clinical trials, it has been shown to have comparable effects to standard pharmaceutical antidepressants and greater effects than placebos in the treatment of major depression. Compared to standard drug treatment, the standardized extract of St. John's wort

Latin Name
- *Hypericum perforatum*

Parts Used
- Flower
- Aerial parts (everything above the ground)

Common Combinations
- **For depression with anxiety:** Passionflower and lavender
- **For genital warts:** Echinacea and propolis
- **For herpes:** Lemon balm and propolis
- **For menopausal symptoms:** Chaste tree and black cohosh
- **For PMS:** Chaste tree

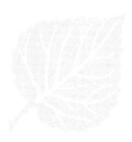

has significantly fewer adverse effects. In Germany, the standardized extract WS 5570 is authorized to be marketed as treatment for mild to moderate major depressive disorder.

Genital Warts

In vitro research supports St. John's wort's antiviral actions. Clinical studies are needed to confirm its potential use in the treatment of genital warts.

Herpes

One open-label trial found that a St. John's wort and copper sulfate formula was just as effective as acyclovir when applied topically to herpes lesions. Sensations of burning and stinging, pain and blistering of lesions were significantly reduced. One study on St. John's wort for depression noted that the oral supplement appeared to reduce herpes breakouts in those taking it. In vitro studies also support the use of St. John's wort for herpes.

Menopause

A recent meta-analysis looked at the use of St. John's wort for menopausal symptoms. The researchers concluded that St. John's wort, either alone or in combination with other herbs, significantly reduced menopausal symptoms, especially hot flushes.

Premenstrual Syndrome

Two randomized controlled clinical trials found that St. John's wort was significantly more effective than a placebo at reducing behavioral and physical premenstrual symptoms. Case reports and preliminary studies also support the use of St. John's wort for premenstrual dysphoric disorder, particularly in cases when standard pharmaceutical antidepressants are intolerable because of undesirable side effects.

Health Condition	Level of Scientific Evidence
Depression	Good
Genital warts	Poor
Herpes	Fair
Menopause	Good
Premenstrual syndrome	Good

Safety

St. John's wort speeds up the metabolism of many pharmaceutical drugs, including oral contraceptives. In some cases, women taking both oral contraceptives and St. John's wort have become pregnant because of this interaction. Before taking St. John's wort, consult with a health-care provider familiar with drug–herb interactions.

St. John's wort appears to be safe during pregnancy and breastfeeding.

Further Reading

Abdali K, Khajehei M, Tabatabaee HR. Effect of St John's wort on severity, frequency, and duration of hot flashes in premenopausal, perimenopausal and postmenopausal women: A randomized, double-blind, placebo-controlled study. *Menopause*, 2010 Mar; 17 (2): 326–31.

Canning S, Waterman M, Orsi N, et al. The efficacy of *Hypericum perforatum* (St. John's wort) for the treatment of premenstrual syndrome: A randomized, double-blind, placebo-controlled trial. *CNS Drugs*, 2010 Mar; 24 (3): 207–25.

Clewell A, Barnes M, Endres JR, et al. Efficacy and tolerability assessment of a topical formulation containing copper sulfate and *Hypericum perforatum* on patients with herpes skin lesions: A comparative, randomized controlled trial. *Journal of Drugs in Dermatology*, 2012 Feb; 11 (2): 209–15.

Dante G, Bellei G, Neri I, Facchinetti F. Herbal therapies in pregnancy: What works? *Current Opinion in Obstetrics & Gynecology*, 2014 Apr; 26 (2): 83–91.

Gastpar M. *Hypericum* extract WS 5570® for depression — An overview. *International Journal of Psychiatry in Clinical Practice*, 2013 Nov; 17 Suppl 1: 1–7.

Linde K, Berner MM, Kriston L. St. John's wort for major depression. *Cochrane Database of Systematic Reviews*, 2008 Oct 8; (4): CD000448.

Liu YR, Jiang YL, Huang RQ, et al. *Hypericum perforatum* L. preparations for menopause: A meta-analysis of efficacy and safety. *Climacteric*, 2014 Aug; 17 (4): 325–35.

Sarris J. St. John's wort for the treatment of psychiatric disorders. *Psychiatric Clinics of North America*, 2013 Mar; 36 (1): 65–72.

van Die MD, Bone KM, Burger HG, et al. Effects of a combination of *Hypericum perforatum* and *Vitex agnus-castus* on PMS-like symptoms in late-perimenopausal women: Findings from a subpopulation analysis. *Journal of Alternative and Complementary Medicine*, 2009 Sep; 15 (9): 1045–48.

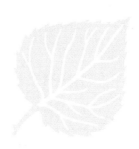

Schisandra

Latin Name
- *Schisandra chinensis*

Part Used
- Berries

Common Combinations
- For sexual dysfunction: Shatavari, ginseng and ginkgo
- For stress: Shatavari, ashwagandha and eleuthero

Did You Know?

Longevity Herb

In TCM, schisandra is considered a longevity herb, helping people lead a fuller, longer life and slowing down the natural aging process.

Current Medicinal Uses

Schisandra is an adaptogenic herb, used to increase resistance to stress. It is also antioxidant and hepato-protective, which makes it useful in reducing the negative effects of hepatitis and cirrhosis of the liver.

History and Energetics

Schisandra has a long history of use in traditional Chinese medicine (TCM). Its Chinese name, *wu wei zi*, means "five-flavored seed," an acknowledgment of the burst of flavors the berries deliver: they are at once bitter, sweet, sour, salty and pungent. In some places, the fresh berries are juiced and used as a drink.

From a TCM perspective, schisandra calms the heart and quiets the spirit. It is often included in formulas for insomnia, night sweats, spontaneous sweating and heart palpitations. Depending on a particular woman's overall health, schisandra may be helpful in reducing menopausal symptoms.

In addition, according to classic TCM texts, schisandra collects and astringes fluids lost in sweating, urination, diarrhea and chronic coughs. It may also be used to treat spermatorrhea and vaginal discharge. In order for this astringent action to work most effectively, it needs to be dispersed. The berries should be crushed beforehand to allow the bitter inner parts to combine with the sour exterior. Otherwise, unhealthy qi may be retained, causing bloating and distention.

Research Evidence
Hepatitis

Preclinical studies on schisandra for hepatitis show that it may significantly decrease liver enzymes. For this reason, it is often added to herbal formulas for treating hepatitis, even though it does not appear to have the antiviral properties necessary to wipe out the hepatitis virus. In an open-label trial looking at people with chronic hepatitis C, a combination of schisandra, licorice, milk thistle, vitamin C and other nutrients reduced liver enzymes in 44% of patients and decreased viral load in 25% of patients. More research is needed.

Stress

In one placebo-controlled trial, a combination of schisandra, eleuthero and rhodiola improved accuracy, speed and attention during stressful cognitive tasks. In a trial on people with depression, schisandra increased energy, physical activity, mood and sleep. Trials on schizophrenic patients have shown schisandra to improve mood, social functioning, hallucinations, catatonia and sleep.

Health Condition	Level of Scientific Evidence
Hepatitis	Poor
Stress	Fair

Did You Know?

Aphrodisiac
Schisandra has long been considered an aphrodisiac, increasing sexual desire by improving overall health.

Safety

Overall, schisandra, like most adaptogens and tonic herbs, is relatively safe. Schisandra is contraindicated in pregnancy, except to induce labor. According to TCM principles, schisandra should be avoided in acute coughs.

Further Reading

Aslanyan G, Amroyan E, Gabrielyan E, et al. Double-blind, placebo-controlled, randomised study of single dose effects of ADAPT-232 on cognitive functions. *Phytomedicine*, 2010 Jun; 17 (7): 494–99.

Melhem A, Stern M, Shibolet O, et al. Treatment of chronic hepatitis C virus infection via antioxidants: Results of a phase I clinical trial. *Journal of Clinical Gastroenterology*, 2005 Sep; 39 (8): 737–42.

Panossian AG. Adaptogens in mental and behavioral disorders. *Psychiatric Clinics of North America*, 2013 Mar; 36 (1): 49–64.

Seaweed

Latin Names

- *Fucus vesiculosus* (bladderwrack)
- *Sargassum* spp.

Parts Used

- Whole plant

Common Combination

- For iodine-deficiency hypothyroidism: Ashwagandha and bacopa

Current Medicinal Uses

Seaweed is a rich source of iodine, a key element in the proper functioning of the thyroid gland. In cases where hypothyroidism is a result of iodine deficiency, seaweed may be helpful.

History and Energetics

Sea vegetables are a mainstay of traditional coastal cuisines in Japan, Korea, the British Isles, Scandinavia and many other places. Bladderwrack and other types of seaweed were also burned to make soda ash, or sodium carbonate.

Iodine was first identified in bladderwrack in 1811 and was used to treat thyroid goiters caused by iodine deficiency. *Sargassum*, a genus of brown seaweeds traditionally used in China, Japan and Korea, also has a history of use in hypothyroidism. Known as *hai zao* in traditional Chinese medicine, sargassum is bitter, salty and cold and has been used to disperse phlegm and shrink goiters. Seaweed is also a good source of calcium, fiber and other minerals.

Research Evidence
Hypothyroidism

Iodine is used by the human body in the production of thyroid hormones. The high content of iodine in bladderwrack and other brown seaweeds formed the basis of its use in treating hypothyroidism. However, based on research on sargassum, there is some evidence that iodine is not the sole constituent responsible for promoting thyroid health. Pharmacological and animal studies suggest that polysaccharides, fucoidans and several other compounds may have effects on the immune system that would support seaweed's use in addressing autoimmune-related thyroid conditions.

More research is definitely needed, as these studies appear to contradict other studies and empirical evidence showing that high consumption of seaweed may, in fact, induce thyroid disease.

Did You Know?

Other Iodine Sources

Land plants are generally poor sources of iodine unless their soil has been fertilized by seaweed. In many countries, table salt is now supplemented with iodine.

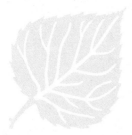

Health Condition	Level of Scientific Evidence
Hypothyroidism	Poor

Safety

Iodine can aggravate or induce hyperthyroidism in some people. When thyroid disease is related to an autoimmune process (as in Graves' disease and Hashimoto's thyroiditis), iodine should be avoided.

Seaweed should be avoided in greater than culinary amounts during pregnancy and breastfeeding, as it can have negative health effects on both women and their babies.

Different seaweeds have vastly different iodine content. In cases of iodine deficiency, standardized herbal extracts are recommended over seaweed ingestion, to prevent toxic levels of iodine.

Further Reading

Leung AM, Braverman LE. Iodine-induced thyroid dysfunction. *Current Opinion in Endocrinology, Diabetes, and Obesity*, 2012 Oct; 19 (5): 414–19.

Liu L, Heinrich M, Myers S, Dworjanyn SA. Towards a better understanding of medicinal uses of the brown seaweed *Sargassum* in Traditional Chinese Medicine: A phytochemical and pharmacological review. *Journal of Ethnopharmacology*, 2012 Aug 1; 142 (3): 591–619.

Rhee SS, Braverman LE, Pino S, et al. High iodine content of Korean seaweed soup: A health risk for lactating women and their infants? *Thyroid*, 2011 Aug; 21 (8): 927–28.

Zimmermann M, Delange F. Iodine supplementation of pregnant women in Europe: A review and recommendations. *European Journal of Clinical Nutrition*, 2004 Jul; 58 (7): 979–84.

Zimmermann MB, Boelaert K. Iodine deficiency and thyroid disorders. *Lancet Diabetes & Endocrinology*, 2015 Jan 12. [Epub ahead of print.]

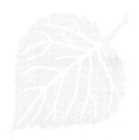

Did You Know?

Alginates and Carrageenan

Alginates (from bladderwrack) and carrageenan (derived from the seaweed Irish moss) — both constituents that give seaweed its gelatinous texture — are widely used in processed foods, jellies, ice creams and even toothpaste.

Shatavari

Latin Name
- *Asparagus racemosus*

Part Used
- Root

Common Combinations
- For low milk supply: Fenugreek
- For sexual dysfunction: Ginseng and ginkgo

Current Medicinal Uses

Shatavari is a tonic herb used to promote lactation and overall fertility. In Ayurvedic and Unani medicine, shatavari is considered an excellent tonic herb and is used as a general rejuvenator and to improve sperm counts.

History and Energetics

The name "shatavari" means either "woman who has a hundred husbands" or "curer of a hundred diseases," according to different sources. It has played a prominent role in women's health, having been used as a rejuvenating uterine tonic for promoting fertility and preventing miscarriage; to help women recover from childbirth; as a galactagogue for low milk supply; to treat menopausal symptoms; and as an aphrodisiac for diminished sexual function. It has also been used for indigestion, stomach ulcers and nervous conditions.

Research Evidence
Low Milk Supply

Early clinical research found that shatavari increased breast milk production in women complaining of low supply. Animal studies support these early studies.

More recently, two randomized trials were conducted to evaluate the effectiveness of shatavari in improving breast milk production. In one study, shatavari in combination with other herbs performed no better than a placebo in increasing prolactin levels or the weight of infants. The other trial, on shatavari alone, found significant increases in both prolactin and infant weight gain compared to a placebo.

Sexual Dysfunction

Some preliminary evidence supports the use of shatavari to promote male sexual function. More research on women is needed.

Health Condition	Level of Scientific Evidence
Low milk supply	Mixed
Sexual dysfunction	Poor

Safety

No major side effects have been noted in the clinical studies on shatavari in breastfeeding women. No studies have been conducted on the safety of shatavari during pregnancy.

Further Reading

Gupta M, Shaw B. A double-blind randomized clinical trial for evaluation of galactogogue activity of *Asparagus racemosus* Willd. *Iranian Journal of Pharmaceutical Research*, 2011 Winter; 10 (1): 167–72.

Mortel M, Mehta SD. Systematic review of the efficacy of herbal galactogogues. *Journal of Human Lactation*, 2013 May; 29 (2): 154–62.

Sharma S, Ramji S, Kumari S, Bapna JS. Randomized controlled trial of *Asparagus racemosus* (shatavari) as a lactogogue in lactational inadequacy. *Indian Pediatrics*, 1996 Aug; 33 (8): 675–77.

Did You Know?

Shatavar Vatika Herbal Park

A park in the state of Haryana, India, designated for the preservation and propagation of endangered Ayurvedic herbal medicinal species, is named after shatavari.

Shepherd's Purse

Latin Name
- *Capsella bursa-pastoris*

Parts Used
- Aerial parts (everything above the ground)

Common Combination
- For acute menorrhagia: Geranium and yarrow

Did You Know?

Culinary Use
A member of the same family of plants as mustard and broccoli, shepherd's purse has also been eaten as a green vegetable.

Current Medicinal Uses

Shepherd's purse is used as an astringent and hemostatic, to stop nosebleeds and passive bleeding in conditions such as menorrhagia, bleeding fibroids and hemorrhoids.

History and Energetics

Historically, shepherd's purse was used to prevent hemorrhaging after childbirth. Like yarrow, it was used during the First World War to stop both external and internal bleeding.

In homeopathic treatment, shepherd's purse is used for excessive bleeding caused by fibroids and accompanied by back pain and a generalized feeling of soreness, or when every other menses is particularly heavy.

Research Evidence
Menorrhagia

Research on shepherd's purse is lacking, but early pharmacological and animal studies support its use in stopping excessive bleeding.

Health Condition	Level of Scientific Evidence
Menorrhagia	Poor

Safety

Shepherd's purse should be avoided during pregnancy and breastfeeding. Large amounts of shepherd's purse may cause heart palpitations.

Further Reading

Kuroda K, Kaku T. Pharmacological and chemical studies on the alcohol extract of *Capsella bursa-pastoris*. *Life Sciences*, 1969 Feb 1; 8 (3): 151–55.

Vermathen M, Glasl H. Effect of the herb extract of *Capsella bursa-pastoris* on blood coagulation. *Plánta Medica*, 1993; 59 (7): A670.

Slippery Elm

Current Medicinal Uses

Slippery elm bark is used as a demulcent to ease symptoms of heartburn, diarrhea, constipation, canker sores, sore throat, irritable bowel syndrome, stomach ulcers and inflammatory bowel disease. The mucilaginous constituents in the bark coat the mucous membranes of the body wherever they are directed, providing a smooth, soothing layer of protection to inflamed tissues.

History and Energetics

Slippery elm bark was historically made into a gruel and eaten as survival food, and it was also used to preserve meats. The Chippewa and Ojibwa peoples used it for sore throats. The Cherokee used it to soothe the stomach and bowels of pregnant women. It has also been used to ease childbirth. Externally, it has been used for eye infections, boils and sores.

The flower essence of elm is beneficial for those who feel overwhelmed by the amount of responsibility they have taken on. They may struggle with feelings of depression and exhaustion, along with a sense that there is too much to do, that a task is too difficult or even that accomplishing a task is not humanly possible.

Research Evidence

The few studies that exist clearly show that slippery elm contains high concentrations of mucilage, which is known to soothe irritated mucous membranes. In one small pilot study, a combination of slippery elm and other nutritional and herbal supplements was found to decrease abdominal symptoms in people with irritable bowel syndrome.

Heartburn

Clinical research hasn't caught up with years of safe traditional use of slippery elm for relieving the pain of heartburn and reflux. Human clinical studies have not yet been conducted, and the phytopharmacological research is extremely dated.

Latin Name
- *Ulmus fulva*

Part Used
- Inner bark

Common Combination
- **For heartburn and stomach ulcers:** Deglycyrrhizinated licorice

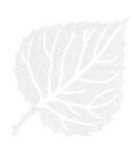

Health Condition	Level of Scientific Evidence
Heartburn	Poor

Safety

As a good source of soluble fiber, slippery elm may interfere with the absorption of medications, so it should be taken at a different time of day than drugs and nutritional supplements. Slippery elm inner bark is likely safe in pregnancy and breastfeeding, although there are no clinical studies to confirm this.

Further Reading

Gill RE, Hirst EL, Jones JK. Constitution of the mucilage from the bark of *Ulmus fulva* (slippery elm mucilage): The sugars formed in the hydrolysis of the methylated mucilage. *Journal of the Chemical Society*, 1946 Nov: 1025–29.

Hawrelak JA, Myers SP. Effects of two natural medicine formulations on irritable bowel syndrome symptoms: A pilot study. *Journal of Alternative and Complementary Medicine*, 2010 Oct; 16 (10): 1065–71.

Hough L, Jones JK, Hirst EL. Chemical constitution of slippery elm mucilage: Isolation of 3-methyl d-galactose from the hydrolysis products. *Nature*, 1950 Jan 7; 165 (4184): 34.

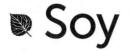# Soy

Current Medicinal Uses

Soy is a great example of food that is used as medicine. Because it contains isoflavones, a class of phytoestrogens, it is most commonly used for menopausal symptoms and to prevent breast cancer and osteoporosis.

History and Energetics

Soy has been cultivated and included as part of the diet in China since the eleventh century BCE. It is now a major food source in East Asian countries and for vegetarians worldwide. Soybeans can be cooked and enjoyed as they are or processed into a wide variety of products, including tofu, tempeh, soy milk, soybean oil, soy sauce and miso. It is also found in other food products, such as lecithin, flour, emulsifying agents and texturized vegetable protein.

From a traditional Chinese medicine perspective, the soybean is very cooling. It is almost always combined with other foods to create a dish that is warming overall, to promote proper digestion. If eaten alone, soybeans are believed to weaken kidney and adrenal function. Fermented soy products, such as tempeh, soy sauce and miso, are considered less cooling and more digestible, but they often contain more salt.

Research Evidence

Initially, researchers believed that phytoestrogens increased estrogen in the body and would therefore be best suited for conditions in which estrogen is decreased, such as menopause. They were concerned that soy's isoflavones would exacerbate conditions in which estrogen levels are already higher than normal, such as estrogen-receptor-positive breast cancer and fibroids. However, phytopharmacological and clinical human studies have led to quite a different conclusion. Phytoestrogens bind estrogen receptors just as biological estrogen does, but the resulting effects are weaker. Because of this difference in strength, in cases where there are high concentrations of circulating biological estrogen, phytoestrogens appear to block estrogen receptors and thus decrease the effects of estrogen. When estrogen is low, on the other hand,

Latin Name
- *Glycine max*

Parts Used
- Whole food
- Isoflavone extracts

Common Combinations
- **For breast cancer:** Green tea and barberry

- **For menopausal symptoms and osteoporosis:** Red clover and black cohosh

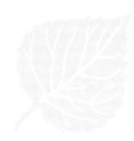

phytoestrogens increase the effects of estrogen by binding to empty receptors. Their overall effect is amphoteric, or balancing.

Breast Cancer

Several recent systematic reviews have concluded that high daily soy intake (two to three servings daily) may be protective against the development of breast cancer and its recurrence, and may also reduce the risk of mortality. No increases in circulating estrogen have been found in women who consume larger amounts of soy.

Menopause

In several meta-analyses of human clinical trials, soy isoflavones have been shown to reduce the frequency and severity of menopausal hot flushes. Although the effects are not quite as good as those seen with synthetic hormone replacement therapy (HRT) with estradiol, soy isoflavones are significantly more effective than a placebo. However, treatment with soy takes substantially longer than treatment with HRT: benefits may not be apparent for several months, and maximum effects may not be felt for up to a year.

Osteoporosis

Studies on the use of soy to prevent osteoporosis are fewer but also very promising. Two recent systematic reviews concluded that soy may increase bone density and decrease markers of bone loss in urine, particularly in postmenopausal women. Benefits to bone mineral density have been observed after six to twelve months of soy isoflavone use. Further research is needed to confirm whether these positive results translate into decreased fracture risk.

> **Did You Know?**
>
> **Soy Production**
>
> Soy is now a major crop worldwide. In 2004, soy accounted for 27% of the United States' agricultural exports to the European Union.

Health Condition	Level of Scientific Evidence
Breast cancer	Good
Menopause	Good
Osteoporosis	Good

Safety

Soy is considered a major allergen, and allergy labeling for soy is required in some countries. People with allergies to peanuts, peas, lentils, rye and/or barley should be cautious about consuming soy products.

Further Reading

Chen M, Rao Y, Zheng Y, et al. Association between soy isoflavone intake and breast cancer risk for pre- and post-menopausal women: A meta-analysis of epidemiological studies. *PLoS One*, 2014 Feb 20; 9 (2): e89288.

Chen MN, Lin CC, Liu CF. Efficacy of phytoestrogens for menopausal symptoms: A meta-analysis and systematic review. *Climacteric*, 2014 Dec 1: 1–10.

Fritz H, Seely D, Flower G, et al. Soy, red clover, and isoflavones and breast cancer: A systematic review. *PLoS One*, 2013 Nov 28; 8 (11): e81968.

Li L, Lv Y, Xu L, Zheng Q. Quantitative efficacy of soy isoflavones on menopausal hot flashes. *British Journal of Clinical Pharmacology*, 2014 Oct 15. [Epub ahead of print.]

Messina M. Soy foods, isoflavones, and the health of postmenopausal women. *American Journal of Clinical Nutrition*, 2014 Jun 4; 100 (Supplement 1): 423S–430S.

Morimoto Y, Maskarinec G, Park SY, et al. Dietary isoflavone intake is not statistically significantly associated with breast cancer risk in the Multiethnic Cohort. *British Journal of Nutrition*, 2014 Sep 28; 112 (6): 976–83.

Taku K, Melby MK, Kronenberg F, et al. Extracted or synthesized soybean isoflavones reduce menopausal hot flash frequency and severity: Systematic review and meta-analysis of randomized controlled trials. *Menopause*, 2012 Jul; 19 (7): 776–90.

Taku K, Melby MK, Nishi N, et al. Soy isoflavones for osteoporosis: An evidence-based approach. *Maturitas*, 2011 Dec; 70 (4): 333–38.

Wei P, Liu M, Chen Y, Chen DC. Systematic review of soy isoflavone supplements on osteoporosis in women. *Asian Pacific Journal of Tropical Medicine*, 2012 Mar; 5 (3): 243–48.

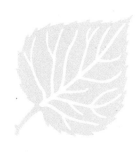

Spearmint

Latin Name
- *Mentha spicata*

Parts Used
- Aerial parts (everything above the ground) before flowering

Common Combination
- For PCOS with hirsutism: Licorice and peony

Current Medicinal Uses

Spearmint is used much like peppermint (which is a hybrid of spearmint and watermint): to relax the digestive system and relieve bloating, gas, stomachaches and nausea. Like peppermint, it is also used topically for headaches and other muscle and nerve pains. More recently, it has been studied for its potential to alleviate hirsutism (male-pattern secondary hair growth) in women.

History and Energetics

Spearmint, although perhaps less well known, predates peppermint and has a much longer history of medicinal use for digestive upset. It was also used to encourage sweating and cool a fever and was strewn across floors and added to bathwater for its clean, energizing scent. The Ancient Romans added it to milk to prevent the milk from souring or curdling in the stomach.

Despite spearmint's long-standing use, peppermint gained favor over it in United States pharmacopeias around the turn of the twentieth century. Spearmint was relegated to use primarily as a flavoring agent rather than a medicinal herb. It was, and still is, popular in candies, toothpaste and gum.

Some sources say spearmint's English name has a similar origin to its Latin species name, *spicata*, meaning "like a spike." The name is a reference to the plant's spire-shaped flower stalks. "Spire mint," some contend, became "spearmint." Others sources suggest that the herb was named after the St. Pierre monks, who grew "St. Pierre mint."

Research Evidence
Polycystic Ovarian Syndrome

Two studies have looked at the use of spearmint tea to decrease androgens in women with hirsutism. In one open-label trial in which women with hirsutism drank 1 cup (250 mL) of spearmint tea for five days during the follicular phase of their menstrual cycle, a significant

decrease in free testosterone was noted, along with an increase in follicle-stimulating hormone, luteinizing hormone and estradiol.

In the second trial, a 2-cup (500 mL) dosage of spearmint tea was compared to a placebo herbal tea in women with polycystic ovarian syndrome (PCOS). After one month of treatment, tests showed a substantial reduction in free and total testosterone and improved luteinizing hormone and follicle-stimulating hormone levels. In addition, the women felt that their hirsutism had improved.

More research is needed — in particular, trials that last longer than thirty days, as hirsutism is likely to take much longer to resolve. In the meantime, spearmint tea is an easy and delicious way to treat hirsutism in PCOS.

Did You Know?

Trans Women
Spearmint might also be useful for trans women, but no studies have been conducted to date.

Health Condition	Level of Scientific Evidence
Polycystic ovarian syndrome	Fair

Safety

Overall, spearmint is a safe herb, especially in normal medicinal doses. Like peppermint, spearmint can relax the lower esophageal sphincter leading into the stomach and aggravate heartburn and acid reflux in some people. Excessive use should be avoided in early pregnancy, as spearmint may act as an emmenagogue.

Further Reading

Akdoğan M, Tamer MN, Cüre E, et al. Effect of spearmint (*Mentha spicata* Labiatae) teas on androgen levels in women with hirsutism. *Phytotherapy Research*, 2007 May; 21 (5): 444–47.

Grant P. Spearmint herbal tea has significant anti-androgen effects in polycystic ovarian syndrome: A randomized controlled trial. *Phytotherapy Research*, 2010 Feb; 24 (2): 186–88.

🍃 Tea Tree Oil

Latin Name
- *Melaleuca alternifolia*

Part Used
- Essential oil made from the leaves of the tea tree

Common Combinations
- **For acne:** Green tea and calendula
- **For infectious vaginitis:** Garlic and calendula

Current Medicinal Uses

Tea tree oil is typically used as a topical antiseptic for skin infections, acne, boils, warts, ringworm, athlete's foot and other fungal and/or bacterial infections. It has also been used to treat vaginal yeast infections and other forms of infectious vaginitis.

History and Energetics

The tea tree is native to Australia and New Zealand. Aboriginals in Oceania used tea tree leaves as infusions or inhaled the volatile oils of the leaves for use in coughs and colds. The Bundjalung rubbed the leaves on cuts, bites, burns and other skin ailments to prevent infection, and they made a paste out of ground leaves that they used for wounds and as an insect repellant.

Captain James Cook, who traveled to Australia from England, named the plant tea tree, as it was the first plant he was given to drink as tea by the indigenous peoples on his initial voyage there in 1770.

Research Evidence

Acne

In a randomized, double-blind study, 5% tea tree oil gel applied topically twice daily to acne outbreaks significantly decreased the number and severity of acne lesions when compared to a placebo. A previous single-blind study found no difference in effect between 5% tea tree oil gel and benzoyl peroxide, a first-line pharmaceutical therapy. Tea tree wasn't as good at reducing oiliness but was more effective than benzoyl peroxide at reducing scaling, itchiness and dryness. With tea tree oil gel, it took longer for the positive effects to be seen, but the treatment was better tolerated and had fewer reported side effects.

Vaginitis

In vitro and pharmacological studies have shown that tea tree oil has antibacterial and antifungal properties against *Escherichia coli*, *Staphylococcus*, *Streptococcus*, *Trichomonas*, *Tinea* (fungi that cause skin infections,

including ringworm and athlete's foot), *Candida albicans* and various microorganisms associated with bacterial vaginosis. In one study of an animal model of vaginal candidiasis, tea tree oil appeared to be effective in resolving the yeast infection. Human studies are lacking, but case studies and the experiential knowledge of clinicians and herbalists suggest that diluted tea tree oil may be useful in addressing bacterial vaginosis.

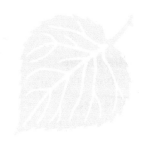

Health Condition	Level of Scientific Evidence
Acne	Good
Vaginitis	Poor

Safety

Essential oils should not be used internally, as they are extremely concentrated extracts of the volatile constituents. When used topically, they must be diluted in a carrier oil to avoid irritation and potential toxicity. Allergic hypersensitivity to tea tree oil is common. Caution is advised.

Since there are no safety studies on the use of tea tree oil during pregnancy or breastfeeding, caution or avoidance is advised.

Further Reading

Bassett IB, Pannowitz DL, Barnetson RS. A comparative study of tea-tree oil versus benzoylperoxide in the treatment of acne. *Medical Journal of Australia*, 1990 Oct 15; 153 (8): 455–58.

Blackwell AL. Tea tree oil and anaerobic (bacterial) vaginosis. *The Lancet*, 1991 Feb 2; 337 (8736): 300.

Carson CF, Hammer KA, Riley TV. *Melaleuca alternifolia* (tea tree) oil: A review of antimicrobial and other medicinal properties. *Clinical Microbiology Reviews*, 2006 Jan; 19 (1): 50–62.

Enshaieh S, Jooya A, Siadat AH, Iraji F. The efficacy of 5% topical tea tree oil gel in mild to moderate acne vulgaris: A randomized, double-blind placebo-controlled study. *Indian Journal of Dermatology, Venereology and Leprology*, 2007 Jan–Feb; 73 (1): 22–25.

Hammer KA, Carson CF, Riley TV. In vitro susceptibilities of lactobacilli and organisms associated with bacterial vaginosis to *Melaleuca alternifolia* (tea tree) oil. *Antimicrobial Agents and Chemotherapy*, 1999 Jan; 43 (1): 196.

🌿 Tribulus

Latin Name
- *Tribulus terrestris*

Parts Used
- Leaf
- Fruit

Common Combination
- For sexual dysfunction: Shatavari, rhodiola and ginseng

Current Medicinal Uses

Tribulus has been used to improve muscle mass, enhance athletic performance, increase sperm count and treat erectile dysfunction in men. More recently, it has been explored for its potential use in improving sexual function in women, particularly postpartum.

History and Energetics

Tribulus is the Latin word for "caltrop," a spiky weapon that slowed down invading forces by puncturing the feet of soldiers and their mounts. In Sanskrit, the plant is called *gokshura*, meaning "cow barb," and one of its English common names is puncture vine. All of its names provide a good reminder to avoid stepping on tribulus's hazardous seeds, which resemble thumbtacks.

Tribulus's use in improving sexual function was noted as early as 1025 CE, when Avicenna extolled its aphrodisiac qualities in his *Canon of Medicine*. It has long had a place in Unani and Ayurvedic medicine as a sexual and fertility tonic, used for spermatorrhea, low sperm count and impotence. It was also used for urinary conditions such as cystitis and urinary tract infections, as well as heart disease and gout. In traditional Chinese medicine, the fruit was used for skin lesions, chest pain and painful, swollen eyes.

Research Evidence

Research on tribulus has primarily centered on increasing muscle mass, energy, libido and sperm counts in men. As the diagnosis of female hypoactive sexual desire disorder became recognized, some researchers began to consider the potential use of tribulus in addressing sexual dysfunction in women as well.

Did You Know?

Bodybuilders

Although the fruit and root are the parts of tribulus that were traditionally used, the leaf and extracts made from the aerial parts of the plant became popular among bodybuilders and were researched for their ability to boost testosterone.

Sexual Dysfunction

A recent randomized, double-blind, placebo-controlled trial on women with hypoactive sexual desire disorder found that tribulus use brought significant improvements in overall female sexual function index, desire, arousal, lubrication, satisfaction and pain. A qualitative study of hospital records came to a similar conclusion. The researchers noted a statistically significant improvement in female sexual function index, an increase in dehydroepiandrosterone (DHEA) and decreased levels of free and total testosterone.

Health Condition	Level of Scientific Evidence
Sexual dysfunction	Fair

Safety

Some tribulus supplements have been adulterated with anabolic steroids. Caution is advised when buying tribulus (and all herbal products). It is important to source botanicals from suppliers who accurately define their products and are known to be compliant with federal agencies.

Tribulus should be avoided during pregnancy and breastfeeding, as safety has not been studied and there have been reports of toxicity when tribulus is taken during pregnancy.

Further Reading

Akhtari E, Raisi F, Keshavarz M, et al. *Tribulus terrestris* for treatment of sexual dysfunction in women: Randomized double-blind placebo-controlled study. *Daru*, 2014 Apr 28; 22: 40.

Gama CR, Lasmar R, Gama GF, et al. Clinical assessment of *Tribulus terrestris* extract in the treatment of female sexual dysfunction. *Clinical Medicine Insights: Women's Health*, 2014 Dec 22; 7: 45–50.

Turmeric

Latin Name
- *Curcuma longa*

Part Used
- Rhizome, frequently standardized to high percentages of curcumin (the main active constituent of turmeric)

Common Combinations
- For rheumatoid arthritis: Boswellia, willow and ginger
- For osteoarthritis: Boswellia and ginger

Current Medicinal Uses

Turmeric is a potent herbal anti-inflammatory, useful in a wide variety of health conditions, including arthritis, sprains, wounds, swellings, asthma, eczema, psoriasis, liver and gallbladder conditions, gastritis, inflammatory bowel disease, hemorrhoids and cancer.

In traditional Chinese medicine, turmeric is known as *jiang huang*, or yellow ginger. It is used to invigorate blood circulation and unblock stagnant qi that is causing pain, as in dysmenorrhea, abdominal pain and joint pain.

History and Energetics

Turmeric has been in use as a spice for over 4,000 years. It was noted in ancient Ayurvedic and Unani medical texts and was used in South Asian and Middle Eastern cooking. It has been compared to other valuable herbs, being called both "Indian saffron" and "yellow ginger."

Research Evidence

Breast Cancer

In vitro and in vivo studies have shown the potential of turmeric to inhibit breast cancer growth, enhance the effects of chemotherapy drugs and reduce the side effects of radiation therapy. A recent randomized, double-blind, placebo-controlled trial found that high-dose curcumin significantly reduced the severity of dermatitis in women receiving radiation therapy for breast cancer.

Endometriosis

In vivo and animal studies show that turmeric may inhibit the growth and development of endometrial tissue. Human clinical studies are needed.

Rheumatoid Arthritis and Osteoarthritis

Preclinical in vitro and animal studies support the use of turmeric in the management of rheumatoid arthritis. A small randomized study on people with rheumatoid arthritis compared curcumin to diclofenac sodium, an NSAID. The people who took turmeric experienced significant improvement in their symptoms, including reduced tenderness and swelling of their rheumatic joints.

Did You Know?

Word Origin
The name "turmeric" refers to the rich yellow color of the root and comes from the Latin words *terra merita*, meaning "meritorious earth." In Sanskrit, turmeric has over fifty names, many referring to its beautiful golden color and specific medicinal uses.

There have been several positive randomized trials on the use of curcumin for osteoarthritis, showing that it significantly improves pain, function and quality of life compared to a placebo. In one trial, curcumin was found to be just as effective as ibuprofen for reducing pain and improving mobility. Another trial showed that curcumin may decrease dependency on NSAIDs.

Health Condition	Level of Scientific Evidence
Breast cancer	Fair
Endometriosis	Poor
Osteoarthritis	Good
Rheumatoid arthritis	Fair

Safety

Turmeric should be avoided during pregnancy or if you have gallstones with a potential for bile duct obstruction.

Further Reading

Chandran B, Goel A. A randomized, pilot study to assess the efficacy and safety of curcumin in patients with active rheumatoid arthritis. *Phytotherapy Research*, 2012 Nov; 26 (11): 1719–25.

Kuptniratsaikul V, Dajpratham P, Taechaarpornkul W, et al. Efficacy and safety of *Curcuma domestica* extracts compared with ibuprofen in patients with knee osteoarthritis: A multicenter study. *Clinical Interventions in Aging*, 2014 Mar 20; 9: 451–58.

Nagaraju GP, Aliya S, Zafar SF, et al. The impact of curcumin on breast cancer. *Integrative Biology* (Cambridge), 2012 Sep; 4 (9): 996–1007.

Panahi Y, Rahimnia AR, Sharafi M, et al. Curcuminoid treatment for knee osteoarthritis: A randomized double-blind placebo-controlled trial. *Phytotherapy Research*, 2014 Nov; 28 (11): 1625–31.

Ryan JL, Heckler CE, Ling M, et al. Curcumin for radiation dermatitis: A randomized, double-blind, placebo-controlled clinical trial of thirty breast cancer patients. *Radiation Research*, 2013 Jul; 180 (1): 34–43.

Sinha D, Biswas J, Sung B, et al. Chemopreventive and chemotherapeutic potential of curcumin in breast cancer. *Current Drug Targets*, 2012 Dec; 13 (14): 1799–819.

Zhang Y, Cao H, Yu Z, et al. Curcumin inhibits endometriosis endometrial cells by reducing estradiol production. *Iranian Journal of Reproductive Medicine*, 2013 May; 11 (5): 415–22.

Uva Ursi

Latin Name
- *Arctostaphylos uva-ursi*

Part Used
- Leaf

Common Combinations
- **For acute UTIs:** Corn silk and goldenseal
- **To prevent recurrence of UTIs:** Cranberry

Current Medicinal Uses

Uva ursi is primarily used for conditions of the genitourinary tract, including urinary tract infections (UTIs), cystitis and prostatitis.

History and Energetics

Native Americans used uva ursi for a variety of conditions, including kidney and bladder infections, back pain relief and eye infections. Uva ursi berries were eaten fresh or were dried or frozen for use throughout the winter months. The leaves were often mixed with other herbs into a product called kinnikinnick, which was smoked ceremonially.

The homeopathic remedy made from uva ursi is used when there is shooting pain that travels from hip to hip, along with burning pain, during a UTI.

Research Evidence
Urinary Tract Infections

Uva ursi's active constituent for treating UTIs is arbutin, which converts to hydroquinone in the body. In the kidneys, hydroquinone acts as a potent antimicrobial that is then excreted through the urine.

In vitro and pharmacological studies support the use of uva ursi for UTIs, and a double-blind study on uva ursi and dandelion leaf reinforces these preclinical results. After one year of use to prevent recurrent bladder infections, none of the people taking uva ursi and dandelion had experienced a UTI, compared to 20% of those taking a placebo.

Health Condition	Level of Scientific Evidence
Urinary tract infections	Fair

Safety

Uva ursi is not safe during pregnancy or breastfeeding. When taken over the long term, uva ursi may irritate the gastrointestinal tract or exacerbate constipation.

Further Reading

de Arriba SG, Naser B, Nolte KU. Risk assessment of free hydroquinone derived from *Arctostaphylos uva-ursi* folium herbal preparations. *International Journal of Toxicology*, 2013 Nov–Dec; 32 (6): 442–53.

Schindler G, Patzak U, Brinkhaus B, et al. Urinary excretion and metabolism of arbutin after oral administration of *Arctostaphylos uvae ursi* extract as film-coated tablets and aqueous solution in healthy humans. *Journal of Clinical Pharmacology*, 2002 Aug; 42 (8): 920–27.

Yarnell E. Botanical medicines for the urinary tract. *World Journal of Urology*, 2002 Nov; 20 (5): 285–93.

Did You Know?

Alkalinity

Uva ursi works best in an alkaline environment. Arbutin is converted to aglycone hydroquinone in the intestines and then conjugated (bound to other compounds) in the liver. In the bladder, conjugated hydroquinone is unbound and is then free to act as an antibacterial. Studies have shown its antibacterial action to be greater in the presence of alkaline urine. If the urine isn't alkaline enough, decreasing acidic foods and supplements and increasing alkalizing foods and supplements can be helpful.

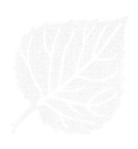

Valerian

Latin Name
- *Valeriana officinalis*

Part Used
- Root

Common Combinations
- **For dysmenorrhea:** Ginger, fennel and cramp bark
- **For insomnia:** Lavender and passionflower
- **For insomnia with depression:** St. John's wort
- **For perimenopausal sleep disturbances:** St. John's wort and passionflower

Folklore

Non-Medicinal Uses

Valerian was an ingredient in love spells and was used to create peace between people who were fighting.

Current Medicinal Uses

Valerian is typically used for insomnia related to anxiety and/or depression. It has also been used to treat gastro-intestinal and menstrual cramps. It is typically added to formulas when a little sedation is desired.

History and Energetics

Valerian has a long history of use as a sedative. It was described in ninth-century Islamic texts recording North African medicinal plants and is thought to be the plant the Greeks and Romans called *phu*, because of its unmistakable smell. The authenticity and quality of valerian was determined by the pungency of its roots.

Native North Americans used different species of valerian for stomach complaints, headaches, seizures, menstrual complaints, colds and tuberculosis, to relieve pain and as a sedative.

Research Evidence

Dysmenorrhea

Preliminary research supports the use of valerian for menstrual cramps. One randomized, placebo-controlled trial of 100 university students with primary dysmenorrhea (where no cause for the pain can be found) found that valerian significantly decreased both the severity and the duration of the pain. The quantity of non-steroidal anti-inflammatory drugs (NSAIDs) used to manage pain also decreased significantly among the women taking valerian.

A second study found that valerian was as effective as the drug mefenamic acid in its ability to decrease pain associated with primary dysmenorrhea.

Insomnia in Menopause

Overall, reviews on the efficacy of valerian for insomnia are generally positive. Several clinical reviews have concluded that valerian improves subjective quality of sleep, as well as the time it takes to fall asleep. A study looking specifically at the impact of valerian on sleep quality in postmenopausal women found a significant improvement in sleep quality with valerian. Thirty percent of the women who took valerian reported improvements in sleep quality, compared with 4% of the women who took a placebo.

A trial that used a combination herbal product containing valerian and lemon balm found that the herbs significantly improved sleep quality in postmenopausal women. In this trial, 36% of women taking the herbs noted improvements in their sleep, compared with only 8% of those taking a placebo.

Health Condition	Level of Scientific Evidence
Dysmenorrhea	Fair
Insomnia in menopause	Fair

Safety

Overall, valerian is a relatively safe herb with limited side effects. The simultaneous use of valerian with benzo-diazepines or other sedative or antianxiety medications may increase both the therapeutic effects and the side effects of the pharmaceutical.

Valerian should be avoided during pregnancy and breastfeeding.

Further Reading

Fernández-San-Martín MI, Masa-Font R, Palacios-Soler L, et al. Effectiveness of valerian on insomnia: A meta-analysis of randomized placebo-controlled trials. *Sleep Medicine*, 2010 Jun; 11 (6): 505–11.

Mirabi P, Alamolhoda SH, Esmaeilzadeh S, Mojab F. Effect of medicinal herbs on primary dysmenorrhoea — A systematic review. *Iranian Journal of Pharmaceutical Research*, 2014 Summer; 13 (3): 757–67.

Mirabi P, Dolatian M, Mojab F, Majd HA. Effects of valerian on the severity and systemic manifestations of dysmenorrhea. *International Journal of Gynaecology and Obstetrics*, 2011 Dec; 115 (3): 285–88.

Salter S, Brownie S. Treating primary insomnia — The efficacy of valerian and hops. *Australian Family Physician*, 2010 Jun; 39 (6): 433–37.

Taavoni S, Ekbatani N, Kashaniyan M, Haghani H. Effect of valerian on sleep quality in postmenopausal women: A randomized placebo-controlled clinical trial. *Menopause*, 2011 Sep; 18 (9): 951–55.

Taavoni S, Nazem Ekbatani N, Haghani H. Valerian/lemon balm use for sleep disorders during menopause. *Complementary Therapies in Clinical Practice*, 2013 Nov; 19 (4): 193–96.

Wild Yam

Latin Names
- *Dioscorea villosa* (wild yam)
- *Dioscorea opposita* (Chinese yam)

Parts Used
- Root
- Rhizome

Common Combinations
- **For intestinal colic:** Ginger and chamomile
- **For menstrual cramps:** Cramp bark, fennel and ginger

Current Medicinal Uses

Wild yam is used as an antispasmodic, especially in cases of colic, menstrual cramps and ovarian pain, and to relieve the pain of gallstones.

Chinese yam, or *shan yao*, is used in traditional Chinese medicine as a qi tonic for the treatment of fatigue, sweating, poor appetite, chronic cough and frequent urination.

History and Energetics

Wild yam was used by the Aztecs and Maya for pain relief during pregnancy and labor and for menstrual cramps and rheumatism. It was also used as an antispasmodic to prevent early miscarriage and for intestinal colic and cramping pains in the abdomen. Wild yam's use for treating pelvic and intestinal spasms may be responsible for one of its alternative names, colic root.

Research Evidence

Dysmenorrhea

There are no human clinical studies to evaluate the effectiveness of wild yam as an antispasmodic or pain reliever. Animal studies, however, suggest that wild yam provides pain relief for inflammation or nerve-related pain.

In vitro studies indicate that Chinese yam, *Dioscorea opposita*, contains antioxidants useful in treating fertility, as well as other compounds that can inhibit cyclooxygenases, a common action of non-narcotic anti-inflammatories and painkillers. More research is needed.

Health Condition	Level of Scientific Evidence
Dysmenorrhea	Poor

Safety

Wild yam is best avoided in cases of intestinal spasm, gallbladder inflammation, potential bile duct obstruction or liver disease without the supervision of a licensed health-care professional.

Further Reading

Ju Y, Xue Y, Huang J, et al. Antioxidant Chinese yam polysaccharides and its pro-proliferative effect on endometrial epithelial cells. *International Journal of Biological Macromolecules*, 2014 May; 66: 81–85.

Lima CM, Lima AK, Melo MG, et al. Bioassay-guided evaluation of *Dioscorea villosa* — An acute and subchronic toxicity, antinociceptive and anti-inflammatory approach. *BMC Complementary and Alternative Medicine*, 2013 Jul 28; 13: 195.

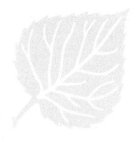

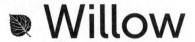 Willow

Latin Names
- *Salix alba*
  (white willow)
- *Salix nigra*
  (black willow)

Part Used
- Bark

Common Combination
- **For arthritis:**
  Ginger, turmeric
  and boswellia

Current Medicinal Uses

Willow is primarily used as an anti-inflammatory and analgesic for muscle and joint pain. It has also been used for fevers, diarrhea and sore throat.

History and Energetics

Willow has been used since at least the Ancient Egyptian era and was well known throughout different cultures for its benefits in alleviating pain and fever. Native North Americans used willow as an analgesic, as did Hippocrates, who wrote about the herbal remedy in the fifth century BCE.

Willow bends easily without breaking, and as a medicinal herb, it imparts this flexibility in strength. Taken internally, willow increases flexibility in once painful, rigid, achy joints. It enhances our physical and emotional pliability and adaptability, without causing us to lose our sense of our authentic identity. In Taoism, willow represents the concept of strength in weakness.

The flower essence of willow is used when someone is stuck in self-pity, feeling bitter and resentful. It helps to restore optimism, playfulness and resilience of spirit.

Willow in any form is an excellent treatment when physical pain is accompanied by, or is a manifestation of, difficulty finding flexibility and optimism in life. Willow works best when someone's thinking is as rigid and stiff as their muscles and joints.

Research Evidence
Osteoarthritis and Rheumatoid Arthritis

In people with osteoarthritis, willow bark has been shown to significantly reduce pain scores compared to a placebo in several randomized, controlled human trials. A systematic review on the use of willow for musculoskeletal pain in general similarly concluded that willow reduces pain scores compared to a placebo.

In a small study specifically studying the use of willow for rheumatoid arthritis, the herb did reduce pain more than a placebo, but the difference was not considered statistically significant. Preclinical trials support the use of willow bark for pain relief in musculoskeletal conditions such as rheumatoid arthritis. More research is needed.

Health Condition	Level of Scientific Evidence
Osteoarthritis	Good
Rheumatoid arthritis	Poor

Safety

Willow should be avoided by people who have a known allergy to salicylates or a genetic glucose-6-phosphate dehydrogenase (G6PD) deficiency. Willow bark may have additive effects with salicylate drugs and should be avoided by those taking warfarin, as the combination may increase bleeding. Safety during pregnancy or breastfeeding has not been established.

Further Reading

Biegert C, Wagner I, Lüdtke R, et al. Efficacy and safety of willow bark extract in the treatment of osteoarthritis and rheumatoid arthritis: Results of 2 randomized double-blind controlled trials. *Journal of Rheumatology*, 2004 Nov; 31 (11): 2121–30.

Schmid B, Lüdtke R, Selbmann HK, et al. Efficacy and tolerability of a standardized willow bark extract in patients with osteoarthritis: Randomized placebo-controlled, double blind clinical trial. *Phytotherapy Research*, 2001 Jun; 15 (4): 344–50.

Uehleke B, Müller J, Stange R, et al. Willow bark extract STW 33-I in the long-term treatment of outpatients with rheumatic pain mainly osteoarthritis or back pain. *Phytomedicine*, 2013 Aug 15; 20 (11): 980–84.

Vlachojannis JE, Cameron M, Chrubasik S. A systematic review on the effectiveness of willow bark for musculoskeletal pain. *Phytotherapy Research*, 2009 Jul; 23 (7): 897–900.

🌿 Witch Hazel

Latin Name
- *Hamamelis virginiana*

Parts Used
- Bark
- Leaf

Common Combination
- For varicose veins and hemorrhoids: Gingko and horse chestnut

Current Medicinal Uses

Witch hazel is a great astringent, used to stop the flow of blood externally but also to treat weakness in the blood vessels, as with hemorrhoids and varicose veins, both of which are frequently experienced during pregnancy or postpartum.

History and Energetics

Witch hazel is a rather unusual shrub, with flowers that bloom in the winter, unlike most plants in North America. The Cherokee, Osage, Iroquois and Chippewa used it to treat sores, scratches and skin ulcers. The Iroquois also used it to prevent hemorrhage after childbirth and to prevent bleeding and miscarriage in pregnant women who had fallen or been hurt. Other Native American uses included treatment for sore throat, colds, sore muscles, diarrhea, tuberculosis and painful menses.

Witch hazel may have gotten its name from the historical use of Y-shaped witch hazel twigs in dowsing, an ancient method of divining for water underground. The "witch" part of the name does not imply that the herb was often used by witches, but rather it comes from the Old English word *wych*, referring to the pliability of the branches. The "hazel" part likely arose because the common hazel (*Corylus* species) was also used for dowsing in Europe.

Witch hazel's ability to find fluids underground is akin to its ability to find unhealthy seepage of blood and fluids within the body. Therapeutically, witch hazel astringes unnecessary or excess fluids, such as those found in hemorrhoids, varicose veins, bruises, diarrhea, weeping wounds and leukorrhea (vaginal discharge). Eclectic herbalists used witch hazel specifically for passive hemorrhages — cases where blood or another fluid slowly leaks, much like the elusive underground springs sought by dowsers.

Research Evidence

Hemorrhoids and Varicose Veins

Research on witch hazel's use in hemorrhoids and varicose veins is limited. It has been shown in laboratory studies to inhibit the enzymes that degrade the integrity of veins and connective tissue in both conditions. Pharmacological studies also demonstrate astringent, vasoconstrictive and anti-inflammatory properties, supported by the presence of tannins and proanthocyanidins in witch hazel's chemistry.

Health Condition	Level of Scientific Evidence
Hemorrhoids	Poor
Varicose veins	Poor

Safety

Witch hazel is generally considered safe when used topically. It may cause skin irritation in some people. Internally, witch hazel is not recommended during pregnancy or breast-feeding, since there is insufficient research.

Further Reading

Abascal K, Yarnell E. Botanical treatments for hemorrhoids. *Alternative and Complementary Therapies*, 2005 Dec; 11 (6): 285–89.

Hughes-Formella BJ, Filbry A, Gassmueller J, Rippke F. Anti-inflammatory efficacy of topical preparations with 10% *Hamamelis* distillate in a UV erythema test. *Skin Pharmacology and Applied Skin Physiology*, 2002 Mar–Apr; 15 (2): 125–32.

MacKay D. Hemorrhoids and varicose veins: A review of treatment options. *Alternative Medicine Review*, 2001 Apr; 6 (2): 126–40.

Did You Know?

Commercial Preparations

Witch hazel alcohol extract or tincture, standardized to at least 5% tannins, is approved for internal and external use for treating hemorrhoids in Europe.

Unfortunately, the clear steam distillate of witch hazel found on pharmacy shelves in North America contains virtually no tannins and is therefore devoid of most of the plant's astringent healing power. Look for witch hazel tinctures or ask a naturopathic doctor or herbalist.

🌿 Yarrow

Latin Name
- *Achillea millefolium* (yarrow)
- *Achillea biebersteinii* Afan. (yellow marabou)

Parts Used
- Aerial parts (everything above the ground)

Common Combinations
- **For menorrhagia, endometriosis or fibroids:** Geranium and shepherd's purse
- **For endometriosis:** Trillium, cinnamon and dang gui
- **For hemorrhoids and varicose veins:** Horse chestnut and witch hazel

Current Medicinal Uses

Yarrow is used to control the proper movement of blood, either to encourage its flow or to stop excessive bleeding, as needed. It reduces excess menstrual blood in menorrhagia, fibroids and endometriosis and helps bring on menstruation when it is late. Externally, yarrow is used to treat hemorrhoids and varicose veins and to staunch bleeding from cuts.

History and Energetics

Native North Americans used yarrow primarily to cool the blood during fever, to relieve a headache by encouraging a nosebleed and, topically, as a poultice to heal cuts, burns and boils. The Blackfoot and Cherokee used yarrow to treat excessive menstrual flow and to help expel the placenta after delivery.

As a flower essence, yarrow protects the user from toxic energetic influences, helping those who are sensitive and vulnerable to outside influences to create a boundary from within. Yarrow flower essence is often used for children with hyperactivity disorders or autistic tendencies, as well as for health-care workers who feel overly affected by the energy of their clients. It provides a protective boundary to stop the "bleeding" of one's personal energy into the external environment.

Research Evidence

Preliminary animal studies show that yarrow protects the gastrointestinal system from the development of ulcers and helps heal stomach and intestinal linings when ulcers already exist. Other studies have demonstrated yarrow's wound-healing effects on the surface of the skin. These studies support the traditional use of yarrow to heal wounds and cuts and to staunch internal bleeding in smooth muscle tissues, such as the stomach.

Amenorrhea/Oligomenorrhea

Although yarrow has traditionally been used to bring on menses and is contraindicated in pregnancy due to its emmenagogue effect, no clinical research currently exists to confirm this use.

Endometriosis

An experimental animal model showed that a related species called yellow marabou (*Achillea biebersteinii* Afan.), traditionally used in Turkey and Iran, significantly decreased the size of endometrial lesions in the abdomen, as well as adhesions associated with endometriosis, when compared to a placebo in one study. More research is needed to confirm these results.

Fibroids

Unfortunately, no scientific research has been conducted on yarrow specifically with respect to the treatment of fibroids.

Hemorrhoids

Clinical trials on the use of yarrow in hemorrhoids are lacking. However, preclinical evidence supports yarrow's ability to heal wounds and astringe hemorrhages and ulcerations in other types of tissue. More research is needed.

High Blood Pressure

In several different studies, yarrow significantly reduced blood pressure in animal models. According to some researchers, yarrow may act in a similar manner to a common class of drugs used for high blood pressure called · ACE inhibitors (angiotensin-converting enzyme inhibitors).

Menorrhagia

Unfortunately, no studies have investigated the use of yarrow in the treatment of menorrhagia, despite a long history of traditional use for this purpose.

Did You Know?

Hops Replacement
Yarrow can be used instead of hops in the making of beer.

Health Condition	Level of Scientific Evidence
Amenorrhea/ oligomenorrhea	Poor
Endometriosis	Poor
Fibroids	Poor
Hemorrhoids	Poor
High blood pressure	Poor
Menorrhagia	Poor

Safety

Yarrow may cause an allergic reaction in people sensitive to other plants in the Asteraceae family. As it may have emmenagogue effects, yarrow should be avoided in pregnancy.

Further Reading

Demirel MA, Suntar I, Ilhan M, et al. Experimental endometriosis remission in rats treated with *Achillea biebersteinii* Afan.: Histopathological evaluation and determination of cytokine levels. *European Journal of Obstetrics, Gynecology, and Reproductive Biology*, 2014 Apr; 175: 172–77.

de Souza P, Gasparotto A Jr, Crestani S, et al. Hypotensive mechanism of the extracts and artemetin isolated from *Achillea millefolium* L. (Asteraceae) in rats. *Phytomedicine*, 2011 Jul 15; 18 (10): 819–25.

Khan AU, Gilani AH. Blood pressure lowering, cardiovascular inhibitory and bronchodilatory actions of *Achillea millefolium*. *Phytotherapy Research*, 2011 Apr; 25 (4): 577–83.

Potrich FB, Allemand A, da Silva LM, et al. Antiulcerogenic activity of hydroalcoholic extract of *Achillea millefolium* L.: Involvement of the antioxidant system. *Journal of Ethnopharmacology*, 2010 Jul 6; 130 (1): 85–92.

Saeidnia S, Gohari A, Mokhber-Dezfuli N, Kiuchi F. A review on phytochemistry and medicinal properties of the genus *Achillea*. *Daru*, 2011; 19 (3): 173–86.

Glossary

adaptogen: A medicine that helps the body adapt to new or stressful situations by building resistance to stress, reducing the stress response and increasing endurance.

allopathic medicine: The system of medicine practiced by medical doctors (MDs), also called conventional or mainstream medicine. Allopathic medicine uses therapies that produce effects different from those of the disease being treated. The term "allopathic medicine" was coined by Samuel Hahnemann, widely regarded as the father of homeopathy.

alterative: A medicine that restores overall function, detoxifies and eliminates waste.

analgesic: A medicine that relives pain.

antibodies: Proteins produced and circulated in the body in response to antigens (bacteria, viruses or other foreign substances) as part of the immune system response.

antihemorrhagic: A medicine that stops bleeding.

anti-inflammatory: A medicine that reduces inflammation locally and/or systemically.

antimicrobial: A medicine that supports innate immune responses and is active against bacteria, viruses, fungi and protozoa.

antipyretic: A medicine that prevents or allays fever.

antispasmodic: A medicine that reduces pain caused by smooth and/or skeletal muscle spasm.

antirheumatic: A medicine that alleviates rheumatism and other conditions characterized by pain and stiffness.

aphrodisiac: A medicine that increases sexual arousal.

astringent: A medicine that constricts and tones tissues and mucous membranes and stops bleeding.

Ayurvedic medicine: The traditional Hindu system of medicine, which originated in India and was based on Vedic texts. Therapies used in Ayurvedic medicine include botanical medicine, diet, exercise, yoga, meditation, mineral supplementation and surgical techniques.

autoimmunity: A condition in which the body produces antibodies in response to normal tissues rather than to foreign substances.

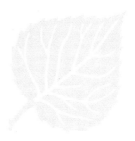

bitter: A medicine that increases digestive secretions, increases appetite and awakens metabolism and consciousness.

bioindividualism: A principle that recognizes the unique biological needs, preferences, challenges and responses of individual people.

botanical medicine: A form of medicine that uses plants and plant preparations as therapeutic agents to prevent or treat disease.

cardioactive: A medicine that stimulates or regulates the heart.

cardiotonic: A medicine that tonifies the heart and cardiovascular system.

cardiovascular system: The body system, also known as the circulatory system, that delivers blood, oxygen and nutrients to the body's tissues.

carminative: A medicine that soothes and relaxes the digestive tract and relieves intestinal gas.

choleretic: A medicine that stimulates the production of bile in the liver.

cholagogue: A medicine that encourages the release of bile from the gallbladder into the intestines to help digest food, especially fats.

clinical trial: A prospective research study on human subjects designed to test whether a strategy, treatment or device is safe and/or effective for preventing, treating or managing a health condition.

cohort study: A type of clinical trial that is designed as an observational study. One group of people who have taken or been exposed to a certain variable is compared to another group of people who are similar overall except for the variable being studied. Cohort studies are often used to evaluate risk factors for disease.

counterirritant: A medicine that activates nerve cells in the skin to alter the perception of pain.

demulcent: A medicine that coats, soothes and protects mucous membranes.

diaphoretic: A medicine that promotes perspiration.

diuretic: A medicine that increases urinary excretion.

double-blind: A study methodology in which neither the researchers nor the participants know whether the participants are in the test group or the control group.

Eclecticism: A system of medicine popular in the United States in the late nineteenth century and first half of the twentieth century. Eclecticism mostly used botanical treatments but also incorporated other substances and physical therapy practices.

edema: Swelling; excess watery fluid trapped in one or more cavities or tissues of the body.

energetics: Subtle properties, or attributes, of herbs, food and other substances. Depending on the medical tradition (e.g., Native American, Ayurvedic, Chinese), energetics may include elements, tastes, digestive effects, humors, doshas, heating/cooling effects, mental-emotional effects and other, non-physical effects.

escharotic: A corrosive or caustic substance capable of producing a scab or slough to shed dead tissue.

flower essence therapy: A therapy in which remedies made from the flowering parts of plants are used to address emotional or mental aspects of health.

galactagogue: A medicine that increases breast milk production.

hemostatic: A medicine that stops bleeding.

hepatic: A medicine that promotes better liver and gallbladder function and/or detoxification through the liver.

homeopathy: A system of medicine that treats a disease by using diluted doses of a remedy that would, in healthy people, produce the same symptoms as those of the disease.

hypnotic: A medicine that promotes sleep.

hypotensive: A medicine that decreases blood pressure.

indication: A symptom or condition that points out the advisability or suitability of using a specific remedy or other treatment.

laxative: A medicine that promotes bowel activity and movement.

lymph: The fluid that collects and removes the waste products that accumulate around cells and puts them back into circulation in the blood, to be metabolized and excreted as necessary.

materia medica: Remedies or substances used in medicine, or a book detailing those remedies.

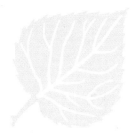

meta-analysis: A statistical method of combining the results of multiple independent studies on the same subject to identify the relationships between the studies (similar effects, opposing effects) and to test for statistical significance, a marker of effectiveness or the validity of the results.

naturopathic medicine: A system of primary health care that blends modern scientific and traditional knowledge to encourage people's inherent self-healing process, treat the underlying causes of disease and emphasize prevention and optimal health. It includes the following therapies, with some variability among legislative jurisdictions: nutrition, botanical medicine, homeopathy, lifestyle counseling, physical medicine, acupuncture, minor surgery, pharmaceuticals and intravenous or injection therapy.

nervine: A medicine that affects the nervous system by relaxing, stimulating, tonifying, combating depression or sedating.

nutritive: A medicine that provides nourishment or nutrients.

open-label: A non-blinded study design in which both researchers and participants know whether they are receiving the treatment or the control/placebo.

parasympathetic nervous system: Also called the "rest and digest" system; the part of the autonomic nervous system that works in opposition to the sympathetic nervous system, slowing down breathing and heart rates and increasing activity in the gastrointestinal system. (*See also* sympathetic nervous system.)

pharmaceutical: Of or relating to a medicinal drug (*adj.*); a medicinal drug (*noun*).

pharmacognosy: A branch of pharmacology that studies medicinal substances obtained from plants and other substances of biological origin.

pharmacopoeia: A book describing drugs and medicinal preparations.

physiomedicalism: A system of herbal medicine that originated as an offshoot from Thomsonian herbalism in the United States. Physiomedicalists believed in the ability of non-toxic herbs to influence broad physiological patterns in the body.

phytochemistry: The chemistry of plants.

phytoestrogen: An estrogen-like compound that occurs naturally in some plants.

phytopharmacology: The study of medicinal substances obtained from plants and their pharmacological action in the human body.

phytotherapy: The use of plants and plant products in medicine.

pilot study: A small-scale preliminary study to evaluate the feasibility, effect size and study methodology of a larger-scale trial.

placebo-controlled: A study methodology in which the control group is given a placebo — an inert treatment that has no inherent physical effect but may have a psychological effect that leads to a physical response.

proximate: Closely related.

randomized controlled trial (RCT): A study in which participants are divided at random into either the experimental or the control group.

renal: Of, or related to, the kidney.

rubefacient: An action or substance that creates redness of the skin by dilating capillaries near the skin's surface.

stagnation: A state of having stopped, ceased to flow, become sluggish or failed to progress. In traditional Chinese medicine, stagnation, or stasis, may be part of a diagnostic pattern (liver qi stagnation, blood stagnation, phlegm stagnation).

sympathetic nervous system: Also called the "fight or flight" system; the part of the autonomic nervous system that is activated under stress, working in opposition to the parasympathetic nervous system. It increases breathing and heart rates, dilates pupils, increases circulation to skeletal muscles and releases glucose into the bloodstream. (*See also* parasympathetic nervous system.)

synergistic: Of, or relating to, the interaction of elements that, when combined, create a total effect that is greater than the sum of the individual elements.

tonic: A medicine that strengthens an organ or a person's overall vitality.

tonifying: Nourishing, replenishing, strengthening or adding tone to something.

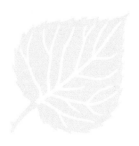

traditional Chinese medicine: A system of medicine that originated in China and is still widely practiced today. Based on the principles of yin and yang, it includes therapies such as herbal medicine, diet, acupuncture, massage (*tui na*) and exercise (*qi gong*).

vasodilating: Widening the diameter of blood vessels.

vis medicatrix naturae: A concept attributed to Hippocrates, literally translated as "the healing power of nature." The phrase has been used to denote both the inherent ability of organisms to heal themselves and the healing powers present within the natural external environment.

vitalism: A doctrine that states that the functions of a living organism are in some part self-determining, not explainable by physiochemical forces alone.

vulnerary: A medicine that heals wounds and skin tissue when used topically.

Resources

Books

Blumenthal M. *The ABC Clinical Guide to Herbs*. Austin, TX: American Botanical Council, 2003.

Bone K, Mills S. *Principles and Practices of Phytotherapy*, 2nd edition. London: Churchill Livingston, 2012.

Boon H, Smith M. *55 Most Common Medicinal Herbs*, 2nd edition. Toronto: Robert Rose, 2009.

Godfrey A, Saunders P, Barlow K, Gilbert C, Gowan M. *Principles and Practices of Naturopathic Botanical Medicine*. Toronto: CCNM Press, 2012.

Herbal Medicines, 4th edition. London: Pharmaceutical Press, 2013.

Hoffmann D. *Medical Herbalism: The Science and Practice of Herbal Medicine*. Rochester, VT: Healing Arts Press, 2003.

PDR for Herbal Medicines, 4th edition. Montvale, NJ: Thomson Healthcare, 2007.

Wichtl M, ed. *Herbal Drugs and Phytopharmaceuticals: A Handbook for Practice on a Scientific Basis*, 3rd edition. Lyttelton, NZ: Medpharm, 2004.

Websites

Educational Resources

American Association of Naturopathic Physicians: www.naturopathic.org

American Botanical Council: abc.herbalgram.org

American Herbalists Guild: www.americanherbalistsguild.com

Canadian Association of Naturopathic Doctors: www.cand.ca

Flora Delaterre: The Plant Detective: www.floradelaterre.com

Henriette's Herbal Homepage: www.henriettes-herb.com

Herb Research Foundation: www.herbs.org

Longwood Herbal Task Force: www.longwoodherbal.org

Southern Cross University, Medicinal Plant Monographs: scu.edu.au/scps/index.php/106

Herbalists and Schools

East West School of Planetary Herbology: www.planetherbs.com

Learning Herbs: learningherbs.com

North American Institute of Medical Herbalism: naimh.com

Sage Mountain: www.sagemountain.com

Susun Weed: susunweed.com

Traditional Roots Institute, National College of Natural Medicine: traditionalroots.org

Wild Rose College of Natural Healing: wrc.net

Herbal Companies

Frontier Co-op: www.frontiercoop.com
Gaia Herbs: www.gaiaherbs.com
Herb Pharm: www.herb-pharm.com
MediHerb: www.mediherb.com
Mountain Rose Herbs: www.mountainroseherbs.com
St. Francis Herb Farm: www.stfrancisherbfarm.com
Wise Woman Herbals: www.wisewomanherbals.com

Herbal Magazines

The Essential Herbal: www.essentialherbal.com
The Herb Quarterly: www.herbquarterly.com
Mother Earth Living: www.motherearthliving.com
Plant Healer Magazine: planthealermagazine.com

Herbs on Film

Herbal Aide: www.cultureunplugged.com/documentary/watch-online/play/12336/Herbal-Aide
Numen: The Healing Power of Plants: www.numenfilm.com

Conservation and Sustainability

Conservation International: www.conservation.org
The Nature Conservancy: www.nature.org
Plant Conservation Alliance: www.nps.gov/plants
Traffic: The Wildlife Trade Monitoring Network: www.traffic.org
United Plant Savers: www.unitedplantsavers.org

Women's Health

Aviva Romm, MD: avivaromm.com
Canadian Foundation for Women's Health: www.cfwh.org
Canadian Women's Health Network: www.cwhn.ca
Center for Young Women's Health: youngwomenshealth.org
Institute of Women's Health & Integrative Medicine: instituteofwomenshealth.com
National Network on Environments and Women's Health: www.nnewh.org
Tieraona Low Dog, MD: www.drlowdog.com
Dr. Tori Hudson, ND: drtorihudson.com
Women's Healthy Environments Network: www.womenshealthyenvironments.ca
Womenshealth.gov: www.womenshealth.gov

Library and Archives Canada Cataloguing in Publication

Gilbert, Cyndi, author
   The essential guide to women's herbal medicine / Cyndi Gilbert, ND.

Includes index.
ISBN 978-0-7788-0506-9 (pbk.)

   1. Herbs—Therapeutic use. 2. Women—Health and hygiene. 3. Women—
Diseases—Alternative treatment. I. Title.

RM666.H33G55 2015   615.3'21082   C2015-901697-5

Index

A

absinthe, 257
acne, 9, 43–46
  barberry, 44, 207
  calendula, 45, 220
  green tea, 45, 277
  tea tree oil, 44, 344
acyclovir, 105, 106, 313, 328
adaptogens, 41, 116, 124,
  182, 364
  varying use of, 188, 252
ADHD, 306
Advil. *See* ibuprofen
alfalfa, 125, 126, 146, 325
alginates, 157, 333
aloe vera, 31, 182, 201, 220
alteratives, 24, 41, 317, 364
amenorrhea, 10, 130–34
  black cohosh, 97, 120,
    132, 213, 228
  chaste tree, 228
  dang gui, 49, 131, 141,
    244
  licorice, 295
  motherwort, 301
  PCOS and, 148, 149, 295
  peony, 308–9
  red clover, 318
  saffron, 323
  yarrow, 360
American Medical
  Association, 27
amla, 61, 204
analgesics, 41, 356, 364.
  See also NSAIDs
androgens
  excessive, 149, 295,
    296–97
  increasing, 182
  reducing, 151–52, 279,
    342–43

andrographis, 102
anemia, 9, 47–50
  dandelion, 49, 241
  dang gui, 49, 244
  nettle, 48, 304
antiandrogens. *See*
  androgens, reducing
antibodies, 364
antidepressants (herbal),
  124. *See also*
  depression
antihemorrhagics, 41, 263,
  364
anti-inflammatories, 41,
  60, 266, 295, 348,
  356, 364
antimicrobials, 41, 193,
  263–64, 344–45, 351,
  364. *See also* antivirals
antioxidants, 83, 85,
  284, 330, 354. *See
  also* flavonoids;
  polyphenols;
  proanthocyanidins
antipyretics, 364
antirheumatics, 364
antispasmodics, 41, 136,
  237, 288, 364
antivirals, 294, 295, 296,
  328
anxiety, 9, 51–57. *See also*
  depression
  Anxiety-Relieving Tea,
    54
  ashwagandha, 204
  chamomile, 53, 226, 227
  hawthorn, 285
  kava, 53–55, 288–89
  lavender, 52–53, 79,
    291–92
  lemon balm, 55, 102,
    293

  motherwort, 112, 301,
    325
  passionflower, 56, 306
  red clover, 318
  teas for, 32, 54
  valerian, 127, 128, 136,
    352
aphrodisiacs, 41, 182, 323,
  331, 364
arbutin, 351
arbutoside, 194
aromatherapy oils
  lavender, 52, 292
  peppermint, 167,
    310–11
arthritis (rheumatoid),
  9, 63–67. *See also*
  osteoarthritis
  boswellia, 218–19
  evening primrose,
    63–64, 253, 254
  ginger, 64, 266–67
  turmeric, 65, 348–49
  willow, 66, 356
ashwagandha (*Withania
  somnifera*), 12, 203–5
  chemotherapy side
    effects, 69, 204
  hypothyroidism, 116,
    204
  stress, 188–89, 204
aspen, 66
Asteraceae family, 25, 217,
  221, 227, 300, 362
astragalus, 243
astringents, 41, 124, 159,
  170, 173, 199, 364
atractylodes, 176
autoimmunity, 63, 248,
  364
Avicenna (Ibn Sina), 19,
  20, 293, 295, 346

mint. *See* peppermint; spearmint

morning sickness, 11, 166–68, 266, 311

motherwort (*Leonarus cardiaca*), 15, 112, 301–2

mu dan pi (*Paeonia suffruticosa*), 308

muira puama, 183, 270

N

Namibia, 61, 246

Native American medicine, 23
  black cohosh, 212
  cramp bark, 237
  geranium, 263
  goldenseal, 274
  nettle, 195, 303
  raspberry, 315
  red clover, 124, 317
  sage, 325
  slippery elm, 337
  uva ursi, 350
  valerian, 352
  willow, 356
  witch hazel, 171, 358
  yarrow, 161, 360

naturopathic medicine, 21, 27–28, 29, 32, 367

nausea and vomiting, 70, 310–11. *See also* chemotherapy
  peppermint, 167, 310–11
  in pregnancy, 11, 166–68, 266, 311

nervines, 41, 53, 173, 188, 367. *See also* anxiety

nervous system, 367, 368

nettle (*Urtica dioica*), 15, 195, 303–5
  anemia, 48, 304
  low milk supply, 164–65, 304

Nettle Tea, 48

nutritive qualities, 146, 164–65, 304

osteoarthritis, 61–62, 304

urinary tract infections, 194, 304

nightshade family (Solanaceae), 24, 205, 224

NSAIDs (non-steroidal anti-inflammatory drugs), 38, 247. *See also specific drugs*

nutritives, 147, 317, 319, 332, 367. *See also* nettle

O

obesity, 82, 148, 186, 279, 282. *See also* metabolic syndrome

obsessive-compulsive disorder (OCD). *See* anxiety

oils
  aromatherapy, 52, 167, 292, 310–11
  essential, 201, 345
  infused, 34, 36
  for sexual activity, 182–83

ointments, 34, 36
  Cayenne Pain-Relief Balm, 59

oligomenorrhea, 10, 130–33
  black cohosh, 132, 213
  chaste tree, 132, 228
  dang gui, 131, 244
  licorice, 132, 295
  peony, 132, 295, 308
  red clover, 133, 318
  yarrow, 133, 360

Open Heart Tea, 111

oregano, 248

Oregon grape (*Mahonia aquifolium*). *See* berberine

osteoarthritis, 9, 58–62
  boswellia, 61, 218–19
  cayenne pepper, 58–60, 224
  dandelion, 60
  devil's claw, 61, 247
  ginger, 60
  nettle, 61–62, 304
  peppermint, 59
  turmeric, 60, 349
  willow, 356
  wintergreen, 60

osteopenia, 144

osteoporosis, 10, 144–47
  black cohosh, 146, 214
  milk thistle, 146, 300
  red clover, 146–47, 319
  soy, 145, 340

oxazepam, 306

P

Pain-Relief Balm, Cayenne, 59

panic disorder. *See* anxiety

Paracelsus, 21, 293

passionflower (*Passiflora incarnata*), 15, 306–7
  anxiety, 54, 56, 306

PCOS (polycystic ovarian syndrome), 11, 148–53
  and amenorrhea, 148, 149, 295
  barberry/berberine, 44, 150, 210
  chaste tree, 150, 229
  cinnamon, 149, 233, 309
  green tea, 151, 279
  licorice, 151, 296–97
  peony, 296–97, 308–9

St. John's wort (*continued*)
  depression, 78, 289, 327–28
  genital warts, 102, 328
  herpes, 105, 328
  menopause, 125–26, 328
  premenstrual syndrome, 177–78, 325
salicylates, 60, 357. *See also* willow
salves, 34, 36
  Cayenne Pain-Relief Balm, 59
Sankaran, Rajan, 24–25
sargassum (*Sargassum* spp.), 332. *See also* seaweed
saw palmetto, 303
schisandra (*Schisandra chinensis*), 15, 189–90, 330–31
Scudder, John, 26
seaweed, 16, 117, 332–33
self-image, 43, 45, 51, 103, 122, 130
sesame oil, 34
sexual activity, 182–83, 192
sexual dysfunction, 11, 180–85
  ashwagandha, 204–5
  dang gui, 182, 244
  evening primrose, 182–83, 254
  gingko, 183, 270, 272
  ginseng, 181–82, 270, 272
  shatavari, 183, 335
  tribulus, 183–84, 347
shan yao (Chinese yam), 354
shao yao. *See* peony
shatavari (*Asparagus racemosus*), 16, 165, 183, 334–35
shen jiang. *See* ginger
Shen Nong, 18, 70, 276

shepherd's purse (*Capsella bursa-pastoris*), 16, 141–42, 336
Siberian ginseng. *See* eleuthero
sildenafil (Viagra), 182, 273
sleep, 127, 306. *See also* insomnia
slippery elm (*Ulmus fulva*), 16, 156, 337–38
smudging, 125, 325
social phobia. *See* anxiety
Solanaceae (nightshade) family, 24, 205, 224
soy (*Glycine max*), 16, 339–41
  breast cancer, 68–69, 340
  menopause, 126, 340
  osteoporosis, 145, 340
spearmint (*Mentha spicata*), 16, 151–52, 342–43
spironolactone, 151, 297
SSRIs (selective serotonin reuptake inhibitors), 79, 323
stagnation, 368
  of blood, 97, 113, 141, 161–62
  of food, 110–11
  of liver qi, 176
Staphylococcus aureus, 194, 344
Steiner, Rudolph, 303
Streptococcus, 344
stress, 11, 186–91
  ashwagandha, 188–89, 204
  eleuthero, 189, 251–52, 331
  rhodiola, 187–88, 321–22, 331
studies
  clinical trial, 365
  cohort, 365

double-blind, 365
meta-analysis, 367
open-label, 367
pilot, 368
placebo-controlled, 368
randomized controlled, 368
sugar, 239. *See also* blood sugar
suppositories, 34, 36
synergy, 29, 369

T

tamoxifen, 70, 72, 277
tannins, 194, 200, 263
TCM (traditional Chinese medicine), 18, 19, 32, 369. *See also specific formulas*
  aphrodisiacs, 182
  berberine, 209
  cinnamon (*guizhi*), 140–41, 232
  corn silk, 235
  dandelion (*pu gong ying*), 177, 240
  dang gui, 49, 124, 131, 141, 182, 243, 245
  eleuthero (*ci wu jia*), 251
  endometriosis, 88, 95–97
  fibroids, 95–97
  geranium (*lao guan cao*), 263
  ginger (*shen jiang*), 135, 265
  gingko (*bai guo*), 269
  ginseng (*ren shen*), 181, 188, 272
  hawthorn, 110–11
  licorice (*gan cao*), 151, 157, 295, 296–97
  menstruation, 129, 131
  motherwort (*yi mu cao*), 301

Wood, Matthew, 28
WS 1442 (hawthorn extract), 284
WS 5570 (St. John's wort extract), 328
wu wei zi. See schisandra

X

xenoestrogens, 129
xiao yao wan, 176
xuefu zhuyu tang, 88

Y

yam. *See* Chinese yam; wild yam
yarrow (*Achillea millefolium*), 16, 360–62

endometriosis, 88–89, 361
fibroids, 98, 361
heart disease, 111, 113
hemorrhoids, 160–61, 361
high blood pressure, 111, 113, 361
menorrhagia, 140, 361
menstrual irregularities, 133, 360
yeast infections, 197, 198–99. *See also Candida albicans*
yellow marabou (*Achillea biebersteinii* Afan.), 16, 361
yi mu cao (*Leonurus japonicus*), 301
yin tonics, 182, 183, 243

Z

zinc, 64, 266